2016

The Year Book of ORTHOPEDICS®

Editor-in-Chief

Bernard F. Morrey, MD

Professor of Orthopedics, Mayo Graduate School of Medicine; Professor of Orthopedics, University of Texas, Health Science Center, San Antonio, Texas

ELSEVIER

MOSBY

ELSEVIER
MOSBY

Senior Clinics Editor: Jennifer Flynn-Briggs
Developmental Editor: Kristen Helm

2016 EDITION

Printed in the United States of America
Composition by TNQ Books and Journals Pvt Ltd, India
Printing/binding by Sheridan Books, Inc.

Editorial Office:
Elsevier, Inc.
Suite 1800
1600 John F. Kennedy Blvd
Philadelphia, PA 19103-2899

International Standard Serial Number: 0276-1092
International Standard Book Number: 978-0-323-44692-1

Editorial Board

Table of Contents

Journals Represented

Journals represented in this YEAR BOOK are listed below.

Academic Emergency Medicine
Acta Orthopaedica
American Journal of Sports Medicine
Annals of Internal Medicine
Annals of Plastic Surgery
Annals of the Rheumatic Diseases
Archives of Physical Medicine and Rehabilitation
Arthroscopy
Bone and Joint Journal
British Journal of Sports Medicine
Canadian Journal of Surgery
Circulation
Clinical Biomechanics
Clinical Journal of Sport Medicine
Clinical Neurology and Neurosurgery
Clinical Orthopaedics and Related Research
Clinical Radiology
Clinical Sarcoma Research
Contact Dermatitis
European Journal of Nuclear Medicine and Molecular Imaging
Foot and Ankle International
Injury
Journal of Athletic Training
Journal of Bone and Joint Surgery (American)
Journal of Clinical Anesthesia
Journal of Clinical Neuroscience
Journal of Hand Surgery (American Volume)
Journal of Orthopaedic and Sports Physical Therapy
Journal of Orthopaedic Research
Journal of Orthopaedic Trauma
Journal of Pediatric Orthopaedics
Journal of Rheumatology
Journal of Trauma and Acute Care Surgery
Journal of Wrist Surgery
Journal of the American Board of Family Medicine
Journal of the American Dental Association
Journal of the American Geriatrics Society
Journal of the American Medical Association surgery
Journal of Vascular Surgery
Medicine (Baltimore)
Neurology
Neurosurgery
New England Journal of Medicine
Orthopedics
Pain
Pediatrics
Plastic and Reconstructive Surgery

Sarcoma
Skeletal Radiology
Skeletal Radiology
Spine
Spine Journal
Transfusion
Wound Repair and Regeneration

Standard Abbreviations

The following terms are abbreviated in this edition: acquired immunodeficiency syndrome (AIDS), anterior cruciate ligament (ACL), anteroposterior (AP), avascular necrosis (AVN), cardiopulmonary resuscitation (CPR), central nervous system (CNS), cerebrospinal fluid (CSF), computed tomography (CT), deoxyribonucleic acid (DNA), electrocardiography (ECG), health maintenance organization (HMO), human immunodeficiency virus (HIV), intensive care unit (ICU), intramuscular (IM), intravenous (IV), magnetic resonance (MR) imaging (MRI), range of motion (ROM), ribonucleic acid (RNA), total hip arthroplasty (THA), total knee arthroplasty (TKA), ultrasound (US), and ultraviolet (UV).

Note

The Year Book of Orthopedics® is a literature survey service providing abstracts of articles published in the professional literature. Every effort is made to assure the accuracy of the information presented in these pages. Neither the editors nor the publisher of the Year Book of Orthopedics® can be responsible for errors in the original materials. The editors' comments are their own opinions. Mention of specific products within this publication does not constitute endorsement.

To facilitate the use of the Year Book of Orthopedics® as a reference tool, all illustrations and tables included in this publication are now identified as they appear in the original article. This change is meant to help the reader recognize that any illustration or table appearing in the Year Book of Orthopedics® may be only one of many in the original article. For this reason, figure and table numbers will often appear to be out of sequence within the Year Book of Orthopedics®.

1 Basic Science

Introduction

The goal of selecting articles for this section has always been to balance emerging techniques of investigation with clinically relevant topics. In this year's edition, there has been an increased emphasis on application. The techniques of investigation continue to reside in the final analysis on the genetic or proteomic control of function. The spectrum of questions that are being addressed and effectively addressed by these techniques holds promise of clinical application in the not too distant future. The clinical application today continues to focus on the impact of ion burden following a metal on metal implant replacement. As a further observation, the discipline of health science research is proving of great value to better understand the effect and the cost benefit impact of our interventions.

Bernard F. Morrey, MD

CRHBP polymorphisms predict chronic pain development following motor vehicle collision

Linnstaedt SD, Bortsov AV, Soward AC, et al (Univ of North Carolina, Chapel Hill; et al)
Pain 157:273-279, 2016

Musculoskeletal pain (MSP) is a common sequela of traumatic stress exposure. While biological factors contributing to chronic MSP after motor vehicle collision (MVC) have traditionally focused on tissue injury, increasing evidence suggests that neuro/stress/immune processes mediated by stress system activation may play a more dominant role. In a previous study, we found that genetic variants in the hypothalamic–pituitary–adrenal (HPA) axis–related gene *FKBP5* influence vulnerability to persistent MSP 6 weeks after MVC. In the present cohort study ($n = 855$), we evaluated whether genetic variants in several other important HPA axis–related genes, including the glucocorticoid receptor (*NR3C1*), corticotropin-releasing hormone receptor R1 (*CRHR1*), and corticotropin-releasing hormone-binding protein (*CRHBP*), influence risk of chronic MSP over time after MVC. Genetic polymorphism rs7718461 in the *CRHBP* gene showed significant association ($P = 0.0012$) with overall pain severity during the year after MVC in regression models controlling for multiple comparisons. Two additional *CRHBP* alleles in high linkage disequilibrium with rs7718461 also showed trend-level significance. In secondary analyses, a significant interaction between this *CRHBP* locus (minor allele frequency = 0.33) and time was observed ($P = 0.015$), with increasing effect observed over time following trauma. A significant *CRHBP* × *FKBP5* interaction was also observed, with substantially increased MSP after MVC in those with a risk allele in both genes compared with either gene alone. The results of this study indicate that genetic variants in 2 different HPA axis genes predict chronic MSP severity following MVC and support the hypothesis that the HPA axis is involved in chronic post-MVC MSP pathogenesis.

▶ Although the science of genetic research is a bit beyond the interest of, and even the relevance to, most orthopedic surgeons, this contribution seemed most interesting. On the basis of prior work by the authors, this follow-up study of a large cohort of patients (n = 855) who had been involved in a motor vehicle accident (MVA) was developed to further understand the genetic relationship to the development of chronic pain associated with MVA. It is sufficient to learn hat there is a statistical relationship of this condition with a genetically determined family of glucocortical hormones that are elaborated by the hypothalamic-pituitary-adrenal axis. The process is activated by stress. This finding may provide some insight into the management of this difficult condition in the future.

B. F. Morrey, MD

Efficacy and Safety of Human Umbilical Cord Blood–Derived Mesenchymal Stem Cells in Anterior Cruciate Ligament Reconstruction of a Rabbit Model: New Strategy to Enhance Tendon Graft Healing

Jang K-M, Lim HC, Jung WY, et al (Korea Univ School of Medicine, Seoul; et al)

Arthroscopy 31:1530-1539, 2015

Purpose.—To investigate whether non-autologous transplantation of human umbilical cord blood–derived mesenchymal stem cells (hUCB-MSCs) could be integrated safely at the bone-tendon junction without immune rejection and could enhance bone-tendon healing effectively during anterior cruciate ligament (ACL) reconstruction in an animal model.

Methods.—ACL reconstructions using hamstring tendons were performed in 30 adult rabbits. The bone tunnels were treated with hUCB-MSCs or were untreated. The specimens were harvested at 4, 8, and 12 weeks. We performed a gross examination of the knee joint; a histologic assessment using H&E staining, as well as immunohistochemical staining, for type II collagen; and an evaluation of bone tunnel widening using micro–computed tomography.

Results.—No evidence of immune rejection was detected. Tendon-bone healing through Sharpey-like fibers was noticed around tendon grafts at

12 weeks in the control group. A smooth transition from bone to tendon through broad fibrocartilage formation was identified in the treatment group, and the interface zone showed abundant type II collagen production on immunohistochemical staining. Histologic scores for bone-tendon healing were significantly higher in the treatment group at all time points ($P < .001$). Micro–computed tomography at 12 weeks showed a significantly smaller tibial ($P = .029$) and femoral ($P = .033$) bone tunnel enlargement in the treated group than in the control group.

Conclusions.—Non-autologous transplantation of hUCB-MSCs was applied in ACL reconstruction without early immune rejection. There was enhanced tendon-bone healing through broad fibrocartilage formation with higher histologic scores and decreased femoral and tibial tunnel widening compared with the control group (79.2% and 80%, respectively, of the control group tunnel area at 12 weeks).

Clinical Relevance.—Non-autologous transplantation of hUCB-MSCs has therapeutic potential in promoting tendon-to-bone healing after ACL reconstruction. Further study in the human model is warranted.

▶ This study clearly states 2 objectives: to demonstrate the safety and efficacy of the use of umbilical mesenchymal stem cells (UC-MSC) on anterior cruciate ligament reconstructive surgery. In this animal model, they were successful in demonstrating a positive effect of UC-MSC in enhancing bone-patella-bone incorporation as evidenced by absence of tunnel narrowing and increased production of type II collagen. Importantly, this enhanced healing occurred without any evidence of an immune rejection response. The authors are careful to point out that the results clearly needs additional study before the concept can be applied to human treatment, but these results might suggest that this proposition may occur sooner than is often the case with applied research efforts.

B. F. Morrey, MD

Cartilage Repair by Human Umbilical Cord Blood-Derived Mesenchymal Stem Cells With Different Hydrogels in a Rat Model

Park Y-B, Song M, Lee C-H, et al (Sungkyunkwan Univ School of Medicine, Seoul, South Korea)

J Orthop Res 33:1580-1586, 2015

This study was carried out to assess the feasibility of human umbilical cord blood-derived mesenchymal stem cells (hUCBMSCs) in articular cartilage repair and to further determine a suitable delivering hydrogel in a rat model. Critical sized full thickness cartilage defects were created. The hUCB-MSCs and three different hydrogel composites (hydrogel A; 4% hyaluronic acid/30% pluronic (1:1, v/v), hydrogel B; 4% hyaluronic acid, and hydrogel C; 4% hyaluronic acid/30% pluronic/chitosan (1:1:2, v/v)) were implanted into the experimental knee (right knee) and hydrogels without hUCB-MSCs were implanted into the control knee (left knee). Defects were evaluated after 8 weeks. The hUCB-MSCs with hydrogels composites resulted in a better repair as seen by gross and histological evaluation compared with hydrogels without hUCB-MSCs. Among the three different hydrogels, the 4% hyaluronic acid hydrogel composite (hydorgel B) showed the best result in cartilage repair as seen by the histological evaluation compared with the other hydrogel composites (hydrogel A and C). The results of this study suggest that hUCB-MSCs may be a promising cell source in combination with 4% hyaluronic acid hydrogels in the in vivo repair of cartilage defects.

▶ This report is of value from several perspectives. It addresses a relevant clinical problem of cartilage damage and introduces the possibility of treatment with mesenchymal stem cells (MSC). The issue is obviously rather complex with subtle variations in preparation and delivery being important variables. In this regard, the investigators demonstrate that the effectiveness is sensitive to the hydrogel composition used for delivery of the stem cells. I have been impressed with the increasing number of investigations that reveal the regenerative potential of mesenchymal stem cells in a spectrum of skeletal pathologies. The findings are important but still a fairly long way from clinical application.

B. F. Morrey, MD

Detrimental Effect of Repeated and Single Subacromial Corticosteroid Injections on the Intact and Injured Rotator Cuff: A Biomechanical and Imaging Study in Rats

Maman E, Yehuda C, Pritsch T, et al (Tel Aviv Univ Sackler Faculty of Medicine, Israel; et al)

Am J Sports Med 44:177-182, 2016

Background.—The effect of corticosteroids on tendons is poorly understood, and current data are insufficient and conflicting.

Purpose.—To evaluate the effects of corticosteroid injections on intact and injured rotator cuffs (RCs) through biomechanical and radiographic analyses in a rat model.

Study Design.—Controlled laboratory study.

Methods.—A total of 70 rats were assigned to 7 groups. Uninjured rats (no tear) received either a single saline injection, a single methylprednisolone acetate (MTA) injection, or triple MTA injections. Injured rats (unilateral supraspinatus injury) received either a single saline injection, triple saline injections, a single MTA injection, or triple MTA injections (injections were subacromial; repeat injections were administered weekly). Rats were sacrificed 1 week after final injection. Shoulders were harvested and grossly inspected, and the supraspinatus tendon was evaluated biomechanically. Bone density at the tendon insertion site on the greater tuberosity was assessed by micro–computed tomography.

Results.—Intact RCs exposed to triple MTA injections had significantly decreased maximal load and stiffness compared with the control group (14.43 vs 21.25 N and 8.21 vs 16.6 N/mm, respectively; $P < .05$). Injured RCs exposed to steroid treatment had significantly lower maximal load (single saline: 10.91 N, single steroid: 8.43 N [$P < .05$]; triple control: 15.77 N, triple steroid: 11.65 N [$P < .05$]) compared with the control at 3 weeks. Greater tuberosity volume density and connectivity density were significantly lower in undamaged rats after triple MTA injection ($P < .05$).

Conclusion.—The study results clearly showed that repeated doses of corticosteroids significantly weaken rat RC and negatively affect bone quality in addition to possibly causing deterioration of the osteotendinous junction. However, data retrieved from animals must be scrupulously analyzed before extrapolation to humans. As such, the potential benefits and harms of subacromial corticosteroid treatment must be considered before administration.

Clinical Relevance.—The potential benefit and detrimental effects of corticosteroid injection should be thoroughly considered before it is administered subacromially in patients with RC injuries (Fig 2).

▶ The main value of this rather simple experiment is that it provides some basis for the emerging concern about the use of cortisone injection in tendons. There are data that clearly show adverse effects on the cellular level. This study primarily assesses the mechanical effect of injection. It should be noted the major effect was in the group with 3 injections at 1-week intervals (Fig 2).

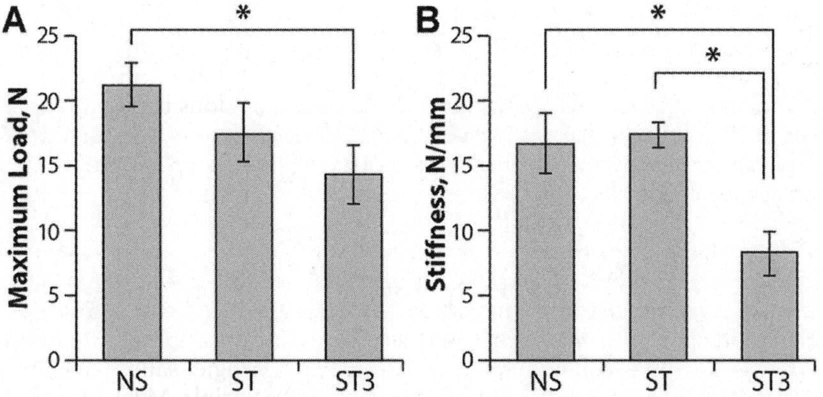

FIGURE 2.—Results of intact rotator cuff (RC) biomechanical testing. No significant difference was observed between groups receiving a single steroid injection (ST) and triple steroid injections (ST3) ($P = .533$) with regard to RC biomechanical strength. (A) A slight decrease in the maximal load was observed. Triple methylprednisolone acetate injections significantly decreased the mean maximal load in the ST3 group compared with the control (NS) group. (B) No significant differences in stiffness were observed between the NS and ST groups. Graphs show mean ± SD. *$P < .05$ (ANOVA). (Reprinted from Maman E, Yehuda C, Pritsch T, et al. Detrimental effect of repeated and single subacromial corticosteroid injections on the intact and injured rotator cuff: a biomechanical and imaging study in rats. *Am J Sports Med.* 2016;44:177-182, with permission from The Author(s).)

The concern one might have is that although the experimental dose of .6 mg/kg is comparable to a typical clinical dosage, the use here is undiluted. More important, 3 intrasubstance injections over a short period is not a realistic clinical practice. Hence, this study shows cortisone in high concentration injected into tendons is associated with definite adverse effects. Extrapolation to the clinical setting should take these factors into consideration.

B. F. Morrey, MD

Effect of Tamoxifen on Fatty Degeneration and Atrophy of Rotator Cuff Muscles in Chronic Rotator Cuff Tear: An Animal Model Study

Cho E, Zhang Y, Pruznak A, et al (Penn State College of Medicine, Hershey, PA)
J Orthop Res 33:1846-1853, 2015

Fatty degeneration of the rotator cuff muscles is an irreversible change resulting from chronic rotator cuff tear and is associated with poor clinical outcomes following rotator cuff repair. We evaluated the effect of Tamoxifen, a competitive estrogen receptor inhibitor, on fatty degeneration using a mouse model for chronic rotator cuff tear. Sixteen adult mice were divided into two diet groups (Tamoxifen vs. Regular) and subjected to surgical creation of a large rotator cuff tear and suprascapular nerve transection in their left shoulder with the right shoulder serving as a control. The rotator cuff muscles were harvested at 16 weeks and subjected to histology and RT-PCR for adipogenic and myogenic markers. Histology showed substantially decreased atrophy and endomysial inflammation in Tamoxifen group, but no significant differences in the amount of intramuscular adipocytes and lipid droplets compared to the Regular group. With RT-PCR, the operated shoulders showed significant upregulation of myogenin and PPAR-γ, and downregulation of myostatin compared to the nonsurgical shoulder. No significant differences of gene expression were found between the two diet groups. Our study demonstrated that tamoxifen diet leads to decreased muscle atrophy and inflammatory changes following chronic rotator cuff tear, but has no apparent effect on adipogenesis.

▶ This work caught my attention because I am currently treating a patient with a massive gluteus medius tear and marked fatty atrophy. The value of this article rests in the concept of attempting to reverse the fatty degeneration, demonstrated to be a negative factor in successful rotator cuff repair. That there was less atrophy and inflammation associated with dietary tamoxifen, an estrogen receptor inhibitor, is consistent with the hypothesis. Unfortunately, there was no effect on the fatty degenerative process. Yet the thought and direction are encouraging.

B. F. Morrey, MD

Effects of Corticosteroids and Hyaluronic Acid on Torn Rotator Cuff Tendons In Vitro and in Rats

Nakamura H, Gotoh M, Kanazawa T, et al (Kurume Univ Med Ctr, Fukuoka, Japan; Kurume Univ, Japan; Kurume Univ School of Medicine, Fukuoka, Japan; et al)

J Orthop Res 33:1523-1530, 2015

Corticosteroids (CS) or hyaluronic acid (HA) is used in subacromial injection for the conservative treatment of rotator cuff tears (RCT); this study addresses the question of how CS and HA affect the tendon tissue and fibroblasts in vitro and in rats. Cell proliferation assays were performed in human tendon fibroblasts from RCT. Rats underwent surgery to create RCT, and the surgical sites were injected with CS or HA. The rotator cuff tendons were subjected to biomechanical testing, microscopic and immunohistochemical analysis of proliferating cell nuclear antigen (PCNA), and ultrastructural analysis. Cell proliferation was significantly decreased with CS in vitro ($p < 0.05$). Maximal load of CS-treated tendons was significantly decreased compared with that of HA-treated tendons ($p < 0.05$), as well as $PCNA^+$ cells at 2 weeks ($p < 0.05$). Ultrastructural observations of the CS-treated rats detected apoptosis of tendon fibroblasts 24 h after surgery. Histological and biomechanical data 4 weeks after surgery were not significant among the three groups. Unlike HA, CS caused cell death, and inhibition of the proliferation of tendon fibroblasts, leading to a delay of tendon healing involved and a subsequent decrease of biomechanical strength at the surgical site.

▶ This study continues to address and attempt to understand the nature of the adverse impact of corticosteroids on tendon healing. In this rat model the study assesses various parameters of tendon healing when subjected to exposure to steroids or hyaluronic acid. The most dramatic finding is the statistical differences in proliferating cell nuclear antigen at virtually all steroid concentrations. This well-done study offers an explanation for the emerging recognition of the harmful effects of steroid injection for tendinopathy.

B. F. Morrey, MD

Adverse Local Tissue Reaction (ALTR) Associated With Corrosion Products in Metal-on-Metal and Dual Modular Neck Total Hip Replacements Is Associated With Upregulation of Interferon Gamma-Mediated Chemokine Signaling

Kolatat K, Perino G, Wilner G, et al (Hosp for Special Surgery, New York, NY)

J Orthop Res 33:1487-1497, 2015

Adverse local tissue reactions (ALTR) associated with tribocorrosion following total hip arthroplasty (THA) have become a significant clinical concern in recent years. In particular, implants featuring metal-on-metal bearing surfaces and modular femoral stems have been reported to result in elevated rates of ALTR. These tribocorrosion-related tissue reactions are characterized by marked necrosis and lymphocytic infiltration, which contrasts sharply with the macrophagic and foreign body giant cell inflammation associated with polyethylene wear particle induced peri-implant osteolysis. In this study, we characterize tribocorrosion-associated ALTR at a molecular level. Gene expression profiling of peri-implant tissue around failing implants identifies upregulation of numerous inflammatory mediators in ALTR, including several interferon gamma inducible factors, most notably the chemokines MIG/CXCL9 and IP-10/ CXCL10. This expression profile is distinct from that associated with polyethylene wear induced osteolysis, which is characterized by induction of markers of alternative macrophage activation, such as chitotriosidase (CHIT-1). Importantly, MIG/CXCL9 and IP-10/ CXCL10 are also elevated at the protein level in the synovial fluid and, albeit more moderately, the serum, of ALTR patients, raising the possibility that these factors may serve as circulating biomarkers for the early detection of ALTR in at-risk patients.

▶ The issue and concern regarding adverse reaction to the metal-on-metal bearing is well recognized. This study is of interest in that it demonstrates potential problems with ion production for nonbearing sources, specifically the interface of modular components. This investigation does add some information, suggesting that the devastating aseptic lymphocyte dominated vasculitis-associated lesions reaction does have a genetic association. In simple terms, it is another expression of host variation. The discussion is thorough and links the development of adverse reactions to a cytokine signing reaction that is mediated by a unique gene expression and results in a toxic tissue reaction. The value of research such as this is in ultimately providing a means of screening at-risk patients before the replacement. These data suggest such an approach is not only viable, but attainable.

B. F. Morrey, MD

Medial and lateral foot loading and its effect on knee joint loading

Schwachmeyer V, Kutzner I, Bornschein J, et al (Charité—Universitätsmedizin Berlin, Germany)

Clin Biomech (Bristol, Avon) 30:860-866, 2015

Background.—The medial knee contact force may be lowered by modified foot loading to prevent the progression of unilateral gonarthrosis but the real effects of such gait modifications are unknown. This study investigates how walking with a more medial or lateral rollover of the foot influences the *in vivo* measured knee contact forces.

Methods.—Five subjects with telemeterized knee implants walked on a treadmill with pronounced lateral or medial foot loading. Acoustic feedback of peak foot pressure was used to facilitate the weight bearing shift. The resultant contact force, F_{res}, the medial contact force, F_{med}, and the force distribution F_{med}/F_{res} across the tibial plateau were computed from the measured joint contact loads.

Findings.—During lateral foot loading, the two maxima of F_{res} during the stance phase, Peak 1 and Peak 2, increased by an average of 20% and 12%, respectively. The force distribution was changed by only −3%/+2%. As a result, F_{med} increased by+16%/+17%. Medial foot loading, on the other hand, changed F_{res} only slightly, but decreased the distribution by −18%/−11%. This led to average reductions of F_{med} by −18%/ −18%. The reductions were realized by kinematic adaptations, such as increases of ankle eversion, step width and foot progression angle.

Interpretation.—Medial foot loading consistently reduced the medial knee compartment, and may be a helpful gait modification for patients with pronounced medial gonarthrosis. The increase of F_{med} during lateral foot loading was most likely caused by muscular co-contractions. Long-term training may lead to more efficient gait and reduce co-contractions.

▶ Despite the wholesale expectation of surgical solutions to knee pain, nonoperative options should continue to be employed if they are in fact effective. Off-loading braces and shoe wedge modifications are commonly used with early medial compartment. This study employs sophisticated gait analysis to document what to me is counterintuitive. Medial loading actually alters the contact center laterally, not medially. The effect was seen in all 5 test subjects and averaged 18% less load on the medial compartment. This had definite clinical implications indicating a medial wedge be employed in the early stages of medial gonarthrosis. Conversely, lateral wedges are to be avoided.

B. F. Morrey, MD

2 General Orthopedics

Introduction

This is one of my favorite sections to develop. We have tried to make it of specific and immediate value to the more general orthopaedic practice. Since all of the content can also be anatomically or otherwise classified, inclusion into the general section is a bit arbitrary. Hence articles relating to arthroplasty topics, such as anticoagulation prophylaxis, are placed here because of the broader application. The section thus covers a broad range of topics, conditions and procedures and for this reason we have expanded the number of reviews over the years. It is hoped this section will be of interest and value to the reader.

Bernard F. Morrey, MD

Aspirin for thromboprophylaxis after primary lower limb arthroplasty: early thromboembolic events and 90 day mortality in 11 459 patients

Ogonda L, Hill J, Doran E, et al (Musgrave Park Hosp, Belfast, UK)

Bone Joint J 98-B:341-348, 2016

Aims.—The aim of this study was to present data on 11 459 patients who underwent total hip (THA), total knee (TKA) or unicompartmental knee arthroplasty (UKA) between November 2002 and April 2014 with aspirin as the primary agent for pharmacological thromboprophylaxis.

Patients and Methods.—We analysed the incidence of deep vein thrombosis (DVT) and pulmonary embolism (PE) then compared the 90-day all-cause mortality with the corresponding data in the National Joint Registry for England and Wales (NJR).

Results.—The incidence of PE was 0.6% after THA, 1.47% after TKA and 1.2% after UKA. The 90-day mortality was 0.39% after THA and 0.44% after TKA. No deaths occurred after UKA. The main causes of death were ischaemic heart disease and respiratory failure. PE was responsible for only 18% of deaths. There was a decline in 90-day mortality, from 0.64% between 2002 and 2007, to 0.21% between 2008 and 2013 after THA, and from 0.47% to 0.39% after TKA for the corresponding period. The standardised mortality ratio (SMR) declined from 86.5

(confidence interval (CI) 63.0 to 137.7) to 39.7 (CI 31.2 to 54.3) $p = 0.024$. The incidence of proximal DVT was 0.3%.

Take Home Message.—With individualised risk assessment and as part of a multimodal approach, Aspirin is safe to use as the main thromboprophylactic agent in primary arthroplasty. It is not associated with an increased incidence of symptomatic DVT, PE or death.

▶ What a great study. There is no topic more confusing in our profession than that of thromboprophylaxis. This is an amazing contribution from a single surgeon doing almost 1000 total hips and knees a year. The study is definitive. Use of 150 mg of aspirin, with early mobilization and mechanical compressive devices can reduce the chance of a pulmonary embolism or mortality to as low a level as any other regimen, but with virtually no morbidity. In addition, it is inexpensive. The secret of this study is the interpretation of the outcome: symptomatic deep vein thrombosis, not that of incidental clots demonstrated by ultrasound or angiogram. The modification of the program as a function of risk should be noted. To be honest, I have used aspirin along with nonmonitored warfarin for 3 weeks for more than 20 years. My clinical impression is similar to the outcomes reported here. Importantly, complications are virtually nonexistent.

B. F. Morrey, MD

From Bench to Bedside: Alpha-defensin—The Biggest Thing in Joint Replacement Infections Since Prophylactic Antibiotics?

Potter BK (Uniformed Services Univ of Health Sciences, Bethesda, MD)
Clin Orthop Relat Res 473:3105-3107, 2015

Background.—Periprosthetic joint infection (PJI) is one of the most dreaded complications after total joint arthroplasty (TJA). Although the infection rates have dropped dramatically, PJI continues to be expensive, to profoundly alter quality of life, and to literally result in death. The diagnosis is often difficult and requires complex interpretation efforts. The Musculoskeletal Infection Society and an international panel recently established a reference standard that may be useful in confirming a diagnosis of PJI and in measuring new diagnostic and therapeutic interventions.

Diagnostic Method.—Synovial fluid alpha-defensin levels have been proposed as an aid in diagnosing PJI in patients who have undergone TJA. Measuring the levels of alpha-defensin in synovial fluid, especially in the context of synovial C-reactive protein levels, has proved quite accurate in diagnosing PJI. One series identified alpha-defensin and several other biomarkers as having 100% sensitivity and specificity in this role. Others have indicated rates of sensitivity and specificity in the range of 97% to 100% and 95% to 96%, respectively. These findings are remarkable because only about half of all preoperative synovial cultures are positive, even when PJI is present.

The studies done thus far include patients who are currently taking antibiotics and/or have systemic inflammatory arthropathies, both of which cause confusion in interpreting routine laboratory results. The test for alpha-defensin is currently available, so it can be employed in patients today.

Disclosures.—The work on alpha-defensin has been done by Dr. Carl Deirmengian and colleagues, who have financial relationships related to the test that is available. Although he hit some roadblocks early on, he eventually saw synovial fluid analysis as the best way to diagnose infection and eventually formed a company and developed the commercial product.

▶ This may be one of the most important articles reviewed this year, simply because it introduces the orthopedic community to the potential dramatic effect of a new laboratory test. I was introduced to this test in England earlier in the year. Given the confusion and difficulty of accurately diagnosing joint replacement infection, I considered this test a godsend. Alpha-defensin is a biomarker found in the synovial fluid in an infected joint replacement. The studies to date reveal a sensitivity and specificity in excess of 95%. If the commercial expression of this test is successful, it will change everything.

B. F. Morrey, MD

Accuracy of in vivo palpation-guided acromioclavicular joint injection assessed with contrast material and fluoroscopic evaluations

Scillia A, Issa K, McInerney VK, et al (Seton Hall Univ, South Orange, NJ)

Skeletal Radiol 44:1135-1139, 2015

Objective.—The purpose of this study was to evaluate the accuracy of in vivo acromioclavicular (AC) joint injections without fluoroscopic guidance and assess whether patient demographics affected the accuracy of injections.

Materials and Methods.—A consecutive cohort of patients who presented with painful acromioclavicular joints was prospectively evaluated. All patients had clinical and radiographic evidence of AC arthritis, had failed conservative measures, and thus had received intraarticular corticosteroid injections. All injections were performed by experienced fellowship-trained musculoskeletal radiologists and by blinded digital palpation technique. Accuracy of injections was assessed with biplanar fluoroscopic views.

Results.—Forty-one AC injections in 22 males and 16 females with a mean age of 51 years (range 18 to 78) were identified. Twenty-three injections were in the right shoulder and 18 in the left. Only 15 injections were confirmed to be in the intraarticular AC joint, yielding an accuracy of 36.5%. There were no significant differences in the mean age (54 vs. 52 years; $p = 0.58$), male-to-female ratio ($p = 0.73$), and side of the injection between the accurate and inaccurate injections, respectively.

Conclusion.—Based on the findings of the present study, the authors encourage the use of image guidance for corticosteroid treatment of the AC joint.

Level of Evidence.—Level IV Therapeutic Case Series.

▶ This is a simple study comparing the accuracy of intraarticular injection of the acromioclavicular (AC) with and without image guidance. The study is straightforward. Comparing fluoroscopy and palpation guidance techniques reveals statistically enhanced accuracy with fluoroscopy. Important additional factors to consider are that placement has been shown to correlate with clinical efficacy. Furthermore, the need for guidance is mainly in the deep or hard to hit joints—hip, sacroiliac, AC, and shoulder joints. We find no added value for the knee or elbow. Finally, we have been using ultrasound guidance for the same reasons defined here. It is as easy, as accurate, and less expensive with no radiation.

B. F. Morrey, MD

Causes and Predictors of 30-Day Readmission After Shoulder and Knee Arthroscopy: An Analysis of 15,167 Cases

Westermann RW, Pugely AJ, Ries Z, et al (Univ of Iowa Hosps and Clinics)

Arthroscopy 31:1035-1040.e1, 2015

Purpose.—To evaluate the incidence, causes, and risk factors for unplanned 30-day readmission after shoulder and knee arthroscopy.

Methods.—A multicenter, prospective clinic registry, the American College of Surgeons National Surgical Quality Improvement Program, was queried for Current Procedural Terminology codes representing the most common shoulder and knee arthroscopic procedures. Unplanned readmissions within 30 days were evaluated dichotomously, and causes of readmission were identified. Univariate and multivariate logistic regression analyses were used to identify variables predictive of readmission.

Results.—In total, we identified 15,167 patients who underwent shoulder and knee arthroscopic procedures in 2012. Overall, 136 (0.90%) were readmitted within 30 days, and the rates were similar after shoulder (0.86%) and knee (0.92%) procedures. Readmissions were most common after arthroscopic debridement of the knee (1.56%) and lowest after rotator cuff and labral repairs (0.68%) and cruciate reconstructions (0.78%). The most common causes of readmission were surgical-site infections (37.1%), deep venous thrombosis and pulmonary embolism (17.1%), and postoperative pain (7.1%). Multivariate analysis identified age older than 80 years (odds ratio [OR], 3.5; 95% confidence interval [CI], 1.5 to 8.1), chronic steroid use (OR, 3.3; 95% CI, 1.5 to 7.2), and elevated American Society of Anesthesiologists class (OR, 4.2; 95% CI, 1.4 to 12.0) as independent risk factors for readmission.

Conclusions.—The rate of unplanned readmissions within 30 days of shoulder and knee arthroscopic procedures is low, at 0.92%, with wound-related complications being the most common cause. In patients with advanced age, with chronic steroid use, and with chronic systemic disease, the risk of readmission may be higher. These findings may aid in the informed-consent process, patient optimization, and the quality-reporting risk-adjustment process.

Level of Evidence.—Level III, prognostic study.

▶ I remember how stunned I was with the first complication I encountered after performing a knee arthroscopy. A deep vein thrombosis (DVT) occurred in an attorney (of course) after arthroscopic meniscectomy. There were virtually no data in the literature about complications of knee arthroscopy. Hence, this submission caught my eye. The easy messages to remember are as follows: the incidence is about 1%; the rate is essentially the same between knee and shoulder; and the causes are also similar, being infection, DVT, and pain. Finally the predisposing factors are similar: comorbidities, older patients, and the use of steroids. The information in this article is simple to remember, and relevant.

B. F. Morrey, MD

High frequency of contact allergy to implant and bone cement components, in particular gentamicin, in cemented arthroplasty with complications: usefulness of late patch test reading

Thomas B, Kulichova D, Wolf R, et al (Ludwig-Maximilians-Univ, Munich, Germany; et al)

Contact Dermatitis 73:343-349, 2015

Background.—Arthroplasty patients with complications may be sensitized to implant components.

Objectives.—To quantify patch test reactions to implant materials in aseptic cemented arthroplasty patients with complications, and to evaluate the benefit of late patch test reading at D6.

Methods.—Analyses of patch test reactions to baseline series and bone cement components and of the questionnaire-aided histories of 250 consecutive patients with suspected implant allergy were performed. Patch tests were read at D2, D3, and D6.

Results.—There were 187 positive reactions to the 29 allergens of the baseline series, and 52 to the seven allergens of the bone cement series. Forty-nine of 250 patients reacted to the bone cement series. In contrast to 'early allergens' such as fragrance mix, late reading at D6 increased the number of positive reactions by 11/32 for nickel, 1/5 for cobalt, and 2/4 for chromium. With bone cement components, most reactions were to gentamicin (25 of 250 patients), and 17 of 25 appeared only at D6.

Conclusion.—Late reading is useful for patch tests with metals and bone cement components. With only D2/D3 readings, 32 reactions to nickel, cobalt, chromium and bone cement components would have been missed. This underlines the utility of late reading in general and in complicated cemented arthroplasty patients, given the unexpectedly high number of gentamicin reactions.

▶ I am really not sure what to make of this report. The issue of contact allergy, especially hypersensitive reactions, is of keen interest to our profession. It is well accepted that a possible allergic reaction may provide an explanation for an otherwise unexplained pain or loosening of an implant. It is also well accepted that the reliability of patch testing is not particularly reliable. The interest in this report was not so much that some reaction was not detected until the 6-day reading, but rather the high rate of positive results. Given that multiple allergens were being investigated, that 187 positive reactions nonetheless occurred in these, albeit selected, patients is greater than I would have anticipated. Of some clinical note is the high relative rate of reaction to the gentamycin as an additive to the cement.

B. F. Morrey, MD

Effectiveness of Botulinum Toxin for Shoulder Pain Treatment: A Systematic Review and Meta-Analysis

Wu T, Fu Y, Song HX, et al (Zhejiang Univ, Hangzhou, People's Republic of China; Alxa League Central Hosp, Hangzhou, People's Republic of China; et al)
Arch Phys Med Rehabil 96:2214-2220, 2015

Objective.—To evaluate the current evidence of the effectiveness of botulinum toxin (BTX) treatment for shoulder pain.

Data Sources.—Ovid MEDLINE In-Process and Other Non-Indexed Citations, Ovid MEDLINE, Ovid EMBASE, Web of Science, and Scopus were searched from inception through week 18 of 2015.

Study Selection.—Randomized controlled trials comparing the clinical efficacy (pain intensity and shoulder range of motion [ROM]) of BTX injection to conventional therapy (steroid or placebo injection) were included.

Data Extraction.—Two reviewers independently screened abstracts and full texts. The results of the pain intensity and shoulder ROM were extracted and presented in the form of mean and SD. We constructed random-effects models and calculated the mean difference (MD) for continuous outcomes. A total of 219 articles were identified, of which 9 articles were eligible for the final analysis.

Data Synthesis.—The analysis indicated a statistically significant decreased pain score in the BTX therapy group compared with the control group, with the MD=1.35 (95% confidence interval [CI], .80=1.91; $P<.001$; $I^2=81\%$). Patients who received BTX therapy were more likely to have a significant increase in shoulder abduction ROM than patients in the control group, with the MD=8.02 (95% CI, 1.17–14.88, P=.02, I^2=89%).

Conclusions.—Compared with conventional (steroid or placebo injection) therapy, BTX injections have beneficial effects for adult patients with shoulder pain, evidenced by improved pain scores and ROM.

▶ I reviewed this article to determine the source of the data, that is, who is treating shoulder pain with botulinum toxin? As is seen, this article emanates from China, where this is clearly a more common practice than in the United States. The authors identified 219 articles on the subject, but after sanction, only 9 remained that were of adequate quality to be of use in this study. This is common with meta-analyses, but the 9 of 219 is a lower useful frequency than is usually seen. All that said, the 9 articles revealed this a useful treatment for shoulder pain. The practical implication is that it may be an alternative, expensive but viable, to those with musculoskeletal pain and numerous allergies to pain medications.

B. F. Morrey, MD

Arthroscopy for Knee Osteoarthritis Has Not Decreased After a Clinical Trial

Adelani MA, Harris AHS, Bowe TR, et al (Washington Univ School of Medicine, Saint Louis, MO; VA Palo Alto Health Care System, Menlo Park, CA)
Clin Orthop Relat Res 474:489-494, 2016

Background.—Multiple clinical trials have shown that arthroscopy for knee osteoarthritis is not efficacious. It is unclear how these studies have affected orthopaedic practice in the USA.

Questions/Purposes.—We questioned whether, in the Veterans Health Administration system, rates of knee arthroscopy in patients with osteoarthritis have changed after publication of the initial clinical trial by Moseley et al. in 2002, and whether rates of arthroplasty within 2 years of arthroscopy have changed during the same period.

Methods.—Patients 50 years and older with knee osteoarthritis who underwent arthroscopy between 1998 and 2010 were retrospectively identified and an annual arthroscopy rate was calculated from 1998 through 2002 and from 2006 through 2010. Patients who underwent knee arthroplasty within 2 years of arthroscopy during each period were identified, and a 2-year conversion to arthroplasty rate was calculated.

Results.—Between 1998 and 2002, the annual arthroscopy rate decreased from 4% to 3%. Of these arthroscopies, 4% were converted to arthroplasty within 2 years. Between 2006 and 2010, the annual arthroscopy rate increased from 3% to 4%. Of these arthroscopies, 5% were converted to arthroplasty within 2 years.

Conclusions.—Rates of arthroscopy in patients with knee osteoarthritis and conversion to arthroplasty within 2 years have not decreased with

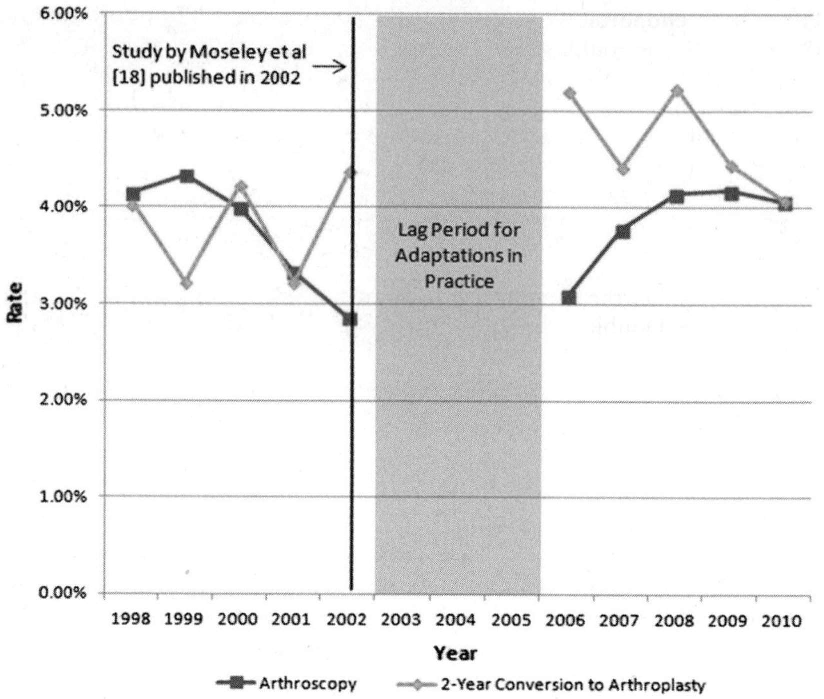

FIGURE 1.—This graph shows the trend in the use of arthroscopy for knee osteoarthritis and 2-year conversion rate to arthroplasty in the Veterans Administration hospital system from 1998 to 2010. (Reprinted from Adelani MA, Harris AHS, Bowe TR, et al. Arthroscopy for knee osteoarthritis has not decreased after a clinical trial. *Clin Orthop Relat Res.* 2016;474:489-494, with permission from The Association of Bone and Joint Surgeons.)

time. It may be that evidence alone is not sufficient to alter practice patterns or that arthroscopy rates for arthritis for patients in the Veterans Health Administration system were already so low that the results of the initial clinical trial had no substantial effect.

Level of Evidence.—Level III, Retrospective cohort study (Fig 1).

▶ I have actually been waiting for this kind of study. I have long been concerned about the apparent lack of impact of studies that question or even prove the ineffectiveness of certain practice policies. The classic article by Moseley et al is now almost 15 years old. This study clearly demonstrates the well-constructed and legitimate analysis has had little or no effect on the clinical practice of managing osteoarthritis of the knee. This in fact is just 1 of many examples of the apparent agnostic attitude of the surgeon to legitimate and clinical relevant data (Fig 1). My concern is that if our profession does not begin to practice according to legitimate data, we will continue to lose the ability to manage our patients in a manner that is in their best interest.

B. F. Morrey, MD

Combined chondroitin sulfate and glucosamine for painful knee osteoarthritis: a multicentre, randomised, double-blind, non-inferiority trial versus celecoxib

Hochberg MC, on behalf of the MOVES Investigation Group (Univ of Maryland School of Medicine, Baltimore; et al)

Ann Rheum Dis 75:37-44, 2016

Objectives.—To compare the efficacy and safety of chondroitin sulfate plus glucosamine hydrochloride (CS+GH) versus celecoxib in patients with knee osteoarthritis and severe pain.

Methods.—Double-blind Multicentre Osteoarthritis interVEntion trial with SYSADOA (MOVES) conducted in France, Germany, Poland and Spain evaluating treatment with CS+GH versus celecoxib in 606 patients with Kellgren and Lawrence grades 2–3 knee osteoarthritis and moderate-to-severe pain (Western Ontario and McMaster osteoarthritis index (WOMAC) score ≥301; 0–500 scale). Patients were randomised to receive 400 mg CS plus 500 mg GH three times a day or 200 mg celecoxib every day for 6 months. The primary outcome was the mean decrease in WOMAC pain from baseline to 6 months. Secondary outcomes included WOMAC function and stiffness, visual analogue scale for pain, presence of joint swelling/effusion, rescue medication consumption, Outcome Measures in Rheumatology Clinical Trials and Osteoarthritis Research Society International (OMERACT-OARSI) criteria and EuroQoL-5D.

Results.—The adjusted mean change (95% CI) in WOMAC pain was −185.7 (−200.3 to −171.1) (50.1% decrease) with CS+GH and −186.8 (−201.7 to −171.9) (50.2% decrease) with celecoxib, meeting the non-inferiority margin of −40: −1.11 (−22.0 to 19.8; $p = 0.92$). All sensitivity analyses were consistent with that result. At 6 months, 79.7% of patients in the combination group and 79.2% in the celecoxib group fulfilled OMERACT-OARSI criteria. Both groups elicited a reduction >50% in the presence of joint swelling; a similar reduction was seen for effusion. No differences were observed for the other secondary outcomes. Adverse events were low and similarly distributed between groups.

Conclusions.—CS+GH has comparable efficacy to celecoxib in reducing pain, stiffness, functional limitation and joint swelling/effusion after 6 months in patients with painful knee osteoarthritis, with a good safety profile.

Trial registration number.—NCT01425853 (Fig 2).

► This is a most impressive study largely due to the impressive study structure: a multicenter (N = 42) European multicountry prospective randomized assessment of 465 patients. In short, the use of 400 mg of chondroitin sulfate and 500 mg glucosamine three times a day is effective. However, it is no more, or less effective, than 200 mg of Celebrex each day.

The detailed comparative outcomes are depicted in Fig 2. There is a clear therapeutic effect of this over-the-counter combined therapy, so it may be a

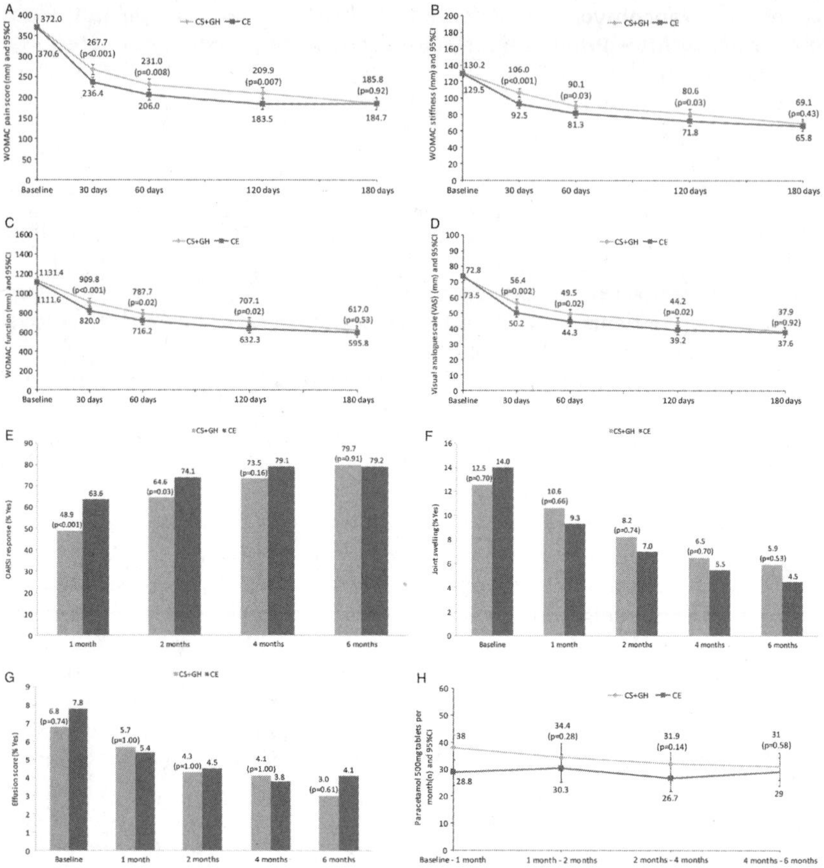

FIGURE 2.—Western Ontario and McMaster osteoarthritis index (WOMAC) (A) pain, (B) stiffness and (C) function subscales, and (D) visual analogue scale by visit; (E) Outcome Measures in Rheumatology Clinical Trials and Osteoarthritis Research Society International (OMERACT-OARSI) responder criteria, (F) joint swelling, (G) joint effusion and (H) consumption of rescue medication, by visit. The *p* values compare values between treatments. Data are least-square means ± SEM. CE, celecoxib; CS+GH, chondroitin sulfate plus glucosamine hydrochloride. (Reprinted from Hochberg MC, on behalf of the MOVES Investigation Group. Combined chondroitin sulfate and glucosamine for painful knee osteoarthritis: a multicentre, randomised, double-blind, non-inferiority trial versus celecoxib. *Ann Rheum Dis.* 2016;75:37-44.)

reasonable alternative to other agents based on patient tolerance and cost considerations.

B. F. Morrey, MD

Addition of Vancomycin to Cefazolin Prophylaxis Is Associated With Acute Kidney Injury After Primary Joint Arthroplasty

Courtney PM, Melnic CM, Zimmer Z, et al (Univ of Pennsylvania, Philadelphia)

Clin Orthop Relat Res 473:2197-2203, 2015

Background.—With increasing prevalence of methicillin-resistant *Staphylococcus aureus* (MRSA) in patients undergoing hip and knee arthroplasty, some have advocated a dual-antibiotic regimen including vancomycin as prophylaxis against surgical site infections. However, routine administration of vancomycin may result in impaired renal functions in susceptible patients.

Questions/Purposes.—The purpose of this study was to determine whether patients receiving antibiotic prophylaxis with cefazolin and vancomycin have a higher risk of postoperative acute kidney injury (AKI) compared with patients receiving cefazolin alone before elective primary hip and knee arthroplasty. We also aimed to compare severity and recovery of AKI in these two cohorts and to determine independent risk factors for AKI.

Methods.—We retrospectively evaluated a series of 1828 patients undergoing primary hip and knee arthroplasty over a 2-year period who received either cefazolin ($n = 500$) or cefazolin and vancomycin ($n = 1328$) as perioperative antibiotic prophylaxis. During the study period, a perceived high prevalence of MRSA infections at our institution led some surgeons to add vancomycin to the prophylactic antibiotic regimen. The patient characteristics, case mix, and preoperative renal function and baseline creatinine clearance were similar between the two groups. We defined AKI according to the published Acute Kidney Injury Network (AKIN) criteria, and the risk of AKI in both groups was compared. We also compared the proportions of patients by AKIN severity stage and assessed recovery as defined by creatinine levels showing kidney function reaching 50% baseline. The American Society of Anesthesiologists (ASA) classification, preoperative chronic kidney disease, intraoperative fluid requirements, and estimated blood loss were recorded. We analyzed the data using a multivariate logistic regression model to identify potential independent risk factors, including dual antibiotic therapy.

Results.—Patients receiving dual antibiotics were more likely to develop AKI compared with those receiving cefazolin alone (13% versus 8%, $p = 0.002$). Dual-antibiotic prophylaxis also was associated with greater severity; patients in the dual antibiotic group had higher rates of Grade II and III acute kidney injury (3% versus 0%, $p = 0.003$). There was no difference in the rate of return to baseline renal function (2 ± 1.4 days versus 3 ± 3.4 days; mean difference, 0.5 days; 95% confidence interval [CI], −0.2 to 1.2 days; $p = 0.155$). Controlling for confounding variables, dual antibiotic prophylaxis (adjusted odds ratio [OR], 1.82; 95% CI, 1.25–2.64; $p = 0.002$), ASA class (adjusted OR, 1.64; 95% CI, 1.24–2.17; $p = 0.001$), and preoperative kidney disease (adjusted OR,

1.81; 95% CI, 1.30–2.52; $p = 0.001$) were independent risk factors for AKI after primary total joint arthroplasty.

Conclusions.—Without a clear advantage in reducing surgical site infections, the utility and safety of routine addition of vancomycin to the prophylactic regimen in all patients undergoing primary hip and knee arthroplasty should be avoided. Further prospective studies should look at the efficacy of preoperative MRSA screening, decolonization, and selective use of vancomycin in high-risk patients.

Level of Evidence.—Level III, therapeutic study.

▶ There are 2 reasons this work was reviewed. The first is the finding that the addition of vancomycin to cefazolin is well documented to have adverse effects on renal function. This finding is contained in the very title of the article. I noted the publication is by a highly regarded peer reviewed journal, and the sample size and methodology fully supports the conclusion. The second reason is that it is a great example of the unintended consequence that are so prevalent in our profession. We simply cannot assume anything, for example, that if a little is good, more is better. Going forward we are going to be held even more to the concept of the "scientific basis of clinical practice." The data simply must support the action.

B. F. Morrey, MD

Is a questionnaire and radiograph-based follow-up model for patients with primary hip and knee arthroplasty a viable alternative to traditional regular outpatient follow-up clinic?

Kingsbury SR, Dube B, Thomas CM, et al (NIHR Leeds Musculoskeletal Biomedical Res Unit, UK)

Bone Joint J 98-B:201-218, 2016

Aims.—Increasing demand for total hip and knee arthroplasty (THA/TKA) and associated follow-up has placed huge demands on orthopaedic services. Feasible follow-up mechanisms are therefore essential.

Methods.—We conducted an audit of clinical follow-up decision-making for THA/TKA based on questionnaire/radiograph review compared with local practice of Arthroplasty Care Practitioner (ACP)-led outpatient follow-up. In all 599 patients attending an ACP-led THA/TKA follow-up clinic had a pelvic/knee radiograph, completed a pain/function questionnaire and were reviewed by an ACP. An experienced orthopaedic surgeon reviewed the same radiographs and questionnaires, without patient contact or knowledge of the ACP's decision. Each pathway classified patients into: urgent review, annual monitoring, routine follow-up or discharge.

Results.—In total, 401 hip and 198 knee patients were included. There was substantial agreement between the ACP and surgeon for both hip (kappa = 0.69, 95% confidence interval (CI) 0.62 to 0.76) and knee (kappa = 0.81, 95% CI 0.74 to 0.88). Positive agreement was very high for discharge and routine follow-up; however the ACP was more likely to select annual monitoring and the surgeon urgent review.

Discussion.—Review of the questionnaire/radiograph together identified all patients in need of increased surveillance, with good agreement for on-going patient management. However, review of the radiograph or questionnaire alone missed some patients with potential problems. A radiograph in conjunction with a questionnaire as a review may represent a cost effective THA/TKA follow-up mechanism.

Take Home Message.—A questionnaire and radiograph-based remote review may represent a cost-effective total joint arthroplasty follow-up mechanism; thereby reducing the considerable burden that follow-up currently places on the NHS.

▶ This article was placed in the general category because I think the message can be applied to procedures other than hip and knee replacement. The findings are clear: the patient need not be seen to adequately provide appropriate recommendation for the mature of ongoing assessments. There are a couple of caveats, however. The first is this finding is specific to the questionnaire instrument. The second is that the accuracy is dependent on both questionnaire and radiographic information. Finally, it is noteworthy that the physician was more inclined to identify urgent surveillance, whereas the non—visit assessment recommended annual monitoring. This is an important study as we drive toward more cost-effective, high-quality management strategies.

B. F. Morrey, MD

Kaplan-Meier Survival Analysis Overestimates the Risk of Revision Arthroplasty: A Meta-analysis

Lacny S, Wilson T, Clement F, et al (Univ of Calgary, Alberta, Canada; et al)

Clin Orthop Relat Res 473:3431-3442, 2015

Background.—Although Kaplan-Meier survival analysis is commonly used to estimate the cumulative incidence of revision after joint arthroplasty, it theoretically overestimates the risk of revision in the presence of competing risks (such as death). Because the magnitude of overestimation is not well documented, the potential associated impact on clinical and policy decision-making remains unknown.

Questions/Purposes.—We performed a meta-analysis to answer the following questions: (1) To what extent does the Kaplan-Meier method overestimate the cumulative incidence of revision after joint replacement compared with alternative competing-risks methods? (2) Is the extent of overestimation influenced by followup time or rate of competing risks?

Methods.—We searched Ovid MEDLINE, EMBASE, BIOSIS Previews, and Web of Science (1946, 1980, 1980, and 1899, respectively, to October 26, 2013) and included article bibliographies for studies comparing estimated cumulative incidence of revision after hip or knee arthroplasty obtained using both Kaplan-Meier and competing-risks methods. We excluded conference abstracts, unpublished studies, or studies using simulated data sets. Two reviewers independently extracted data and evaluated the quality of reporting of the included studies. Among 1160 abstracts identified, six studies were included in our meta-analysis. The principal reason for the steep attrition (1160 to six) was that the initial search was for studies in any clinical area that compared the cumulative incidence estimated using the Kaplan-Meier versus competing-risks methods for any event (not just the cumulative incidence of hip or knee revision); we did this to minimize the likelihood of missing any relevant studies. We calculated risk ratios (RRs) comparing the cumulative incidence estimated using the Kaplan-Meier method with the competing-risks method for each study and used DerSimonian and Laird random effects models to pool these RRs. Heterogeneity was explored using stratified meta-analyses and metaregression.

Results.—The pooled cumulative incidence of revision after hip or knee arthroplasty obtained using the Kaplan-Meier method was 1.55 times higher (95% confidence interval, 1.43–1.68; $p < 0.001$) than that obtained using the competing-risks method. Longer followup times and higher proportions of competing risks were not associated with increases in the amount of overestimation of revision risk by the Kaplan-Meier method (all $p > 0.10$). This may be due to the small number of studies that met the inclusion criteria and conservative variance approximation.

Conclusions.—The Kaplan-Meier method overestimates risk of revision after hip or knee arthroplasty in populations where competing risks (such as death) might preclude the occurrence of the event of interest (revision). Competing-risks methods should be used to more accurately estimate the cumulative incidence of revision when the goal is to plan healthcare services and resource allocation for revisions.

▶ Wow. I must say, this article caught my attention because of the title and because we have grown to rely so heavily on the Kaplan-Meier (KM) estimate to define expected outcomes. So any suggestion that this method may not be accurate is really important not just for joint replacement surgery but because it is used to estimate the efficacy of other surgical interventions. I had not heard of the concept of competing variables, but it makes sense when it is recognized the assumption with the KM model is the patient is followed to death. However, other variables may intervene that shorten the life span, and hence changes the KM conclusion. The important high-level message is that the KM survival curve overestimates failure due to the fact that the method does not consider other factors that influence survival. Thus, the failure may be less than estimated in a person's actual lifetime. It seems it is accurate to reflect the implant's survival, but not that of the patient.

B. F. Morrey, MD

Age-Related Trends in Hip Arthroscopy: A Large Cross-Sectional Analysis

Sing DC, Feeley BT, Tay B, et al (Univ of California-San Francisco)

Arthroscopy 31:2307-2313.e2, 2015

Purpose.—To analyze a large national private payer population in the United States for trends over time in hip arthroscopy by age groups and to determine the rate of conversion to total hip arthroplasty (THA) after hip arthroscopy.

Methods.—We performed a retrospective analysis using the PearlDiver private insurance patient record database from 2007 through 2011. Hip arthroscopy procedures including newly introduced codes such as osteochondroplasty of cam and pincer lesions and labral repair were queried. Hip arthroscopy incidence and conversion rates to THA were stratified by age. Chi-squared analysis was used for statistical comparison. Conversion to THA was evaluated using Kaplan-Meier analysis.

Results.—From 2007 through 2011, 20,484,172 orthopaedic patients were analyzed. Hip arthroscopy was performed in 8,227 cases (mean annual incidence, 2.7 cases per 10,000 orthopaedic patients). The incidence of hip arthroscopies increased over 250% from 1.6 cases per 10,000 in 2007 to 4.0 cases per 10,000 in 2011 ($P < .0001$). Patients in the 40 to 49 age group made up 28% of cases, followed by patients ages 30 to 39 (22%) and 50 to 59 (19%). Patients under 30 years old showed the greatest increase in incidence from 2007 to 2011 (335%), but patients over 60 still had over a 200% increase. Labral debridement was the most common procedure (6,031 cases), and approximately 1.6 procedural codes were billed for every case performed. Labral repair

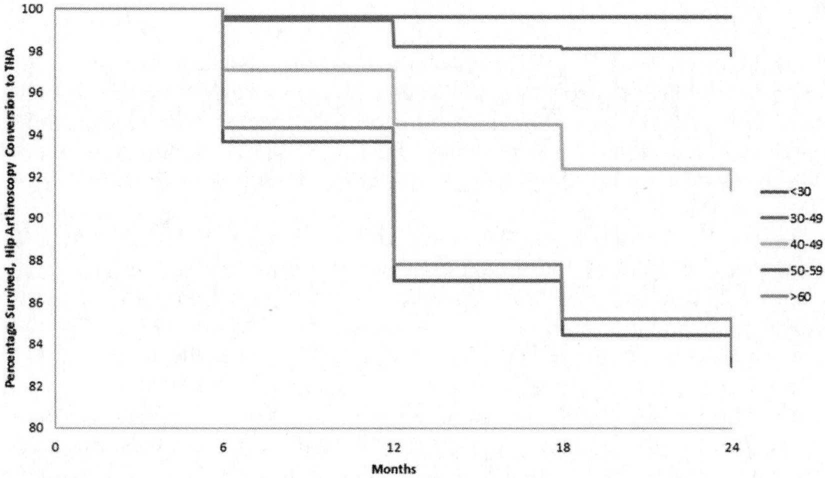

FIGURE 5.—Kaplan-Meier survival curves for conversion to THA by age group within 24 months after hip arthroscopy. (THA, total hip arthroplasty.) (Reprinted from Sing DC, Feeley BT, Tay B, et al. Age-related trends in hip arthroscopy: a large cross-sectional analysis. *Arthroscopy.* 2015;31:2307-2313.e2, with permission from Arthroscopy Association of North America.)

was more common in patients under 30, while labral debridement was more common in older age groups ($P = .046$). Within 24 months of hip arthroscopy, 17% of patients older than 50 required conversion to THA, compared with <1% of patients under 30 ($P < .0001$).

Conclusions.—Hip arthroscopy procedures are increasing in popularity across all age groups, with patients ages 40 to 49 having the highest incidence in this large cross-sectional population, despite a high rate of early conversion to THA within 2 years in patients over 50.

Level of Evidence.—IV, cross-sectional study (Fig 5).

▶ This study addresses an issue that is on my and others minds: What is happening to the practice of arthroscopy of the hip, and what is its impact? This assessment of a practice pattern over a 5-year period quantifies what is known; the use of arthroscopy of the hip is rising exponentially. The indication evolves around the diagnosis and treatment of impingement. The key question is answered in Fig 5. The impact is to avoid surgery by diagnosing and treating the effects of dysplasia. The ability of arthroscopy to avoid hip replacement in those over 50 years is questionable. This might, and should, help refine indications and treatment, but I doubt it will.

B. F. Morrey, MD

A regime of two intravenous injections of tranexamic acid reduces blood loss in minimally invasive total hip arthroplasty: a prospective randomised double-blind study

Hsu C-H, Lin P-C, Kuo F-C, et al (Chang Gung Univ, College of Medicine, Kaohsiung City, Taiwan)

Bone Joint J 97-B:905-910, 2015

Tranexamic acid (TXA), an inhibitor of fibrinolysis, reduces blood loss after total knee arthroplasty. However, its effect on minimally invasive total hip arthroplasty (THA) is not clear. We performed a prospective, randomised double-blind study to evaluate the effect of two intravenous injections of TXA on blood loss in patients undergoing minimally invasive THA.

In total, 60 patients (35 women and 25 men with a mean age of 58.1 years; 17 to 84) who underwent unilateral minimally invasive uncemented THA were randomly divided into the study group (30 patients, 20 women and ten men with a mean age of 56.5 years; 17 to 79) that received two intravenous injections 1 g of TXA pre- and post-operatively (TXA group), and a placebo group (30 patients, 15 women and 15 men with a mean age of 59.5 years; 23 to 84). We compared the peri-operative blood loss of the two groups. Actual blood loss was calculated from the maximum reduction in the level of haemoglobin. All patients were followed clinically for the presence of venous thromboembolism.

The TXA group had a lower mean intra-operative blood loss of 441 ml (150 to 800) *versus* 615 ml (50 to 1580) in the placebo ($p = 0.044$), lower mean post-operative blood loss (285 ml (120 to 570) *versus* 392 ml (126 to 660) ($p = 0.002$), lower mean total blood loss (1070 ml (688 to 1478) *versus* 1337 ml (495 to 2238) ($p = 0.004$) and lower requirement for transfusion ($p = 0.021$). No patients in either group had symptoms of venous thromboembolism or wound complications.

This prospective, randomised controlled study showed that a regimen of two intravenous injections of 1 g TXA is effective for blood conservation after minimally invasive THA.

▶ This study is included in the general orthopedics section because I feel it has broad-reaching implications. The use of tranexamic acid to control operative blood loss is a true game changer. It is routinely used at the Mayo Clinic and is becoming adopted as the standard of care for arthroplasty cases. This prospective, well-done study, shows that the specific regimen of 1 g administered 10 minutes before and 3 hours after a minimally invasive hip replacement is effective to control blood loss. The implication is that this technique is useful in trauma, spine, and in a host of procedures in which blood loss may require transfusion.

B. F. Morrey, MD

Efficacy of Hip Arthroscopy for the Management of Septic Arthritis: A Systematic Review

de SA D, Cargnelli S, Catapano M, et al (McMaster Univ, Hamilton, Ontario, Canada; et al)

Arthroscopy 31:1358-1370, 2015

Purpose.—This systematic review assessed the role of hip arthroscopic irrigation and debridement for eradication of infection in native joints to ascertain outcomes and complications associated with this surgical approach.

Methods.—The Medline, Embase, and PubMed databases were searched on July 20, 2014, for English-language studies that addressed arthroscopic treatment of native septic hip arthritis. The studies were systematically screened and data abstracted in duplicate, with qualitative findings presented.

Results.—There were 11 eligible studies (1 case-control study, 8 case series, and 2 case reports) reporting on 65 patients (65 hips) treated by arthroscopic irrigation and debridement for septic hip arthritis. The mean length of patient follow-up was 19.1 months (range, 6 to 84 months). The indications for surgery were as follows: pyrexia, anterior groin or hip pain with limited hip range of motion and an inability to bear weight, associated leukocytosis, an elevated erythrocyte sedimentation rate or C-reactive protein level, and/or hip imaging or aspiration results consistent with infection.

Specific contraindications for surgery reported across studies included tuberculous of fungal infection, coexistence of osteomyelitis, immunocompromised individuals, and pre-existing surgery on the affected hip. The initial rate of infection eradication was 100%. All studies reported significant improvements in patient pain and function. Improvements were also observed in range of motion, as well as across both the Bennett radiographic and clinical assessments and Harris Hip Score. No complications, major or minor, were reported, and only 1 of 65 hips (1.5%) required revision arthroscopy for recurrence because of a methicillin-resistant *Staphylococcus aureus* infection.

Conclusions.—Arthroscopic native hip irrigation and debridement for septic arthritis appear to comprise a safe and effective treatment option for selected patients (e.g., no deformity, no bacterial infections, and not immunocompromised). Timely diagnosis and intervention, however, remain the most critical prognostic factors for successful outcomes.

Level of Evidence.—Level IV, systematic review of Level IV and V studies.

▶ Arthroscopic debridement and lavage is a logical treatment option for the septic hip. It is attractive as a means of achieving the effect of a surgical procedure without the morbidity. This study of the literature assessed a rather small number of patients ($n = 65$), but it clearly shows that this approach is comparable in effectiveness without the complications associated with open procedures. We have adopted this mode of treatment for the elbow over the past 20 years. Unfortunately, in this study the distribution between the pediatric and adult hip was poorly assessed, and there was no direct comparison to arthrotomy. Regardless, the bottom line is, this treatment is safe and effective.

B. F. Morrey, MD

Are Normal Hips Being Labeled as Pathologic? A CT-based Method for Defining Normal Acetabular Coverage

Larson CM, Moreau-Gaudry A, Kelly BT, et al (Minnesota Orthopedic Sports Medicine Inst at Twin Cities Orthopedics, Edina; Grenoble Univ Hosp, France; New York-Presbyterian Hosp; et al)

Clin Orthop Relat Res 473:1247-1254, 2015

Background.—Plain radiographic measures of the acetabulum may fail to accurately define coverage or pathomorphology such as impingement or dysplasia. CT scans might provide more precise measurements for overcoverage and undercoverage. However, a well-defined method for such CT-based measurements and normative data regarding CT-based acetabular coverage is lacking.

Questions/Purposes.—The purposes of the study were (1) to develop a method for evaluation of percent coverage of the femoral head by the acetabulum and (2) to define normative data using a cohort of asymptomatic patient hip and pelvic CT scans and evaluate the variability in acetabular version for asymptomatic patients with normal lateral coverage (lateral center-edge angle [LCEA] 20°–40°) that has previously been defined as abnormal based on radiographic parameters.

Methods.—Two-hundred thirty-seven patients (474 hips) with hip CT scans obtained for reasons other than hip-related pain were evaluated. The scans were obtained from a hospital database of patients who underwent CT evaluation of abdominal trauma or pain. In addition, hips with obvious dysplasia (LCEA < 20°) or profunda (LCE > 40°) were excluded resulting in a final cohort of 222 patients (409 hips [115 men, 107 women]) with CT scans and a mean age of 25 ± 3 years. CT scan alignment was corrected along the horizontal and vertical axis and percent acetabular coverage around the clockface (3 o'clock = anterior), and regional (anterior, superior, posterior) and global surface area coverage was determined. Percent coverage laterally was correlated with the LCEA and the presence and prevalence of cranial retroversion (crossover sign) and a positive posterior wall sign were determined.

Results.—The mean regional percent femoral head surface area coverage for the asymptomatic cohort was 40% ± 2% anteriorly, 61% ± 3% superiorly, and 48% ± 3% posteriorly. Mean global coverage of the femoral head was 40% ± 2%. The local coverage anteriorly (3 o'clock) was 38% ± 3%, laterally (12 o'clock) was 67% ± 2%, and posteriorly (9 o'clock) was 52% ± 3%. The mean lateral coverage represented a mean LCEA of 31° (± 1 SD). Fifteen percent of hips demonstrated cranial retroversion that would correlate with a crossover sign, and 30% had < 50% posterior coverage that would correlate with a positive posterior wall sign on an anteroposterior pelvis radiograph. In addition, male hips had a higher prevalence of a crossover sign (19% 95% confidence interval [CI], 14%–25% versus 11% 95% CI, 7%–16% $p = 0.03$) and posterior wall sign (46% 95% CI. 39%–53% versus 13% 95% CI, 9%–19% $p < 0.001$) compared with women. A positive crossover sign or posterior wall sign was present for 113 male hips (53% 95% CI, 46%–60%) compared with 39 female hips (20% 95% CI, 15%–26% $p < 0.001$).

Conclusions.—This study provides normative coverage data and a reproducible method for evaluating acetabular coverage. Cranial acetabular retroversion (crossover sign) and a positive posterior wall sign were frequent findings in a young asymptomatic cohort and might be a normal variant rather than pathologic in a significant number of cases.

Level of Evidence.—Level III, diagnostic study.

▶ Given the ever-increasing recognition of femoral acetabular impingement (FAI), this information is extremely important. The need for an intervention is based in part on the combination of symptoms and radiographic findings. The radiographic characteristics are well established with the crossover sign, indicative of acetabular retroversion, as one of the most reliable. The positive posterior wall sign is an additional feature to confirm the presence of dysplasia. This interesting study that appears to be adequately powered, reveals the most important insight that upward of 15% and 30% of normal individuals would have "abnormal" measurements of the crossover and posterior wall signs. The risk of misinterpretation is greater in males. This is important, placing an increased burden on the physician to correctly and carefully document the clinical symptoms and features of FAI.

B. F. Morrey, MD

3 Forearm, Wrist, and Hand

Introduction

The selections for the Forearm, Wrist and Hand section this year are diverse. Common conditions including distal radius fractures, management of wrist ganglia, hand fractures, and effect wrist fusion on function are reviewed. The treatment of entrapment neuropathies including cubital and carpal tunnel are also highlighted. New treatments in the management of Dupuytren's contracture are also reflected in this year's selections. I also wanted to share an article examining and comparing different forearm flaps. There is also an interesting review of efficacy of anesthesia associated with reduction of pediatric distal radius and forearm fractures. Finally, some selections related to the observations associated with complex regional pain syndrome, catastrophic thinking of patients and physician empathy round out the list.

I respectfully submit this year's group of articles for your review. I hope you find them to be as educational as I did.

Marco Rizzo, MD

Triggering of the Digits After Carpal Tunnel Surgery

Acar MA, Kütahya H, Güleç A, et al (Med School of Selcuk Univ, Konya, Turkey; Beyhekim State Hosp, Konya, Turkey; et al)

Ann Plast Surg 75:393-397, 2015

Introduction.—Carpal tunnel syndrome (CTS) and trigger finger may be seen simultaneously in the same hand. The development of trigger finger in patients undergoing CTS surgery is not rare, but the relationship between these conditions has not been fully established.

The aims of this prospective randomized study were to investigate the incidence of trigger finger in patient groups undergoing transverse carpal ligament releasing (TCL) or TCL together with distal forearm fascia releasing and to identify other factors that may have an effect of these conditions.

Materials and Method.—This prospective randomized study evaluated 159 hands of 113 patients for whom CTS surgery was planned. The patients were separated into 2 groups: group 1 (79 hands of 57 patients) undergoing TCL releasing only and group 2 (80 hands of 56 patients) undergoing TCL and distal forearm fascia releasing together. The age and gender of the patients, dominant hand, physical examination findings, visual analogue scale (VAS), and electromyography (EMG) results were recorded. Follow-up examinations were made at 1, 3, 6, 12, and 24 months for all patients. We noted development of trigger finger in the surgical groups, and its location and response to treatment.

Results.—The incidence of trigger finger development was statistically significantly different between group 1 and group 2 (13.9% and 31.3%, respectively). The logistic regression analysis of factors affecting the development of trigger finger posttreatment found that the surgical method and severity of EMG were significant, whereas the effects of the other factors studied were not found to have any statistical significance.

Conclusion.—There was an increased risk of postoperative trigger finger development in patients undergoing TCL and distal forearm fascia releasing surgery for CTS compared to those undergoing CTL only. There is a need for further studies to support this result and further explain the etiology.

▶ Carpal tunnel syndrome and trigger fingers are both common, and they commonly coexist. The authors evaluated 2 groups of patients who underwent carpal tunnel release (one group with transverse carpal ligament release alone and the other with both distal forearm fascia and transverse carpal ligament release). The study was performed prospectively with the aim of identifying differences in postoperative trigger finger between groups.

The results were interesting in that significant differences were found. The cohort that underwent both fascia and ligament release had a higher incidence of trigger finger than the group that underwent ligament release alone. The overall incidence of triggering following carpal tunnel release was 36 of 123 with more than double being in the group that underwent transverse carpal ligament release + distal antebrachial fascia release (25) versus the transverse carpal ligament release alone group (11).

For me, these findings are difficult to definitively explain, and further study is necessary. It seems likely that the positional changes of the tendons when the fascia is released may increase the tension downstream at the a-1 pulley, resulting in increased likelihood of developing a trigger finger. Although the results with respect to outcome of carpal tunnel release were similar between groups, I would caution against the temptation not to completely release the transverse carpal ligament. I believe that complete release of the carpal tunnel should be the priority in these patients, so as not to compromise the release due to concern of developing a postoperative trigger finger. In addition, postoperative wrist immobilization may stabilize the tendons to minimize the risk of triggering postoperatively. Again, further study will help shed better light on this finding.

M. Rizzo, MD

Malunited Fractures in the Hand

Bot AGJ, Jupiter JB (Massachusetts General Hosp, Boston)

J Hand Surg Am 39:378-384, 2014

Posttraumatic deformity of a tubular bone in the hand after malunion can impact function due to alteration in mobility, strength, or associated pain. Surgical intervention is often indicated, with the surgical options based on both the type and location of the deformity, as well as any associated articular, tendon, or soft tissue constraints. This article provides a management approach based on the deformity classification, location, and any associated conditions.

▶ This article is a nice review and update on the current concepts regarding malunions of the hand and their treatment. The authors provide a nice overview of the types of injuries leading to malunion and the clinical presentations associated with malunited fractures.

Case-based examples illustrating concepts and considerations for treatment as well as techniques used help reinforce fundamental principles in the treatment of these often difficult problems.

M. Rizzo, MD

Catastrophic Thinking Is Associated With Finger Stiffness After Distal Radius Fracture Surgery

Teunis T, Bot AGJ, Thornton ER, et al (Harvard Med School, Boston, MA; Univ of Amsterdam, the Netherlands)

J Orthop Trauma 29:e414-e420, 2015

Objectives.—To identify demographic, injury-related, or psychologic factors associated with finger stiffness at suture removal and 6 weeks after distal radius fracture surgery. We hypothesize that there are no factors associated with distance to palmar crease at suture removal.

Design.—Prospective cohort study.

Setting.—Level I Academic Urban Trauma Center.

Patients.—One hundred sixteen adult patients underwent open reduction and internal fixation of their distal radius fractures; 96 of whom were also available 6 weeks after surgery.

Intervention.—None.

Main Outcome Measurements.—At suture removal, we recorded patients' demographics, AO fracture type, carpal tunnel release at the time of surgery, pain catastrophizing scale, Whiteley Index, Patient Health Questionnaire-9, and disabilities of the arm, shoulder, and hand questionnaire, 11-point ordinal measure of pain intensity, distance to palmar crease, and active flexion of the thumb through the small finger. At 6 weeks after surgery, we measured motion, disabilities of the arm, shoulder, and hand,

and pain intensity. Prereduction and postsurgery radiographic fracture characteristics were assessed.

Results.—Female sex, being married, specific surgeons, carpal tunnel release, AO type C fractures, and greater catastrophic thinking were associated with increased distance to palmar crease at suture removal. At 6 weeks, greater catastrophic thinking was the only factor associated with increased distance to palmar crease.

Conclusions.—Catastrophic thinking was a consistent and major determinant of finger stiffness at suture removal and 6 weeks after injury. Future research should assess if treatments that ameliorate catastrophic thinking can facilitate recovery of finger motion after operative treatment of a distal radius fracture.

Level of Evidence.—Prognostic Level I. See Instructions for Authors for a complete description of levels of evidence.

► A small percentage of patients will have difficulty after operative or nonoperative treatment of distal radius fracture. This article ambitiously attempts to identify patient factors associated with finger stiffness following surgical treatment of distal radius fractures.

The authors reviewed 116 cases of adult distal radius fractures that underwent open reduction and internal fixation. Demographic factors were assessed. Additional factors included fracture type, concomitant carpal tunnel release, catastrophizing scale, Whiteley Index, Patient Health Questionnaire-9, Disabilities of the Arm, Shoulder and Hand (DASH) score, 11-point ordinal measure of pain, distance to distal palmar crease flexion lag, and active motion of all digits.

Through multivariate analysis, the authors found that catastrophic thinking was the lone variable associated with limited finger flexion after surgery.

M. Rizzo, MD

Biomechanical Comparison of Volar Fixed-Angle Locking Plates for AO C3 Distal Radius Fractures: Titanium Versus Stainless Steel With Compression

Marshall T, Momaya A, Eberhardt A, et al (Univ of Alabama at Birmingham; et al)
J Hand Surg Am 40:2032-2038, 2015

Purpose.—To determine biomechanical differences between a fixed-angle locking volar titanium plate (VariAx; Stryker, Kalamazoo, MI) and a fixed-angle compression locking volar stainless steel plate (CoverLoc Volar Plate; Tornier, Amsterdam, Netherlands) in the fixation of simulated AO C3 distal radius fractures.

Methods.—Eighteen cadaveric upper extremities (9 matched pairs) with an average age of 54 years were tested. A 4-part AO C3 fracture pattern was created in each specimen. The fractures were reduced under direct vision and fixed with either the fixed-angle locking volar titanium plate or the fixed-angle compression locking volar stainless steel plate. Motion tracking analysis was then performed while the specimens underwent cyclic loading. Changes in displacement, rotation, load to failure, and mode of failure were recorded.

Results.—The fragments, when secured with the fixed-angle compression locking stainless steel construct, demonstrated less displacement and rotation than the fragments secured with the fixed-angle locking titanium plate under physiological loading conditions. In the fixed-angle compression locking stainless steel group, aggregate displacement and rotation of fracture fragments were 5 mm and 3° less, respectively, than those for the fixed-angle locking titanium group. The differences between axial loads at mechanical failure and stiffness were not statistically significant. The compression locking stainless steel group showed no trend in mode of failure, and the locking titanium plate group failed most often by articular fixation failure (5 of 9 specimens).

Conclusions.—The fixed-angle compression locking stainless steel volar plate may result in less displacement and rotation of fracture fragments in the fixation of AO C3 distal radius fractures than fixation by the fixed-angle locking volar titanium plate. However, there were no differences between the plates in mechanical load to failure and stiffness.

Clinical Relevance.—Fixation of distal radius AO C3 fracture patterns with the fixed-angle compression locking stainless steel plate may provide improved stability of fracture fragments.

▶ There has been a long-standing debate regarding the optimal material for plates. Each material has its advantages. Titanium is a better load-sharing material, but steel is stronger. The aim of this study was to compare the plates with respect to maintenance of reduction as well as load to failure. They used 11 cadaver specimens and recreated AO C-3 fractures for the analysis.

While the load to failure was not statistically different between plates, the stainless steel plates had only 1 of 9 fail at the articular fixation, compared with 5 of 9 in the titanium group. In addition, the stainless steel plates fared better with maintenance of reduction. The wrists treated with stainless steel plates had less fragment displacement and rotation than those of titanium.

This study helps surgeons better understand the mechanical considerations in plating distal radius fractures. Although it may not be as relevant in extra-articular or less comminuted fractures, it does appear to have implications in AO-C3 fracture patterns.

M. Rizzo, MD

Outcomes of Open Dorsal Wrist Ganglion Excision in Active-Duty Military Personnel

Balazs GC, Donohue MA, Drake ML, et al (Walter Reed Natl Military Med Ctr, Bethesda, MD)

J Hand Surg Am 40:1739-1747, 2015

Purpose.—To examine the most common presenting complaints of active-duty service members with isolated dorsal wrist ganglions and to determine the rate of return to unrestricted duty after open excision.

Methods.—Surgical records at 2 military facilities were screened to identify male and female active duty service members undergoing isolated open excision of dorsal wrist ganglions from January 1, 2006 to January 1, 2014. Electronic medical records and service disability databases were searched to identify the most common presenting symptoms and to determine whether patients returned to unrestricted active duty after surgery. Postoperative outcomes examined were pain persisting greater than 4 weeks after surgery, stiffness requiring formal occupational therapy treatment, surgical wound complications, and recurrence.

Results.—A total of 125 active duty military personnel (Army, 54; Navy, 43; and Marine Corps, 28) met criteria for inclusion. Mean follow-up was 45 months. Fifteen percent (8 of 54) of the Army personnel were given permanent waivers from performing push-ups owing to persistent pain and stiffness. Pain persisting greater than 4 weeks after surgery was an independent predictor of eventual need for a permanent push-up waiver. The overall recurrence incidence was 9%. No demographic or perioperative factors were associated with recurrence.

Conclusions.—Patients whose occupation or activities require forceful wrist extension should be counseled on the considerable risk of residual pain and functional limitations that may occur after open dorsal wrist ganglion excision.

Type of Study/Level of Evidence.—Therapeutic IV.

► Dorsal wrist ganglia are common and often require intervention. The authors reviewed their outcomes in active duty military personnel after open excision. The average follow-up period was nearly 4 years. Interestingly, 15% of patients necessitated permanent restrictions due to pain and/or stiffness. The overall recurrence rate was 9%.

Many articles laud minimal recurrence rates and excellent outcomes from dorsal ganglion excision, but most are in civilians. However, over the years, I have noted some of the findings experienced by the authors, especially in active individuals. I concur with the authors' conclusion that patients who are very active need to be advised of the risk of pain or difficulty with strenuous activities, especially activities requiring forceful wrist extension.

M. Rizzo, MD

Donor-Site Morbidity of the Radial Forearm Free Flap versus the Ulnar Forearm Free Flap

Hekner DD, Abbink JH, van Es RJ, et al (Univ Med Ctr Utrecht, The Netherlands)
Plast Reconstr Surg 132:387-393, 2013

Background.—Donor-site morbidity following harvest of the radial forearm free flap was compared with that following harvest of the ulnar forearm free flap.

Methods.—Twenty-eight radial forearm and 27 ulnar forearm flaps were harvested in 55 patients with head and neck defects. Pressure perception was measured with Semmes-Weinstein monofilaments. Cold perception was tested with chloroethyl. Donor-site healing was evaluated. Patients were interviewed about grip and pinch strength and donor-site appearance.

Results.—In the radial forearm free flap group, pressure perception and cold perception were reduced in the donor hand, whereas in the ulnar group, no differences were observed between the donor and unoperated hands. In the radial forearm group, 15 percent of patients experienced reduced strength in the donor hand, whereas in the ulnar forearm group, none of the patients reported reduced strength in the donor hand. In the radial forearm group, 14 percent had partial or complete loss of the skin graft, whereas in the ulnar forearm group, 4 percent had partial loss of the skin graft. In the radial forearm group, 18 percent of patients were dissatisfied with the appearance of the donor site, and no complaints were reported in the ulnar forearm group.

Conclusions.—The authors' study shows less donor site-morbidity following harvest of the ulnar forearm free flap than following harvest of the radial forearm free flap. These results emphasize that the ulnar forearm free flap should be considered as an alternative for the radial forearm free flap for reconstruction of soft-tissue defects.

Clinical Question/Level of Evidence.—Therapeutic, III.

▶ Although the radial forearm flap is a commonly used technique for wound coverage, donor site morbidity including aesthetic appearance, radial nerve irritation, flexor tendon adhesions, and limited skin graft take are a known problem. The ulnar forearm flap is a less commonly used alternative to the radial forearm flap. The aim of this study was to compare donor site complications between these 2 flaps.

The authors compare the 2 flaps among 55 patients with essentially equal distribution between groups. Five of 18 radial forearm flap patients complained of the donor site appearance compared to none in the ulnar forearm flap group. In addition, the radial forearm flap group had a higher rate of weakness with grip and pinch compared with the ulnar cohort. The rate of split thickness skin graft sloughing was higher in patients that underwent radial forearm flap procedures.

This study reflects a nice comparison between these 2 flaps. Some surgeons may be less comfortable with the ulnar artery flap, but it is worth considering it as good alternative to the radial forearm flap.

M. Rizzo, MD

Operative Treatment of Unstable Long Oblique Proximal Phalanx Fractures

Nuland K, Charette R, Rodner CM (Univ of Connecticut Health Ctr, Farmington)

J Hand Surg Am 41:120-121, 2016

Background.—Currently, closed reduction and percutaneous pinning (CRPP) is often chosen to address unstable long oblique fractures of the proximal phalanx with malrotation because it limits extensor tendon damage. However, the finger must be immobilized postoperatively and infection is a risk. Motion can begin earlier with screw fixation, but this method has been linked to stiffness and flexion contracture caused by scarring. Use of a plate and screws to fix these fractures requires additional dissection and is relatively more prominent than the CRPP and screw-only choices. A review of the current evidence and current practice, as well as areas to be explored in future research, was offered.

Current Evidence.—Nine studies evaluated the fixation of proximal phalanx fractures, with most patients treated with CRPP. A comparison of surgery and Kirschner wire fixation in 48 patients found good results for all but 4 patients, whereas the treatment of 100 consecutive proximal phalanx fractures within 5 days of injury with CRPP reported 61 excellent results, 29 good results, and 10 poor results related to stiffness. Fifty proximal phalanx fractures treated with CRPP had an 80% excellent or good result and a 20% fair or poor result, with no malunions and a mean time to union of 35 days.

Plate fixation was used for 6 patients to increase fracture stability and permit earlier postoperative movement, but half of these patients developed complications, which the authors attributed to the initial degree of injury severity. Of 55 proximal phalanx fractures treated with open reduction internal fixation with plates, complications, principally stiffness, occurred in 62%, and just 21% had excellent or good results after 43 weeks. A nonrandomized study of 43 patients with oblique and spiral metacarpal and proximal phalangeal fractures with plate and screw fixation or screw-only fixation showed better range of motion and disability scores in patients receiving screw-only fixation for their proximal phalangeal fractures. Fifteen patients with long oblique proximal phalanx fractures received open reduction internal fixation with screws and 17 underwent CRPP. No difference in patient perception of the outcome was noted between the groups. Three who had Kirschner wires placed required a second surgery for stiffness. Of 40 proximal phalangeal fractures managed with nonlocking intrameduallary nails and proximally locking intramedullary nails, total final average finger motion was 219 degrees for the nonlocking and 226 degrees for the locking groups. The most common complication was loss of proximal interphalangeal joint extension of 17 to 20 degrees.

Overall, these studies are small to moderate in size and combine various fracture types, making generalizations difficult. Because most are retrospective case series, they are subject to selection bias. The outcomes are also prone to subjective interpretation.

Conclusions and Future Research.—CRPP with Kirschner wires or open reduction internal fixation with screws using a small dorsal or midaxial incision is the current approach of choice for these patients. Plates and screws do not appear to be supported by the literature, although they may be the right choice in certain circumstances. CRPP and screw-only fixation appear to achieve comparable results, leaving the decision of which to use in the hands of the surgeon. Future studies need to be larger, randomized trials that focus on digital motion, patient symptoms, and disability and document adverse events and costs associated with the various approaches to treatment.

▶ Treatment of long oblique fractures of the phalanges pose challenges to the surgeon. Common complications include loss of reduction, limited motion, and malrotation and malangluation. Debate persists between closed treatment versus open reduction and fixation.

The authors reviewed the current literature regarding treatment of these injuries. They concluded that closed reduction and pinning fares similarly to open reduction and screw fixation. There is no role for plate/screw fixation for these injuries.

Given that closed reduction and pinning fares just as well as open reduction and screw fixation, my preference is to go with closed reduction and pinning as plan A. However, it is also important for the surgeon to individualize each case and be comfortable with and prepared to use all necessary treatment options.

M. Rizzo, MD

Defining the role of intramedullary nailing for fractures of the distal radius: a systematic review

Jordan RW, Saithna A (Univ Hosps Coventry and Warwickshire, UK)

Bone Joint J 97-B:1370-1376, 2015

This article is a systematic review of the published literature about the biomechanics, functional outcome and complications of intramedullary nailing of fractures of the distal radius.

We searched the Medline and EMBASE databases and included all studies which reported the outcome of intramedullary (IM) nailing of fractures of the distal radius. Data about functional outcome, range of movement (ROM), strength and complications, were extracted. The studies included were appraised independently by both authors using a validated quality assessment scale for non-controlled studies and the CONSORT statement for randomised controlled trials (RCTs).

The search strategy revealed 785 studies, of which 16 were included for full paper review. These included three biomechanical studies, eight case series and five randomised controlled trials (RCTs).

The biomechanical studies concluded that IM nails were at least as strong as locking plates. The clinical studies reported that IM nailing gave a comparable ROM, functional outcome and grip strength to other fixation techniques.

However, the mean complication rate of intramedullary nailing was 17.6% (0% to 50%). This is higher than the rates reported in contemporary studies for volar plating. It raises concerns about the role of intramedullary nailing, particularly when comparative studies have failed to show that it has any major advantage over other techniques. Further adequately powered RCTs comparing the technique to both volar plating and percutaneous wire fixation are needed.

▶ The authors review and critically analyze the role of intramedullary nailing in the management of distal radius fractures. The review included biomechanical studies. The basic science evaluations demonstrated that they were at least as strong as volar locking plates (the standard that they used for comparison). In addition, the clinical results of intramedullary nailing were adequate and comparable to other methods of open reduction and internal fixation. However, the complication rates of nailing were substantially higher than other methods of fixation. Because most intramedullary nails are inserted from the radial side, superficial branch of the radial nerve irritation and first dorsal compartment tendonitis or tenosynovitis were among the highest complications noted.

Aside from potentially higher complication rates, I feel the indications for nailing are more narrow than those of locked volar plating. In addition, there is less ability to restore volar tilt with intramedullary nailing. Although this study does not compel the reader to embrace intramedullary nailing as a treatment for distal radius fractures, I agree with the authors' assessment that prospective analyses would better assess their potential role in distal radius fracture treatment.

M. Rizzo, MD

Distal Radioulnar Joint Reaction Force Following Ulnar Shortening: Diaphyseal Osteotomy Versus Wafer Resection

Canham CD, Schreck MJ, Maqsoodi N, et al (Univ of Rochester, NY; et al)
J Hand Surg Am 40:2206-2212, 2015

Purpose.—To compare how ulnar diaphyseal shortening and wafer resection affect distal radioulnar joint (DRUJ) joint reaction force (JRF) using a nondestructive method of measurement. Our hypothesis was that ulnar shortening osteotomy would increase DRUJ JRF more than wafer resection.

Methods.—Eight fresh-frozen human cadaveric upper limbs were obtained. Under fluoroscopic guidance, a threaded pin was inserted into the lateral radius orthogonal to the DRUJ and a second pin was placed in the medial ulna coaxial to the radial pin. Each limb was mounted onto a mechanical tensile testing machine and a distracting force was applied across the DRUJ while force and displacement were simultaneously measured. Data sets were entered into a computer and a polynomial was generated and solved to determine the JRF. This process was repeated after ulnar diaphyseal osteotomy, ulnar re-lengthening, and ulnar wafer resection. The JRF was compared among the 4 conditions.

Results.—Average baseline DRUJ JRF for the 8 arms increased significantly after diaphyseal ulnar shortening osteotomy (7.2 vs 10.3 N). Average JRF after re-lengthening the ulna and wafer resection was 6.9 and 6.7 N, respectively. There were no differences in JRF among baseline, relengthened, and wafer resection conditions.

Conclusions.—Distal radioulnar joint JRF increased significantly after ulnar diaphyseal shortening osteotomy and did not increase after ulnar wafer resection.

Clinical Relevance.—Diaphyseal ulnar shortening osteotomy increases DRUJ JRF, which may lead to DRUJ arthrosis.

▶ The authors investigated the joint reaction forces at the distal radioulnar joint between the native wrist, the wrist after ulnar shortening, and the wrist following wafer procedure. The results demonstrated increased forces with ulnar shortening compared with the other cohorts.

Both ulnar shortening and distal ulnar wafer procedures have been shown to be effective in the treatment of ulnocarpal impingement. Ulnar shortening has the advantage of being a joint stabilizing procedure. Therefore, the findings of this article would be consistent with that observation, and one should be wary of the long-term effects of shortening and the potential of inviting arthritis later in life.

M. Rizzo, MD

The Unstable Distal Radius Fracture—How Do We Define It? A Systematic Review

Walenkamp MMJ, Vos LM, Strackee SD, et al (Univ of Amsterdam, The Netherlands; Maasstad Hosp, Rotterdam, The Netherlands)

J Wrist Surg 4:307-316, 2015

Background.—Unstable distal radius fractures are a popular research subject. However, to appreciate the findings of studies that enrolled patients with unstable distal radius fractures, it should be clear how the authors defined an *unstable distal radius fracture*.

Questions.—In what percentage of studies involving patients with unstable distal radius fractures did the authors define *unstable distal radius fracture*? What are the most common descriptions of an unstable distal radius fracture? And is there one preferred evidence-based definition for future authors?

Methods.—A systematic search of literature was performed to identify any type of study with the term *unstable distal radius fracture*. We assessed whether a definition was provided and determined the level of evidence for the most common definitions.

Results.—The search yielded 2,489 citations, of which 479 were included. In 149 studies, it was explicitly stated that patients with unstable distal radius fractures were enrolled. In 54% (81/149) of these studies, the authors defined an unstable distal radius fracture. Overall, we found 143 different definitions. The seven most common definitions were: displacement following adequate reduction; Lafontaine's definition; irreducibility; an AO type C2 fracture; a volarly displaced fracture; Poigenfürst's criteria; and Cooney's criteria. Only Lafontaine's definition originated from a clinical study (level IIIb).

Conclusion.—In only half of the studies involving patients with an unstable distal radius fracture did the authors defined what they considered an *unstable distal radius fracture*. None of the definitions stood out as the preferred choice. A general consensus definition could help to standardize future research.

▶ This article attempts to answer an important question: How do we define an unstable distal radius fracture? They performed a literature search examining the most commonly accepted definitions used today. The authors reviewed nearly 500 articles that met inclusion criteria and found more than 140 definitions, which they further narrowed to 7 that they considered most relevant or commonly considered. They went on to find that the current literature is grossly inconsistent in defining instability of distal radius. Among the 7 definitions, Lafontaine et al's 1989 article is the only one that is based on some degree of evidence (Level III). All the others are based on expert opinion. Age greater than 60 years, comminution and initial shortening were proposed by the authors to be predictors of instability.

Without a validated, consistent and universally accepted definition for unstable distal radius fractures, a foundation is lacking for sound scientifically based analyses of treatments of these common injuries. I agree with the authors that a universal definition will help standardize future research.

M. Rizzo, MD

The Effect of Midcarpal Versus Total Wrist Fusion on the Hand's Load Distribution During Gripping

Mühldorfer-Fodor M, Reger A, Schoonhoven Jv, et al (Rhön Klinikum AG, Bad Neustadt/Saale, Germany; et al)

J Hand Surg Am 40:2183-2190, 2015

Purpose.—To analyze the total grip force and load distribution of the hand with midcarpal fusion (MCF) and total wrist fusion (TWF).

Methods.—Twelve patients with unilateral TWF and 12 patients with unilateral MCF were assessed at an average 64 months (range, 19-100 months) postoperatively. The total grip force and load distribution of both hands were measured by the Manugraphy system using 3 cylinder sizes. The load applied to 7 anatomical areas of the hand during cylinder grip was analyzed, comparing the operated and the nonsurgical hands.

Results.—For the 100 mm and 150 mm cylinders, a significantly lower total grip force was found in hands operated with either TWF or MCF. For the 200 mm cylinder, there was a significant difference between nonsurgical hands and those with MCF but not between nonsurgical hands and those with TWF. For the 100 mm cylinder, the difference between nonsurgical and operated hands was greater in hands with TWF than those with MCF. For the load distribution of the hand, no differences between the operated and the nonsurgical hand were found for either MCF or TWF.

Conclusions.—MFC and TWF resulted in a reduced cylinder grip force. With respect to the load distribution, neither procedure influenced the relative contribution that each area of the hand produced during cylinder grip.

Type of Study/Level of Evidence.—Therapeutic III.

▶ The authors compared midcarpal fusions with total wrist fusions in the context of total grip force. They found that, compared with the nonoperated hands, both groups had weakness with cylindrical grip strength (at 100 and 150 mm). For the largest cylindrical size (200 mm), the partial wrist fusion fared worse than the nonoperated side, but the total fusion did not have significant difference compared with the nonoperated extremity. The position of total wrist fusion in their cohort was 14 degrees extension and 7 degrees ulnar deviation. The partial wrist fusion group had an average flexion/extension arc of 27/30 degrees and radial/ulnar deviation arc of 14/9 degrees.

Because of some of the difficulties with smaller grip radii with the total wrist fusions, the authors concluded that patients more dependent on grip for work and activities would fare better in more extended positions. Although this may intuitively make sense, the conclusion is less than convincing based on the results. I would think that if greater wrist extension would benefit strength, then the midcarpal fusion group would have fared better than the total wrist fusion group because the wrist would have naturally fallen into the "optimal" extended position when trying to maximize strength (because the partial fusions were, on average, able to generate 30 degrees of extension). That did not appear to be the case. The authors also noted that they did not measure the position of the wrist in the midcarpal fusion group while gripping, which would have been helpful.

M. Rizzo, MD

Dorsal Screw Penetration With the Use of Volar Plating of Distal Radius Fractures: How Can You Best Detect?

Hill BW, Shakir I, Cannada LK (Saint Louis Univ, MO)

J Orthop Trauma 29:e408-e413, 2015

Objectives.—To evaluate the most vulnerable position at which volar plate screws may penetrate the dorsal cortex of the radius and to determine which specific intraoperative fluoroscopic images (lateral, 45 degrees supination, 45 degrees pronation, and dorsal tangential) are most useful to detect dorsal cortex penetration.

Methods.—Four 2.5-mm locking screws were inserted distally using 18-, 20-, or 22-mm screws in 7 cadaveric specimens apiece. The specimens were then evaluated to count the number of screws breaching the dorsal cortex and the amount of penetration. Lateral, 45 degrees supination, 45 degrees pronation, and dorsal tangential fluoroscopic views were taken of each wrist. Sixty-three orthopaedic surgeons of varying experience were then asked to evaluate whether the screws penetrated the dorsal cortex after viewing each image.

Results.—Dorsal cortex screw penetration of at least 1 screw occurred in 3.6% of specimens with 18-mm screws, 25% of specimens with 20-mm screws, and 57% specimens with 22-mm screws. Radial-sided screws more commonly breached the dorsal cortex. The sensitivity was 58% on the lateral view, 88% on the 45 degrees supination view, 53% on the 45 degrees pronation view, and 67% on the dorsal tangential view. Additionally, surgeons with more experience were less accurate in detecting prominent screws.

Conclusions.—Clinicians should consider use of these views to evaluate dorsal screw penetration after volar plating but may opt to subtract a few millimeters from their measured screw lengths to avoid over penetration past the dorsal cortex.

▶ The authors performed a cadaver study examining for dorsal distal radial cortical penetration after distal radius fracture fixation. They used different screw lengths ranging from 18 to 22 mm in 21 different cadaver specimens (7 in each group). The examined the wrists with imaging and direct visualization. The results demonstrated that with the 18-mm screws, the dorsal cortex was breached by at least 1 screw in 3.6% of wrists; with the 20-mm screw, 25% of specimens; and with the 22-mm screw, there was 57% incidence of dorsal cortex penetration.

I applaud the study because it is another fairly simplified way of helping us appreciate the risks associated with dorsal radial breaching of distal screws. We appreciate the value of avoiding penetration of the dorsal cortex with respect to minimizing tendon rupture and irritation risk.

In addition, the authors reiterated that there is a higher risk of cortical breach on the radial side of the distal radius. Radiograph sensitivity was fair. The best view was with the 45-degree supination view, which makes sense given the radial screws were most commonly too long. They conclude that subtracting

4 mm from the measurement would likely be helpful in mitigating the possibility of dorsal screw penetration.

M. Rizzo, MD

Complex Regional Pain Syndrome Type I: Incidence and Risk Factors in Patients With Fracture of the Distal Radius

Jellad A, Salah S, Ben Salah Frih Z (Univ of Monastir, Tunisia)

Arch Phys Med Rehabil 95:487-492, 2014

Objective.—To examine the incidence and predictors of complex regional pain syndrome type I (CRPS I) after fracture of the distal radius.

Design.—Prospective study.

Setting.—University hospital.

Participants.—A consecutive sample of patients (N = 90) with fracture of the distal radius treated by closed reduction and casting.

Interventions.—Not applicable.

Main Outcome Measures.—Occurrence of CRPS I, occurrence of pain, wrist and hand range of motion, radiographic measures, Patient-Rated Wrist Evaluation, Hospital Anxiety and Depression Scale, and Medical Outcomes Study 36-Item Short-Form Health Survey at baseline and 1, 3, 6, and 9 months follow-up.

Results.—CRPS I occurred in 29 patients (32.2%) with a mean delay ± SD of 21.7 ± 23.7 days from cast removal. Univariate analyses found significant differences between patients with CRPS I and patients without CRPS I at baseline for sex ($P = .021$), socioeconomic level ($P = .023$), type of trauma ($P = .05$), pain at rest and activity ($P = .006$ and $P < .001$, respectively), wrist dorsiflexion and pronation ($P = .002$ and $P = .001$, respectively), finger flexion ($P = .047$), thumb opposition ($P = .002$), function of the hand ($P < .001$), and physical quality of life (QOL) ($P = .013$). Logistic regression showed that risk for CRPS I was higher in cases of women (odds ratio [OR]=5.774; 95% confidence interval [CI], 1.391–23.966), medium and low energy trauma patients (OR = 7.718; 95% CI, 1.136–52.44), patients with a Medical Outcomes Study 36-Item Short-Form Health Survey physical functioning score <40 (OR = 4.931; 95% CI, 1.428–17.025), and patients with Patient-Rated Wrist Evaluation pain subscale score >16 (OR = 12.192; 95% CI, 4.484–43.478).

Conclusions.—CRPS I occurs frequently during the third and fourth week after cast removal, especially in women who report severe pain and impairment of physical QOL. Additional prospective studies are required to verify these findings in comminuted and operated fractures of the distal radius.

► Complex regional pain syndrome (CRPS) associated with distal radius fractures can lead to significant morbidity. Identifying risk factors or predictors of "patients at risk" of complex regional pain syndrome would be most helpful to clinicians.

Ninety consecutive patients were treated with closed reduction and casting following distal radius fractures in a university hospital. The incidence of complex regional pain syndrome was 32%. Several demographic variables were linked to pain syndromes, including female sex and lower socioeconomic status. Interestingly, lower or medium energy trauma was related to the development of complex regional pain syndrome.

Most cases of complex regional pain syndrome occurred at the third or fourth week after cast removal.

While the incidence of CRPS in this study seemed high compared with my personal experience, I think the study helps provide a good foundation for future study.

M. Rizzo, MD

Collagenase Clostridium Histolyticum for Dupuytren Contracture: Patterns of Use and Effectiveness in Clinical Practice

Peimer CA, Skodny P, Mackowiak JI (Michigan State Univ, Lansing; Marquette General Healthcare, MI; Auxilium Pharmaceuticals, Inc., Malvern, PA; et al)

J Hand Surg Am 38:2370-2376, 2013

Purpose.—To collect data on the real-world effectiveness of collagenase clostridium histolyticum (CCH) during its first year of use following U.S. Food and Drug Administration approval and compare those results with clinical trial efficacy data.

Methods.—This retrospective chart review was conducted at 10 U.S. community and academic practice sites with major experience using CCH. Charts of patients treated with CCH between February and December 2010 were abstracted, and anonymized data were analyzed. Clinical use, including number of injections per cord and effectiveness outcomes (joint contracture and range of motion) were compared with results from 2 registration trials.

Results.—Data were collected from 501 patients (74% male; 48% employed; mean [SD] age, 65 [10] y); 463 patients had sufficient data for analysis. We found that 1.08 CCH injections were used per treated joint, compared with a mean of 1.7 injections in registration trials. Ninety-three percent of joints received only 1 injection. The mean (SD) number of visits per injection was 2.92 (1.0). Mean (SD) contracture was reduced by 75% from 49° (21) at baseline to 12° (17), similar to the 71% to 79% reduction in clinical trials. Mean (SD) range of motion was improved by 37° from 44° (20) at baseline to 81° (14), similar to the increase of 35° and 37° in the 2 clinical trials; and 67% of first injections resulted in full correction to 0° to 5°, compared with the clinical trial rate of 39%.

Conclusions.—Despite a lower injection rate, correction of joint contracture and range of motion was similar to findings from clinical trials.

Effectiveness reports using this kind of surveillance design could provide patients, physicians, and payers with the information needed to make better treatment and reimbursement decisions.

Type of Study/Level of Evidence.—Therapeutic III.

▶ Since receiving US Food and Drug Administration approval in 2010, clostridial collagenase has been increasingly used in the management of Dupuytren contracture. It has the advantages of being an office-based procedure with arguably less risk than surgery. The disadvantages include cost, 2 separate visits for the patient (1 for the injection and another 1–7 days later for the release), risk of possible tendon and/or skin tears, and recurrence. Prospective randomized studies established its efficacy, and the average number of injections per patient was 1.7. However, the study guidelines did not allow for injections of anesthesia the day of release, and it is common to anesthetize the digit at the time of release. It is also understood that we have had better success with release as a result of being able to eliminate pain.

This article is a review of 463 fingers treated in the first year of use with Xiaflex and confirms that assumption. In addition, there was no discernable difference in functional outcomes and range of motion in this experience compared with the Collagenase Option for the Reduction of Dupuytren's studies. No significant adverse events were experienced in the series.

Clostridial collagenase has established itself as a viable treatment for Dupuytren contracture. The ability to anesthetize patients at the time of release has reduced the need for future injections.

M. Rizzo, MD

Physician Empathy as a Driver of Hand Surgery Patient Satisfaction

Menendez ME, Chen NC, Mudgal CS, et al (Harvard Med School, Boston, MA)

J Hand Surg Am 40:1860-1865, 2015

Purpose.—To examine the relationship between patient-rated physician empathy and patient satisfaction after a single new hand surgery office visit.

Methods.—Directly after the office visit, 112 consecutive new patients rated their overall satisfaction with the provider and completed the Consultation and Relational Empathy Measure, the Newest Vital Sign health literacy test, a sociodemographic survey, and 3 Patient-Reported Outcomes Measurement Information System-based questionnaires: Pain Interference, Upper-Extremity Function, and Depression. We also measured the waiting time in the office to see the physician, the duration of the visit, and the time from booking until appointment. Multivariable logistic and linear regression models were used to identify factors independently associated with patient satisfaction.

Results.—Patient-rated physician empathy correlated strongly with the degree of overall satisfaction with the provider. After controlling for confounding effects, greater empathy was independently associated with patient satisfaction, and it alone accounted for 65% of the variation in satisfaction scores. Older patient age was also associated with satisfaction. There were no differences between satisfied and dissatisfied patients with regard to waiting time in the office, duration of the appointment, time from booking until appointment, and health literacy.

Conclusions.—Physician empathy was the strongest driver of patient satisfaction in the hand surgery office setting. As patient satisfaction plays a growing role in reimbursement, targeted educational programs to enhance empathic communication skills in hand surgeons merit consideration.

Type of Study/Level of Evidence.—Prognostic II.

▶ The authors address an important area of our current health care climate. My experience has been consistent with their conclusions. Most patients tolerate longer waiting times, delays in getting appointments, and logistical hurdles associated with getting to the appointments if their surgeon is empathetic.

Interestingly, older patients were more tolerant and had a greater sense of satisfaction than younger patients.

Advantages of improved patient satisfaction go beyond potential increased reimbursements. I feel strongly that patient satisfaction helps grow your practice through word of mouth. Finally, improved patient satisfaction is likely associated with improved physician satisfaction.

M. Rizzo, MD

Manipulation and reduction of paediatric fractures of the distal radius and forearm using intranasal diamorphine and 50% oxygen and nitrous oxide in the emergency department: a 2.5-year study

Kurien T, Price KR, Pearson RG, et al (Queen's Med Centre, Nottingham, United Kingdom; et al)

Bone Joint J 98-B:131-136, 2016

A retrospective study was performed in 100 children aged between two and 16 years, with a dorsally angulated stable fracture of the distal radius or forearm, who were treated with manipulation in the emergency department (ED) using intranasal diamorphine and 50% oxygen and nitrous oxide. Pre- and post-manipulation radiographs, the final radiographs and the clinical notes were reviewed. A successful reduction was achieved in 90 fractures (90%) and only three children (3%) required remanipulation and Kirschner wire fixation or internal fixation.

The use of Entonox and intranasal diamorphine is safe and effective for the closed reduction of a stable paediatric fracture of the distal radius and forearm in the ED.

By facilitating discharge on the same day, there is a substantial cost benefit to families and the NHS and we recommend this method.

Take home message: Simple easily reducible fractures of the distal radius and forearm in children can be successfully and safely treated in the ED using this approach, thus avoiding theatre admission and costly hospital stay.

▶ Successful closed reduction of distal radius fractures will reduce the need for operative intervention. In addition, there is an added advantage in avoidance of surgery whenever possible in children and patients with open physes. Performing closed reduction of these fractures in the emergency department poses additional challenges in children compared with adult patients.

This study retrospectively examined the efficacy of anesthesia using intranasal diamorphine and 50% oxygen and nitrous oxide in 100 children between 2 and 16 years of age.

The preparation for reduction is initiated with administration of the intranasal diamorphone (0.1 mg/kg). After approximately 20 minutes, the reduction can begin. The child then inhales at least 10 breaths of the Entonox (50% nitrous oxide/50% oxygen) before manipulation. Closed reduction is then performed. After reduction, the child is observed for 30 minutes.

The results demonstrated that successful reduction was achieved in 90% of cases. In the 10% of cases that did not meet the preset standards, only 1 necessitated surgery.

This method of achieving reduction of displaced distal radius and diaphyseal radius fractures in the ED is safe efficient and effective.

M. Rizzo, MD

Fixation Options for the Volar Lunate Facet Fracture: Thinking Outside the Box

Harness NG (Univ of California Irvine, Anaheim)
J Wrist Surg 5:9-16, 2015

Background.—Fractures of the distal radius with small volar ulnar marginal fracture fragments are difficult to stabilize with standard volar locking plates. The purpose of this study is to describe alternative techniques available to stabilize these injuries.

Materials and Methods.—Five patients were identified retrospectively with unstable volar lunate facet fracture fragments treated with supplemental fixation techniques. The demographic data, pre- and postoperative radiographic parameters, and early outcomes data were analyzed. The AO classification, preoperative and final postoperative ulnar variance, articular step-off, volar tilt, radial inclination, and teardrop angle were measured. The lunate subsidence and length of the volar cortex available for fixation were measured from the initial injury films.

Description of Technique.—Lunate facet fixation was based on the morphology of the fragment, and stabilization was achieved with headless compression screws in three patients, a tension band wire construct in one, and two cortical screws in another.

Results.—Five patients with a mean age of 58 years (range: 41–82) were included. There were two AO C3.2 and three B3.3 fractures. Preoperative radiographic measurements including radial inclination, tilt, and ulnar variance all improved after surgery and were maintained within normal limits at 3-month follow-up. There was no change in the teardrop angle at final follow-up (70–64 degrees; $p = 0.14$). None of the patients had loss of fixation or volar carpal subluxation. The mean visual analog scale pain score at 3 months was 1 (range: 0–2).

Conclusions.—The morphology of volar lunate facet fracture fragments is variable, and fixation must be customized to the particular pattern. Small fragments may preclude the use of plates and screws for fixation. These fractures can be managed successfully with tension band wire constructs and headless screws. These low-profile implants may decrease the risk of tendon irritation that might accompany distally placed plates.

▶ It can be challenging to reduce and maintain reduction for lunate facet fractures of the distal radius. Smaller fragments are more difficult to secure. Through 5 cases, the author shares insights regarding the morphology of these injuries and illustrates methods of fixation that have been successful. The presentation of these injuries can be variable and requires versatility from the surgeon. Some of the more distal extending volar rim plates are unable to captures smaller fragments and invite hardware prominence and potential tendon irritation.

The author demonstrates a variety of fixation methods including k-wires, tension band, headless screws, and cortical screws. This article highlights this often challenging problem and is a nice contribution to the literature.

M. Rizzo, MD

Comparison of a New Intramedullary Scaffold to Volar Plating for Treatment of Distal Radius Fractures

Van Kampen RJ, Thoreson AR, Knutson NJ, et al (Mayo Clinic, Rochester, MN; Conventus Orthopaedics, Inc, Maple Grove, MN; et al)

J Orthop Trauma 27:535-541, 2013

Objectives.—To compare the biomechanical properties of a new nitinol intramedullary (IM) scaffold implant with those of volar plates for the treatment of dorsally comminuted extra-articular distal radius fractures using an established model.

Methods.—A dorsal wedge osteotomy was performed on a bone model to simulate a dorsally comminuted extra-articular distal radius fracture. This model was used to compare stiffness of 3 different distal radius fixation devices—an IM scaffold implant, a commercially available titanium volar locking plate, and a stainless steel non-locking T-plate. Six constructs were tested per group. Tolerance for physiological loading was assessed by applying 10,000 cycles of axial loading up to 100 N applied at 2 Hz. Axial and eccentric load stiffness were assessed before cyclic loading and axial stiffness again after cyclic loading. Groups were compared using analysis of variance.

Results.—Initial axial stiffness (in Newton per millimeter) was significantly ($P = 0.011$) different only between the volar locking plate (427 ± 43) and non-locking T-plate (235 ± 69). After cyclic loading, axial stiffness was not significantly different between the volar locking plate (392 ± 67) and IM scaffold implant (405 ± 108), but both were significantly ($P < 0.001$) stiffer than the non-locking T-plate (187 ± 53). Eccentric loading stiffness was not significantly different between the IM scaffold implant (67 ± 140) and volar locking plate (63 ± 5), but both were significantly ($P < 0.001$) stiffer than the non-locking T-plate (25 ± 4).

Conclusions.—Stiffness of the IM scaffold implant and volar locking plate fracture model constructs was equivalent. Biomechanical testing suggests that this novel IM scaffold provides sufficient stability for clinical use, and further testing is warranted.

▶ The authors biomechanically assessed an intramedullary scaffold used in the treatment of distal radius fractures. They compared its strength of supporting the reduction to a titanium volar locking plate and a nonlocking stainless steel t-plate. The results demonstrated comparable superior strength with the scaffold and the titanium locking plate, which is very encouraging.

Locked volar plating has become the preferred operative treatment for unstable distal radius fractures over the past 15 years. I appreciate that complications may arise with their use, and I appreciate the attraction of an intramedullary device. Although I have never placed one, I have concerns about the quality of fixation of the percutaneous headless compression screws in the generally poor distal bone, unless the fixation through the nitinol cage "locks" the screws into place. However, for younger patients with better bone quality, it appears that it would hold up well. It would have been interesting to have compared the device to a dorsal plate or stainless steel volar locking plates as well.

M. Rizzo, MD

Complications after volar locking plate fixation of distal radius fractures

Johnson NA, Cutler L, Dias JJ, et al (Leicester Royal Infirmary, United Kingdom)

Injury 45:528-533, 2014

Volar locking plates are an increasingly popular treatment for distal radius fractures. We reviewed complications observed after volar locking plate fixation in a busy teaching hospital. The purpose of the study was to assess whether complication rates after volar locking plate use in general, routine trauma practice were higher than published literature from expert users.

A retrospective review was carried out of patients treated with a volar locking plate between January 2009 and December 2010. The series included 206 procedures in 204 patients (77 males and 127 females) with mean age of 55 years (range 16-94). Surgery was performed by 18 different consultant surgeons and 11 registrars.

A total of 22 complications were observed in 20 patients with an overall complication rate of 9.7%. Seven (3.4%) patients developed tendon problems including four (1.9%) tendon ruptures. Four (1.9%) patients required re-operation for metalwork problems; four patients developed complex regional pain syndrome (CRPS). Three fracture reduction problems were noted. A total of 16 further operations were carried out for complications.

The overall complication rate was low even when surgery was done by many surgeons, suggesting that this is a safe and reproducible technique. This study provides information which can be used to counsel patients about risks, including those of tendon and metalwork problems. This allows patients to make an informed decision. Surgeons must have specific strategies to avoid these complications and remain vigilant so that these can be identified and managed early.

▶ The authors describe a retrospective analysis of 1 year's worth of distal radius fracture treated with volar locking plates. Among 206 procedures, the overall complication rate (22 complications in 20 patients) was nearly 10%, most related to tendon irritation/rupture, and 4 patients had complex regional pain syndrome. Sixteen required reoperation (4 for tendon ruptures, 4 for hardware problems), and 3 patients lost reduction.

An interesting point of the article is the heterogeniety of the treating surgeons. Eighteen different consultants and 11 registrars performed the surgeries. Intuitively, this would lend itself to higher rates of possible complications, but the complication rates reflect others in the literature. I agree with the authors that the outcomes suggest that volar plating is fairly reproducible in the treatment of distal radius fractures. On a personal note, although it continues to be debated, I have observed that titanium plates carry a higher risk of flexor tendon ruptures compared with stainless steel.

M. Rizzo, MD

4 Elbow

Introduction

While of particular interest to me, this is, appropriately, the smallest section of the YEAR BOOK. As in years past, the main focus is on the most frequently encountered problems seen at the elbow – trauma and tennis elbow. There have been considerable strides in the management of these conditions over the last few years. The selections this year highlight some of these insights that will hopefully be of value to the surgeon.

Bernard F. Morrey, MD

Factors Associated With Failure of Nonoperative Treatment in Lateral Epicondylitis

Knutsen EJ, Calfee RP, Chen RE, et al (George Washington Univ School of Medicine and Health Sciences, DC; Washington Univ School of Medicine, St Louis, MO)
Am J Sports Med 43:2133-2137, 2015

Background.—Lateral epicondylitis is a common cause of elbow pain that is treated with a variety of nonoperative measures and often improves with time. Minimal research is available on patients in whom these nonoperative treatments fail.

Purpose.—To identify baseline patient and disease factors associated with the failure of nonoperative treatment of lateral epicondylitis, defined as surgery after a period of nonoperative treatment.

Study Design.—Case control study; Level of evidence, 3.

Methods.—A total of 580 patients treated for lateral epicondylitis at a tertiary center between 2007 and 2012 were analyzed. Disease-specific and patient demographic characteristics were compared between patient groups (nonoperative vs surgical treatment). A multivariable logistic regression model was created based on preliminary univariate testing to determine which characteristics were associated with failure of nonoperative treatment.

Results.—Of the 580 patients, 92 (16%) underwent surgical treatment at a mean of 6 months (range, 0-31 months) from their initial visit. Univariate analysis demonstrated a potential association ($P < .10$) between

TABLE 2.—Baseline Characteristics Predictive of Failure of Nonoperative Treatment by Multivariate Analysis

Risk Factor	Regression Coefficient, B	Wald Statistic (*P* Value)	Standard Error of B	Odds Ratio (95% CI)
Workers' compensation claim	2.086	25.2 (.000)	0.416	8.1 (3.6-18.2)
Prior injection	1.716	20.1 (.000)	0.378	5.6 (2.7-11.7)
Radial tunnel syndrome	1.119	10.3 (.001)	0.349	3.1 (1.5-6.1)
Prior orthopaedic surgery	1.167	13.1 (.000)	0.323	3.2 (1.7-6.1)
Duration of symptoms >12 mo	0.897	4.0 (.045)	0.447	2.5 (1.0-5.8)

Reprinted from Knutsen EJ, Calfee RP, Chen RE, et al. Factors associated with failure of nonoperative treatment in lateral epicondylitis. *Am J Sports Med.* 2015;43:2133-2137, with permission from The Author(s).

operative management and the following factors at initial diagnosis: increased age, body mass index, duration of symptoms, presence of radial tunnel syndrome, prior injection, physical therapy, splinting, smoking, workers' compensation, a labor occupation, use of narcotics, use of antidepressant medications, and previous orthopaedic surgery. In the final multivariable model, a workers' compensation claim (odds ratio [OR], 8.1), prior injection (OR, 5.6), the presence of radial tunnel syndrome (OR, 3.1), previous orthopaedic surgery (OR, 3.2), and duration of symptoms >12 months (OR, 2.5) remained significant independent predictors of surgical treatment.

Conclusion.—This study identifies risk factors for surgical treatment for lateral epicondylitis. While these findings do not provide information regarding causal factors associated with surgery, these patient and disease-specific considerations may be helpful when counseling patients regarding treatment options and the likelihood of the success of continued nonoperative treatment (Table 2).

▶ This is a nice study supplying helpful information to manage the most common elbow condition requiring a physician's attention. Even though this is a referral center, I found the 16% rate of surgery a little more than I might expect. Of additional note is the relatively short duration of time before surgery is offered. However, the meat of the study is summarized in Table 2. The correlates to surgery are a bit surprising because most try to avoid surgery on worker's compensation patients. That prior orthopedic surgery was also a predictor might suggest either and underlying predilection to musculoskeletal injuries or simply selects a patient willing to undergo surgery to address their complaint.

B. F. Morrey, MD

Corticosteroid and platelet-rich plasma injection therapy in tennis elbow (lateral epicondylalgia): a survey of current UK specialist practice and a call for clinical guidelines

Titchener AG, Booker SJ, Bhamber NS, et al (Royal Derby Hosp, United Kingdom)

Br J Sports Med 49:1410-1413, 2015

Background.—Tennis elbow is a common condition with a variety of treatment options, but little is known about which of these options specialists choose most commonly. Corticosteroid injections in tennis elbow may reduce pain in the short-term but delay long-term recovery. We have undertaken a UK-wide survey of upper limb specialists to assess current practice.

Methods.—Cross-sectional electronic survey of current members of the British Elbow and Shoulder Society (BESS) and the British Society for Surgery of the Hand (BSSH).

Results.—271 of 1047 eligible members responded (25.9%); consultant surgeons constituted the largest group (232/271, 85%). 131 respondents (48%) use corticosteroid injections as their first-line treatment for tennis elbow. 206 respondents (77%) believed that corticosteroid injections are not potentially harmful in the treatment of tennis elbow, while 31 (11%) did not use them in their current practice. In light of recent evidence of the potential harmful effects of corticosteroid therapy, 136 (50%) had not changed their practice while 108 (40.1%) had reduced or discontinued their use. 43 respondents (16%) reported having used platelet-rich plasma injections.

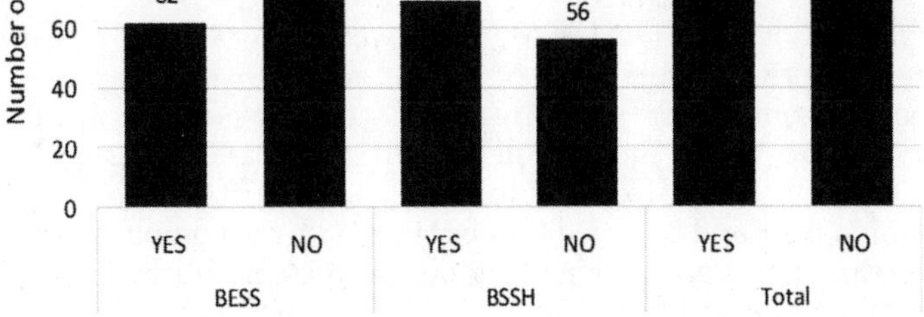

FIGURE 1.—Use of corticosteroid injections as first-line treatment for tennis elbow. (Reprinted from Titchener AG, Booker SJ, Bhamber NS, et al. Corticosteroid and platelet-rich plasma injection therapy in tennis elbow (lateral epicondylalgia): a survey of current UK specialist practice and a call for clinical guidelines. *Br J Sports Med.* 2015;49:1410-1413.)

Conclusions.—Recent high-quality evidence that corticosteroids may delay recovery in tennis elbow appears to have had a limited effect on current practice. Treatment is not uniform among specialists and a proportion of them use platelet-rich plasma injections (Fig 1).

▶ Despite my admitted interest in the elbow, this article was primarily reviewed because of the more important issue: that of the use of steroids to treat tendinopathy. I personally have discontinued the use of steroid in tendon disease, but not for intra-articular pathology. It is interesting to note that, despite clear and growing evidence of the potential harmful effects of steroid injection, the orthopedic community has shown little recognition or practice impact of these data (Fig 1). Too bad, but not surprising.

B. F. Morrey, MD

Demographic Trends and Complication Rates in Arthroscopic Elbow Surgery

Leong NL, Cohen JR, Lord E, et al (Univ of California, Los Angeles; et al)
Arthroscopy 31:1928-1932, 2015

Purpose.—To investigate demographic trends in elbow arthroscopy over time, as well as to query complication rates requiring reoperation associated with these procedures.

Methods.—The Current Procedural Terminology (CPT) billing codes of patients undergoing elbow arthroscopy were searched using a national insurance database. From the years 2007 to 2011, over 20 million orthopaedic patient records were present in the database with an orthopaedic *International Classification of Diseases, Ninth Revision* diagnosis code or CPT code. Our search for procedures and the corresponding CPT codes for the elbow included diagnostic arthroscopy, loose body removal, synovectomy, and debridement. The type of procedure, date, gender, and region of the country were identified for each patient. In addition, the incidence of reoperation for infection, stiffness, and nerve injury was examined.

Results.—There was a significant increase in arthroscopic elbow procedures over the study period. Male patients accounted for 71% of patients undergoing these procedures. Of the elbow arthroscopy patients, 22% were aged younger than 20 years, 25% were aged 20 to 39 years, 47% were aged 40 to 59 years, and 6% were aged 60 years or older. Other than synovectomy, there were regional variations in the incidence of each procedure type. The overall rate of reoperation was 2.2%, with specific rates of 0.26% for infection, 0.63% for stiffness, and 1.26% for nerve injury. It should be noted that because only the complications requiring reoperation are recorded in the database, these numbers are lower than the overall complication rate.

Conclusions.—Overall, the incidence of elbow arthroscopy in this patient population is relatively low and appears to be increasing slightly over time. In the database used in this study, elbow arthroscopy procedures were most commonly performed in male patients and in patients aged 40 to 59 years, with regional variation in the incidence of the different procedures. Furthermore, the rate of complications requiring reoperation was low, with a nerve operation being the most common reoperation performed.

Level of Evidence.—Level IV, therapeutic case series.

▶ The information in this article is very straightforward, and it is included purely for information. The frequency of elbow arthroscopy increased in a linear fashion over the decade studied. As anticipated, loose body and debridement/synovectomy are the most frequent procedures. The point to highlight is that the frequency of complication is not common, but this report is only of those requiring additional surgery. Note that the 1.2% nerve injury is not trivial; further, the .25% infection rate is low, and some are able to be treated without additional surgery. The 2 points to understand are that the nerve injury can be catastrophic, and the elbow is at greater risk than other joints. Finally, note that a whopping 20% of surgeries are performed on those less than 20 years of age; only 5% are on those older than 59 years. These demographics are dramatically different from what occurs with the knee, shoulder, and ankle.

B. F. Morrey, MD

Epidemiology of Medial Ulnar Collateral Ligament Reconstruction: A 10-Year Study in New York State

Hodgins JL, Vitale M, Arons RR, et al (Columbia Univ Med Ctr, NY; Greenwich Hosp, CT)

Am J Sports Med 44:729-734, 2016

Background.—Despite an increase in the prevalence of medial ulnar collateral ligament (UCL) reconstruction of the elbow in professional baseball and popularity within the media, there are no population-based studies examining the incidence of UCL reconstruction.

Purpose.—To examine the epidemiological trends of UCL reconstruction on a statewide level over a 10-year period. The primary endpoint was the yearly rate of UCL reconstruction over time; secondary endpoints included patient demographics, institution volumes, and concomitant procedures on the ulnar nerve.

Study Design.—Descriptive epidemiology study.

Methods.—The New York Statewide Planning and Research Cooperative System (SPARCS) database contains records for each ambulatory discharge in New York State. This database was used to identify all UCL reconstructions in New York State from 2002 to 2011 using the outpatient CPT-4 (*Current Procedural Terminology, 4th Revision*) code. Assessed were patient age, sex, ethnicity, insurance status, and associated procedures, as well as hospital volume.

Results.—There was a significant yearly increase in the number of UCL reconstructions ($P < .001$) performed in New York State from 2002 to 2011. The volume of UCL reconstructions increased by 193%, and the rate per 100,000 population tripled from 0.15 to 0.45. The mean ± SD age was 21.6 ± 8.89 years, and there was a significant trend for an increased frequency in UCL reconstruction in patients aged 17 to 18 and 19 to 20 years ($P < .001$). Male patients were 11.8 times more likely to have a UCL reconstruction than female patients ($P < .001$), and individuals with private insurance were 25 times more likely to have a UCL reconstruction than those with Medicaid ($P = .0014$). There was a 400% increase in concomitant ulnar nerve release/transposition performed over time in the study period, representing a significant increase in the frequency of ulnar nerve procedures at the time of UCL reconstruction ($P < .001$).

Conclusion.—The frequency of UCL reconstruction is steadily rising in New York State and becoming more common in adolescent athletes. Emphasis on public education on the risks of overuse throwing injuries and the importance of adhering to preventative guidelines is essential in youth baseball today (Fig 1).

▶ This is a very useful contribution. What has been documented in New York is not just occurring around the country, it is occurring around the world! In

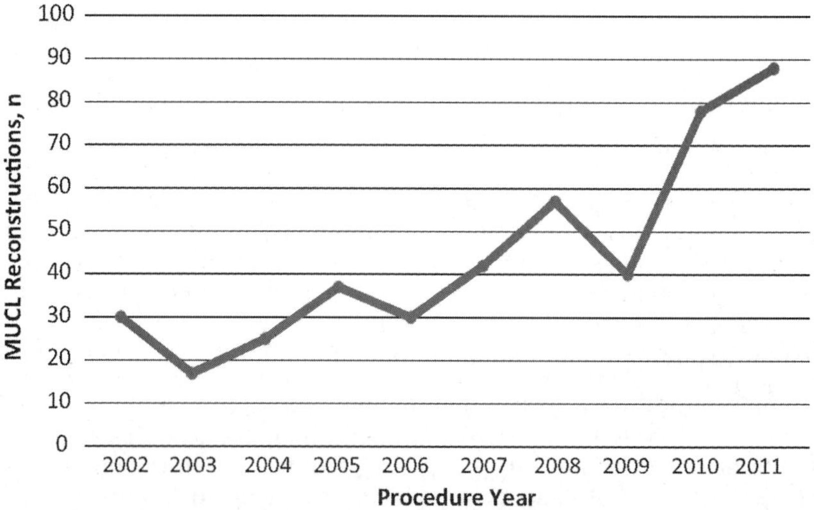

FIGURE 1.—The number of medial ulnar collateral ligament (MUCL) reconstructions performed in New York State by year. There is a significant trend for a greater number of reconstructions performed over time ($P < .001$). (Reprinted from Hodgins JL, Vitale M, Arons RR, et al. Epidemiology of medial ulnar collateral ligament reconstruction: a 10-year study in New York State. *Am J Sports Med.* 2016;44:729-734, with permission from The Author(s).)

addition, the implication that this article references is that one component of the markedly increasing frequency of surgery (Fig 1) is that many are in the younger, even high school, age group. This really is a concern because, believe it or not, there is a perception that the medial collateral ligament reconstruction can actually enhance one's performance. Oh my! The point is that only we can reverse this perverse trend. We simply have to resist the pressure from parents, patients, coaches, and society to operate on this lesion. Some will heal without surgery. The real problem is we have little information to distinguish who will heal and who will not. This information must be provided, but is difficult to elicit.

B. F. Morrey, MD

CORR Insights®: Good Functional Recovery of Complex Elbow Dislocations Treated With Hinged External Fixation: A Multicenter Prospective Study

Hoffmeyer P (Univ Hosp of Geneva, Switzerland)

Clin Orthop Relat Res 473:1462-1463, 2015

Background.—Conservative treatment of complex fracture dislocations of the elbow involves prolonged immobilization, which can produce a stiff, paradoxically unstable, painful joint. Therefore surgery is the best choice for patients who can undergo it. Diagnosis must include meticulous neurovascular evaluation and a combination of standard radiographs plus computed tomography (CT) scanning with 3-D reconstructions to prepare adequately for surgery. The surgical considerations and recommendations were outlined.

Surgical Considerations.—Collateral ligaments tend to heal in simple dislocations when the joint is properly reduced and stabilized. The primary stabilizing influence after dislocation is the osseous elements. Displaced fractures require reduction, fixation, or replacement of the radial head along with restoration of the integrity of the ulnohumeral joint, including the coronoid. The operation should preserve triceps muscle function and securely fix olecranon fractures. Surgery should also preserve the option of performing additional surgery should it be needed.

For radial head excision, the coronoid can be approached through a lateral incision. If it can be reconstructed, a medial incision should be used. If olecranon fracture is included, a special posterior approach may be required. The incisions must allow for visualization of the nerves in the area when the external fixator is applied around the elbow. Early mobilization is critical for a stabilized joint.

Recommendations.—Anatomical restoration is achieved through coronoid reconstruction and radial head stabilization. With complex dislocations, the reconstructed coronoid and restored radial head must be protected to permit ligamentous as well as bony healing. Use of a protective external fixator is advised. An image intensifier will help to determine proper guide pin positioning and set the center or rotation for the hinged fixator. Fixator pins should be inserted through direct vision using 4-cm incisions so that the nerves are protected. A unilateral fixator is required to avoid the need for a bilateral transfixing frame. This will permit early motion and avoid lengthy immobilization of the elbow.

Conclusions.—The challenge in repair of complex fracture dislocations of the elbow is to achieve exact positioning of the external fixator with respect to the elbow's center of rotation. Ulnohumeral flexion-extension is a combination of spiral and translational motion, so any asymmetrical tensions on the collateral ligaments must be minimized. Hinges should permit the complex flexion-extension elbow motion that is needed for proper healing and eventual function. A future development that may lead to better results is a computer-driven, motorized, hinged fixator to provide the active mobilization needed.

▶ Complex instability along with severe C3 distal humeral fractures is the most difficult elbow injury to manage and carries the poorest prognosis. The author clearly summarizes the principles of treatment, emphasizing the absolute requirement to stabilize the ulnohumeral joint. The principles are not debated, but the incidentals and the means of accomplishing the goals remain under investigation. It is interesting to note that the articulated external fixator is recommended as an important adjunct. Although this is widely accepted in Europe, its use in North America is less common. Personally, I continue to favor the use of an external fixator, as suggested by the author, for the reasons he articulated.

B. F. Morrey, MD

Endoscopic vs Open Decompression of the Ulnar Nerve in Cubital Tunnel Syndrome: A Prospective Randomized Double-Blind Study

Schmidt S, Kleist Welch-Guerra W, Matthes M, et al (Ernst Moritz Arndt Univ, Greifswald, Germany)

Neurosurgery 77:960-971, 2015

Background.—Prospective randomized data for comparison of endoscopic and open decompression methods are lacking.

Objective.—To compare the long- and short-term results of endoscopic and open decompression in cubital tunnel syndrome.

Methods.—In a prospective randomized double-blind study, 54 patients underwent ulnar nerve decompression for 56 cubital tunnel syndromes from October 2008 to April 2011. All patients presented with typical clinical and neurophysiological findings and underwent preoperative nerve ultrasonography. They were randomized for either endoscopic (n = 29) or open (n = 27) surgery. Both patients and the physician performing the follow-up examinations were blinded. The follow-up took place 3, 6, 12, and 24 months postoperatively. The severity of symptoms was measured by McGowan and Dellon Score, and the clinical outcome by modified Bishop Score. Additionally, the neurophysiological data were evaluated.

Results.—No differences were found regarding clinical or neurophysiological outcome in both early and late follow-up between both groups. Hematomas were more frequent after endoscopic decompression ($P = .05$). The most frequent constrictions were found at the flexor carpi ulnaris (FCU) arch and the retrocondylar retinaculum. We found no compressing structures more than 4 cm distal from the sulcus in the endoscopic group. The outcome was classified as "good" or "excellent" in 46 out of 56 patients (82.1%). Eight patients did not improve sufficiently or had a relapse and underwent a second surgery.

Conclusion.—The endoscopic technique showed no additional benefits to open surgery. We could not detect relevant compressions distal to the FCU arch. Therefore, an extensive far distal endoscopic decompression is not routinely required. The open decompression remains the procedure of choice at our institution.

▶ Management of cubital tunnel syndrome has changed significantly over the past 15 years. Before this time, many surgeons preferred transposition as their treatment of choice. With the science indicating that in situ decompression fares as well and is generally safer, many have moved to in situ being the treatment of choice.

The advent of endoscopic techniques has been lauded by some investigators as a preferred method over open (or simple) decompression. The authors of this article attempted to compare these 2 methods in a Level 1, prospective randomized study. The study included 29 endoscopically treated patients and 27 open and the patients were followed postoperatively for 2 years. Clinical and electrodiagnostic outcomes were similar between groups. Complications rates were similar except that the endoscopic group had a greater number of hematomas.

Based on this study, there is no compelling reason to consider endoscopic cubital tunnel release over the open simple decompression. My personal experience reflects this conclusion.

M. Rizzo, MD

5 Shoulder and Elbow

Introduction

Several years ago I was embarrassed to realize this section was almost entirely related to rotator cuff topics. I have since guarded against this mistake. However, the predominant theme of the current literature regarding the shoulder is related to the rotator cuff, so there are several articles reviewed which are considered particularly relevant to this subject. While the reverse total shoulder is also much discussed, we have avoided too much coverage as this remains a procedure that is still largely done by fellowship trained shoulder surgeons. This year's selections are intended to provide a fairly broad and balanced coverage of important contributions in the area of shoulder pathology and surgery.

Bernard F. Morrey, MD

ArtiFacts: The Case of Jules Pedoux

Hawk AJ (Defense Health Agency, Silver Spring, MD)

Clin Orthop Relat Res 474:302-303, 2016

Background.—The development of joint arthroplasty in the mid-twentieth century can be traced back to a patient named Jules Pedoux who required treatment of a tuberculosis-related abscess in his shoulder in 1893.

> *Case Report.*—Pedoux contracted a tuberculosis infection, which included the shoulder abscess, and his physician recommended disarticulating the shoulder, but the patient refused. Jules Emile Pean, his surgeon, commissioned J. Porter Michaels, a dentist, to fabricate a shoulder prosthesis that would allow Pedoux to keep his shoulder intact. Michaels used vulcanite and platinum, materials commonly used to make dentures, to create the prosthesis because these materials did not oxidize and were unlikely to cause tissue inflammation.
>
> The shoulder joint prosthesis allowed full arm range of motion (ROM). Muscles were attached through holes on the sides of the

shaft. The pivot joint allowed medial arm rotation. The prosthesis was attached to the humerus with screws and to the scapula with platinum wire. Pean removed the synovium and humeral head and placed the prosthesis. Pedoux was fully ambulatory 12 days later and discharged after 20 days. He was able to work as a waiter because the joint worked so well. However, fistulas developed along the line of incision, leading to removal of the prosthesis in 1895.

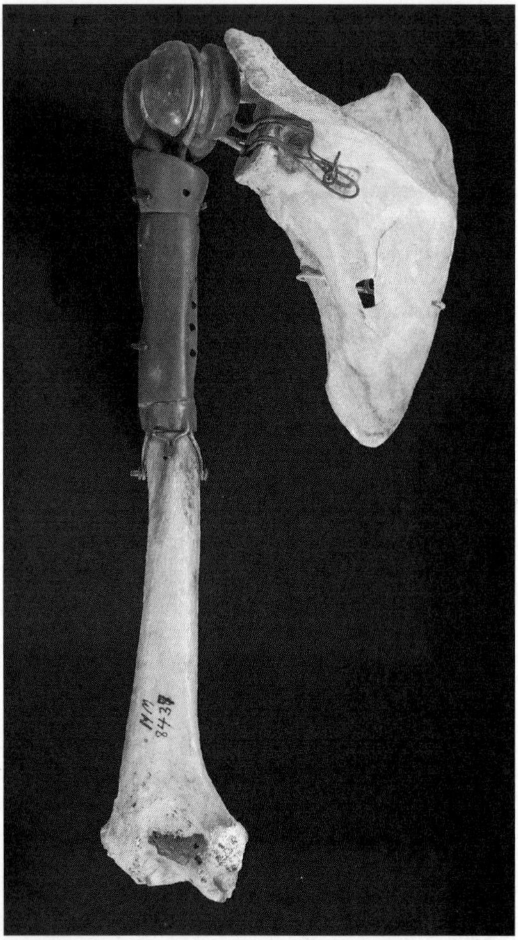

FIGURE 1.—In 1893, the surgeon Jules Emile Pean commissioned J. Porter Michaels, a dentist, to craft a shoulder prosthesis for his patient, Jules Pedoux. Mr. Michaels crafted the prosthesis from materials he commonly used to make dentures—vulcanite and platinum. (This image has been manipulated by using dodging and burning techniques. It has been cropped to emphasize the subject. National Museum of Health and Medicine photo illustration by Matthew Breitbart/Released). (Reprinted from Hawk AJ. Arti-Facts: the case of jules pedoux. *Clin Orthop Relat Res*. 2016;474:302-303, with permission from The Association of Bone and Joint Surgeons.)

Results.—This early use of a shoulder prosthesis showed that the body can tolerate artificial implants. As a result, the course toward modern shoulder arthroplasty was begun (Fig 1).

▶ This may be the only time I have ever included such an article in the 17 years that I have served as editor of the YEAR BOOK, but I just could not resist. The article speaks for itself, and I would encourage the reader to read the whole thing because it is only 2 pages long. It is just amazing to me that such a sophisticated design with materials known to be relatively inert could have been envisioned and successfully executed in 1893 (Fig 1). It is too bad the etiology was an infection; otherwise this may have lasted a lifetime.

B. F. Morrey, MD

Management and functional outcomes following sternoclavicular joint dislocation

Kirby JC, Edwards E, Kamali Moaveni A (Alfred Hosp, Melbourne, Victoria, Australia)

Injury 46:1906-1913, 2015

Introduction.—The aim of this study is to describe the demographics, management and functional outcomes of patients presenting with a sternoclavicular joint (SCJ) dislocation.

Methods.—A retrospective medical record review was conducted examining patients with SCJ dislocation admitted to an adult level 1 trauma centre between 2004 and 2012. Patient demographics, symptoms, associated injuries, imaging technique used in diagnosis, surgical data and neurovascular complications were recorded. Patients received a single-page questionnaire to assess physical function using two validated shoulder questionnaires.

Results.—A total of 22 patients were identified, out of which 77% sustained a posterior dislocation. Mean age was 30 years (range 16–65), and the most common cause of injury was a direct blow during sport (n = 11). Open reduction and internal fixation were performed in 13 patients, definitive closed reduction used in seven and two patients were managed expectantly. Functional outcomes for patients were excellent, with American Shoulder and Elbow Society (ASES) and Subjective Shoulder Value (SSV) scores >80 in 87.5% of cases. There were preoperative symptoms consistent with mediastinal compression in 50% and one delayed presentation with thoracic outlet syndrome. No patient had neurovascular compromise or functional deficit post-operatively, regardless of joint congruency.

Conclusion.—This is the largest case series from a single institution currently available examining SCJ dislocation. We recommend an initial trial of closed reduction, followed by open reduction and internal fixation if

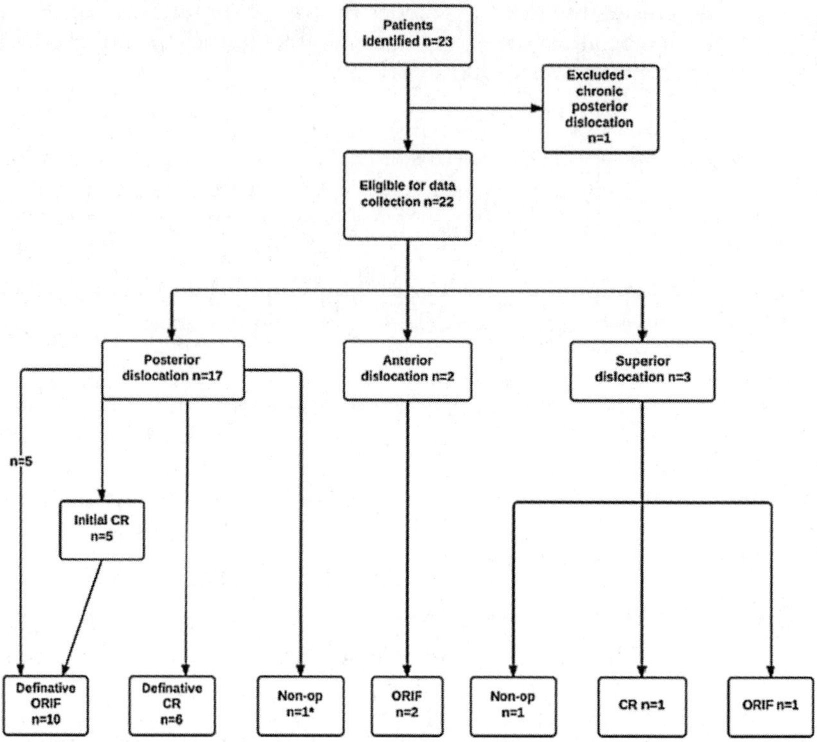

FIGURE 7.—Flowchart of patient selection and management. *Physeal fracture dislocation. Managed with figure-of-eight brace fitted with good result with follow-up of 6 months in outpatients. CR, closed reduction; ORIF, open reduction and internal fixation. (Reprinted from Kirby JC, Edwards E, Kamali Moaveni A. Management and functional outcomes following sternoclavicular joint dislocation. *Injury.* 2015;46:1906-1913, with permission from Elsevier.)

there is joint instability or malreduction. Functional outcome following both closed and open reduction of the SCJ is excellent (Fig 7).

▶ There is little written regarding this injury, so there is little other than opinion to guide treatment. The intimacy of the cervical structures prompts a more serious consideration of the management of the posterior dislocation of the sternoclavicular joint. I found it interesting that both nonoperative and surgical stabilization can be considered indicated, depending, as always, on the pathophysiology (Fig 7). Although a sample of 20 is not large, it is relatively so. The almost 90% success rate achieved by following the logic presented in this article would seem be provide a useful clinical guide to the surgeon.

B. F. Morrey, MD

An evidence-based review of current perceptions with regard to the subacromial space in shoulder impingement syndromes: Is it important and what influences it?

Mackenzie TA, Herrington L, Horlsey I, et al (Salford Univ, Manchester, United Kingdom; English Inst of Sport, Manchester, United Kingdom; et al)

Clin Biomech (Bristol, Avon) 30:641-648, 2015

Background.—Reduction of the subacromial space as a mechanism in the etiology of shoulder impingement syndromes is debated. Although a reduction in this space is associated with shoulder impingement syndromes, it is unclear if this observation is cause or consequence.

Method.—The purposes of this descriptive review are to provide a broad perspective on the current perceptions with regard to the pathology and pathomechanics of subacromial and internal impingement syndromes,

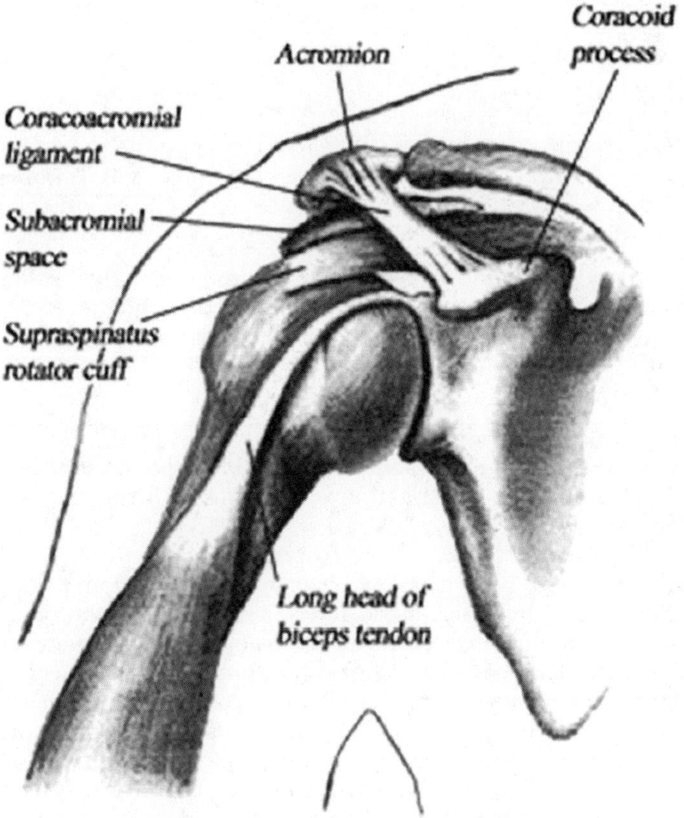

FIGURE 1.—Coronal cross-section of the subacromial space. (Reprinted from Mackenzie TA, Herrington L, Horlsey I, et al. An evidence-based review of current perceptions with regard to the subacromial space in shoulder impingement syndromes: is it important and what influences it? *Clin Biomech.* 2015;30:641-648, with permission from Elsevier Ltd.)

consider the role of the subacromial space in impingement syndromes, describe the intrinsic and extrinsic mechanisms considered to influence the subacromial space, and critique the level of evidence supporting these concepts.

Finding.—Based on the current evidence, the hypothesis that a reduction in subacromial space is an extrinsic cause of impingement syndromes is not conclusively established and the evidence permits no conclusion.

Interpretation.—If maintenance of the subacromial space is important in impingement syndromes regardless of whether it is a cause or consequence, research exploring the correlation between biomechanical factors and the subacromial space, using the later as the outcome measure, would be beneficial (Fig 1).

▶ I must admit that I have been following this particular subject for years. It has been difficult to resolve the conflicting reports. I never quite bought into the concept of the morphologic basis of impingement, which justifies arthroscopic decompression. The substantive literature that clearly indicates comparable resolution with nonoperative treatment is in some conflict with the widespread practice of arthroscopic decompression. This is a nice review of the evidence to explain the pathophysiology of the impingement process (Fig 1). The authors conclude that the information currently in the literature does not provide a compelling explanation for the etiology of the process.

B. F. Morrey, MD

A comparison of magnetic resonance arthrography and arthroscopic findings in the assessment of anterior shoulder dislocations

Jordan RW, Naeem R, Srinivas K, et al (Birmingham Heartlands Hosp, United Kingdom)

Skeletal Radiol 44:653-657, 2015

Objective.—The aim of this study is to establish the sensitivity and specificity of MRA in the investigation of patients with traumatic anterior shoulder dislocations.

Materials and Methods.—A retrospective analysis of consecutive patients undergoing both magnetic resonance arthrography and arthroscopic assessment after a traumatic anterior shoulder dislocation between January 2011 and 2014 was performed. Demographic data were collected from electronic records. Images were interpreted by 8 musculoskeletal radiologists and patients were treated by 8 consultant orthopaedic surgeons. Arthroscopic findings were obtained from surgical notes and these findings were used as a reference for MRA. The sensitivity, specificity, and positive predictive value were calculated for the different injuries.

Results.—Sixty-nine patients underwent both an MRA and shoulder arthroscopy during the study period however, clinical notes were unavailable in 9 patients. Fifty-three patients (88%) were male, the mean age was

28 years (range 18 to 50) and 16 subjects (27%) had suffered a primary dislocation. The overall sensitivity and specificity of MRA to all associated injuries was 0.9 (CI 0.83–0.95) and 0.94 (CI 0.9–0.96) retrospectively. The lowest sensitivity was seen in osseous Bankart 0.8 (CI 0.44–0.96) and superior labral tear (SLAP) lesions 0.5 (CI 0.14–0.86). The overall positive predictive value was 0.88 (CI 0.76–0.91) with the lowest values found in rotator cuff 0.4 (CI 0.07–0.83) and glenohumeral ligament (GHL) lesions 0.29 (CI 0.05–0.7).

Conclusion.—Magnetic resonance angiography has a high sensitivity when used to identify associated injuries in shoulder dislocation, although in 8 patients (13%) arthroscopy identified an additional injury. The overall agreement between MRA and arthroscopic findings was good, but the identification of GHL and rotator cuff injuries was poor.

▶ Validating the accuracy of MR imaging has always been considered both essential and often lacking in many applications. As we have become so dependent on MRI to assist in the diagnosis of shoulder pathology, any insight as to its accuracy is highly desirable. Thus, although this study suffers from multiple participants, 8 radiologist and 8 surgeons, and a relatively small sample stratified by several diagnoses, the findings are quite interesting. Considering arthroscopic findings to be "truth," the overall accuracy of the MRI was quite good. However, in those very clinical settings that we have come to rely on this imaging modality—labral tears, superior labral tear lesions, and cuff tears, the readings were unreliable. Surgeon, take heed.

B. F. Morrey, MD

Operative Management Options for Traumatic Anterior Shoulder Instability in Patients Younger Than 30 Years

Davis DE, Abboud JA (Thomas Jefferson Univ, Philadelphia, PA)
Orthopedics 38:570-576, 2015

Anterior instability of the glenohumeral joint is a relatively common problem in the young population. Identification and treatment is essential to reduce the risk of recurrent instability, whether that is re-dislocation or subluxation events. Non-operative treatment for first-time dislocations was the classic option; however, a relatively high rate of recurrent dislocations has led to earlier operative management in some cases. Surgical treatment through either an open or arthroscopic approach has continued to be an area of research and debate. The decision depends partly on the exact etiology of the instability and the extent of soft tissue or bony deficiency. As arthroscopic techniques and experience improve, surgical procedures for arthroscopic anterior shoulder instability continue to evolve. This review serves as an in-depth overview of the treatment options for traumatic anterior shoulder instability in the patient younger than 30 years, generally focusing on non-rotator cuff–associated etiologies for recurrent instability.

▶ This article summarizes a large body of literature on this common and debated problem. The issue of assessment is being modified in recent years with the MRI that accurately reveals the extent of soft tissue injury but with well-developed standards can tend to overread the extent of damage. Managing the initial episode is one of the most discussed issues in this context. A recent literature review documented a recurrence rate of 7% in those undergoing repair, either arthroscopic or open, and an almost 50% recurrence rate in the nonoperated patient. Strong evidence exists to recommend repair of a Bankart lesion if it is present. In very broad terms, osseous lesions involving more than 30% of either the glenoid or of the humeral head should be addressed with surgery. The important feature to appreciate in older individuals is the presence of a concurrent rotator cuff injury, in which initial treatment is rehabilitation. If surgery is required, both the cuff and capsular deficiencies should be addressed.

B. F. Morrey, MD

Multidirectional Instability of the Shoulder: A Systematic Review

Longo UG, Rizzello G, Loppini M, et al (Campus Bio-Medico Univ, Rome, Italy; et al)

Arthroscopy 31:2431-2443, 2015

Purpose.—To analyze outcomes of surgical and conservative treatment options for multidirectional instability (MDI).

Methods.—A systematic review of the literature according to the Preferred Reporting Items for Systematic Reviews and Meta-Analyses (PRISMA) guidelines was performed. A comprehensive search of the PubMed, MEDLINE, CINAHL, Cochrane, EMBASE, and Google Scholar databases using various combinations of the keywords "shoulder," "multidirectional instability," "dislocation," "inferior instability," "capsulorrhaphy," "capsular plication," "capsular shift," "glenoid," "humeral head," "surgery," and "glenohumeral," over the years 1966 to 2014 was performed.

Results.—Twenty-four articles describing patients with open capsular shift, arthroscopic treatment, and conservative or combined management in the setting of atraumatic MDI of the shoulder were included. A total of 861 shoulders in 790 patients was included. The median age was 24.3 years, ranging from 9 to 56 years. The dominant side was involved in 269 (58%) of 468 shoulders, whereas the nondominant side was involved in 199 (42%) shoulders. Patients were assessed at a median follow-up period of 4.2 years (ranging from 9 months to 16 years). Fifty-two of 253 (21%) patients undergoing physiotherapy required surgical intervention for MDI management, whereas the overall occurrence of redislocation was seen in 61 of 608 (10%) shoulders undergoing surgical procedures. The redislocation event occurred in 17 of 226 (7.5%) shoulders with open capsular shift management, in 21 of 268 (7.8%) shoulders with arthroscopic plication management, in 12 of 49 (24.5%) shoulders undergoing arthroscopic thermal shrinkage, and in 11 of 55 (22%) shoulders undergoing arthroscopic laser-assisted capsulorrhaphy.

Conclusions.—Arthroscopic capsular plication and open capsular shift are the best surgical procedures for treatment of MDI after failure of rehabilitative management. Arthroscopic capsular plication shows results comparable to open capsular shift.

Level of Evidence.—Level IV, systematic review of Level I to IV studies.

▶ The single value of this well-done literature review is that it demonstrates that, based on current reported experience, open and arthroscopic surgery is equally effective to treat multidirectional instability. Both are about 93% effective to treat nontraumatic instability. The quality of orthopaedic data on the subject is reflected by the fact only about 2.5% of the database-identified articles could pass the review criteria. Even at that level, the surveillance is quite variable: 9 months to 15 years. It is worth noting the existence of a standard according to which these literature reviews should be conducted: the Preferred Reporting Items for Systematic Reviews and Meta-Analyses (PRISMA). I was not aware of this, and it represents development of the growing tendency to perform such reviews.

B. F. Morrey, MD

Dextrose Prolotherapy Versus Control Injections in Painful Rotator Cuff Tendinopathy

Bertrand H, Reeves KD, Bennett CJ, et al (Univ of British Columbia, Vancouver, Canada; Univ of Kansas; Private Practice, West Vancouver, British Columbia, Canada; et al)

Arch Phys Med Rehabil 97:17-25, 2016

Objective.—To compare the effect of dextrose prolotherapy on pain levels and degenerative changes in painful rotator cuff tendinopathy against 2 potentially active control injection procedures.

Design.—Randomized controlled trial, blinded to participants and evaluators.

Setting.—Outpatient pain medicine practice.

Participants.—Persons (N = 73) with chronic shoulder pain, examination findings of rotator cuff tendinopathy, and ultrasound-confirmed supraspinatus tendinosis/tear.

Interventions.—Three monthly injections either (1) onto painful entheses with dextrose (Enthesis-Dextrose), (2) onto entheses with saline (Enthesis-Saline), or (3) above entheses with saline (Superficial-Saline).

All solutions included 0.1% lidocaine. All participants received concurrent programmed physical therapy.

Main Outcome Measures.—Primary: participants achieving an improvement in maximal current shoulder pain ≥2.8 (twice the minimal clinically important difference for visual analog scale pain) or not. Secondary: improvement in the Ultrasound Shoulder Pathology Rating Scale (USPRS) and a 0-to-10 satisfaction score (10, completely satisfied).

Results.—The 73 participants had moderate to severe shoulder pain (7.0 ± 2.0) for 7.6 ± 9.6 years. There were no baseline differences between groups. Blinding was effective. At 9-month follow-up, 59% of Enthesis-Dextrose participants maintained ≥2.8 improvement in pain compared with Enthesis-Saline (37%; $P = .088$) and Superficial-Saline (27%; $P = .017$). Enthesis-Dextrose participants' satisfaction was 6.7 ± 3.2 compared with Enthesis-Saline (4.7 ± 4.1; $P = .079$) and Superficial-Saline (3.9 ± 3.1; $P = .003$). USPRS findings were not different between groups ($P = .734$).

Conclusions.—In participants with painful rotator cuff tendinopathy who receive physical therapy, injection of hypertonic dextrose on painful entheses resulted in superior long-term pain improvement and patient satisfaction compared with blinded saline injection over painful entheses, with intermediate results for entheses injection with saline. These differences could not be attributed to a regenerative effect. Dextrose prolotherapy may improve on the standard care of painful rotator cuff tendinopathy for certain patients.

▶ We desperately seek randomized controlled trials to provide a scientific basis for our clinical practice. This is such a study and addresses a common and difficult problem of the symptomatic rotator cuff. The conclusion that prolotherapy is safe and effective "long term" is asserted. However, it should be noted the diagnosis was by ultrasound and included a spectrum of cuff pathology from calcific tendinosis to frank tear. However, the small sample size does not allow stratification according to specific pathology. Furthermore, the conclusion is based on a 59% positive response rate with surveillance of 6 months. The control is against 2 versions of saline injections, not other recognized or accepted therapies. So, in conclusion, prolotherapy is better than saline at 6 months. And it is safe.

B. F. Morrey, MD

Prognostic Factors Affecting Rotator Cuff Healing After Arthroscopic Repair in Small to Medium-sized Tears

Park JS, Park HJ, Kim SH, et al (Korea Univ Anam Hosp, Seoul, South Korea; Seoul Natl Univ Hosp, South Korea; et al)

Am J Sports Med 43:2386-2392, 2015

Background.—Small and medium-sized rotator cuff tears usually have good clinical and anatomic outcomes. However, healing failure still occurs in some cases.

Purpose.—To evaluate prognostic factors for rotator cuff healing in patients with only small to medium-sized rotator cuff tears.

Study Design.—Case-control study; Level of evidence, 3.

Methods.—Data were prospectively collected from 339 patients with small to medium-sized rotator cuff tears who underwent arthroscopic repair by a single surgeon between March 2004 and August 2012 and who underwent magnetic resonance imaging or computed tomographic arthrography at least 1 year after surgery. The mean age of the patients was 59.8 years (range, 39-80 years), and the mean follow-up time was 20.8 months (range, 12-66 months). The functional evaluation included the visual analog scale (VAS) for pain, American Shoulder and Elbow Surgeons score, Constant-Murley score, and Simple Shoulder Test.

Results.—Postoperative VAS for pain and functional scores improved significantly compared with preoperative values ($P < .001$). Forty-five healing failures occurred (13.3%), and fatty degeneration of the infraspinatus muscle, tear size (anteroposterior dimension), and age were significant factors affecting rotator cuff healing ($P < .001$, $=.018$, and $=.011$, respectively) in multivariate logistic regression analysis. Grade II and higher infraspinatus fatty degeneration correlated with a higher failure rate. The failure rate was also significantly higher in patients with a tear >2 cm in size (34.2%) compared with patients with a tear ≤2 cm (10.6%) ($P < .001$). A receiver operating characteristic curve was used to determine the predictive cut-off value for the oldest age and the largest tear size for successful healing, which were calculated as 69 years and 2 cm, respectively, with a specificity of 90%.

Conclusion.—In small to medium-sized rotator cuff tears, grade II fatty degeneration of the infraspinatus muscle according to the Goutallier classification could be a reference point for successful healing, and anatomic outcomes might be better if repair is performed before the patient is 69 years old and the tear size exceeds 2 cm.

▶ This is one of many excellent studies originating from Asia. The study confirms the prognostic value of fatty degeneration, indicating chronicity, tear size, and patient age as influencing healing and outcome. These factors have been demonstrated in the past, but it is of great, and frankly disappointing, interest to note that these variable were given little consideration by a consensus panel trying to determine the appropriate indications for surgical intervention. The findings of this study should be seriously factored into the surgical decision-making process; the findings of the consensus panel reflect that this methodology has a way to go to become relevant to our practice.

B. F. Morrey, MD

Does Early Versus Delayed Active Range of Motion Affect Rotator Cuff Healing after Surgical Repair? A Systematic Review and Meta-analysis

Kluczynski MA, Isenburg MM, Marzo JM, et al (The State Univ of New York, Buffalo)

Am J Sports Med 44:785-791, 2016

Background.—The timing of passive range of motion (ROM) after surgical repair of the rotator cuff (RC) has been shown to affect healing. However, it is unknown if early or delayed active ROM affects healing.

Purpose.—To determine whether early versus delayed active ROM affects structural results of RC repair surgery.

Study Design.—Systematic review and meta-analysis.

Methods.—A systematic review of articles published between January 2004 and April 2014 was conducted. Structural results were compared for early (<6 weeks after surgery) versus delayed (≥6 weeks after surgery) active ROM using chi-square and Fisher exact tests, as well as relative risks (RRs) and 95% CIs. The analyses were stratified by tear size and repair method.

Results.—A total of 37 studies (2251 repairs) were included in the analysis, with 10 (649 repairs) in the early group and 27 (1602 repairs) in the delayed group. For tears ≤3 cm, the risk of a structural tendon defect was higher in the early versus delayed group for transosseous plus single-row suture anchor repairs (39.7% vs 24.3%; RR, 1.63 [95% CI, 1.28-2.08]). For tears >3 cm, the risk of a structural tendon defect was higher in the early versus delayed group for suture bridge repairs (48% vs 17.5%; RR, 2.74 [95% CI, 1.59-4.73]) and all repair methods combined (40.5% vs 26.7%; RR, 1.52 [95% CI, 1.17-1.97]). For tears >5 cm, the risk of structural tendon defect was higher in the early versus delayed group for suture bridge repairs (100% vs 16.7%; RR, 6.00 [95% CI, 1.69-21.26]). There were no statistically significant associations for tears measuring ≤1, 1-3, or 3-5 cm.

Conclusion.—Early active ROM was associated with increased risk of a structural defect for small and large RC tears, and thus might not be advisable after RC repair.

▶ This is a good study with useful insights regarding a continuously debated issue: when to move the rotator cuff repair. Note the use of 1.5% of the referenced literature, which is pretty typical for these kinds of analyses of the literature. I was a bit surprised to see the cohort with early motion faired less well. In reference to confounding variables, the analysis focused much more on early and late intervention than arthroscopic versus open procedures; I was also concerned that this was true for large tears, as to be expected, but also the case for small, < 3-cm tears. So the issue is, how much of a problem is it to regain motion? Does it justify risks of early motion? The final arc of motion was not much different regardless of timing of motion Final analysis: it's up to the surgeon's judgment to weigh these 2 variables.

B. F. Morrey, MD

Factors associated with hospital admission after rotator cuff repair: the role of peripheral nerve blockade

Danninger T, Stundner O, Rasul R, et al (Weill Cornell Med College, NY; et al)
J Clin Anesth 27:566-573, 2015

Study Objective.—The objective was to analyze the impact of a peripheral nerve block in addition to general anesthesia on hospital admission after surgical rotator cuff repair.

Design.—This was a population-based outcome study. The cost effectiveness of ambulatory rotator cuff repair relies on the discharge of patients on the day of surgery. As the impact of a peripheral nerve block in addition to general anesthesia on this outcome is unknown, we sought to elucidate this subject using population-based data.

Patients and Methods.—Information on patients undergoing rotator cuff surgery under general anesthesia with or without the addition of a peripheral nerve block (GN vs G) from a retrospective database provided by Premier Perspective, Inc, Charlotte, NC (http://www.premierinc.com), was analyzed. Using multilevel multivariable regressions, we evaluated the independent impact of the type of anesthesia on the outcomes hospital admission, combined major complications, and increased hospital costs.

Results.—We identified 27,201 patients who underwent surgical rotator cuff repair. Approximately 89% (24,240) of patients were discharged on the day of surgery, whereas 11% (2961) were admitted to the hospital. The admission rates for the GN group were 9.1% and 11.2% for the G group ($P = .0001$). The multivariable regression models showed that patients with the addition of a peripheral nerve block had 18%less risk of being admitted to the hospital (relative risk [RR] = 0.82; 95% confidence interval [CI], 0.74-0.91; $P = .0003$) compared with those without this intervention. Differences in risk for combined major complications (RR = 1.00; 95% CI, 0.83-1.20; $P = .9751$) or increased hospital costs (RR = 0.97; 95% CI, 0.93-1.02; $P = .2538$) were nonsignificant.

Discussion.—For patients undergoing surgical rotator cuff repair under general anesthesia, the addition of a peripheral nerve block may be

TABLE 4.—Multivariable regression results and absolute risk reduction

	RR				ARR			
Outcome	RR	95% CI of RR		*P* Value	ARR	95% CI of ARR		*P* Value
Admission status	0.82	0.74	0.91	.0003	−0.02	−0.03	−0.01	<.0001
Combined major complications	1.00	0.83	1.20	.9751	0.00	−0.01	0.01	.9201
Increased hospital costs	0.97	0.93	1.02	.2538	0.00	−0.02	0.01	.8153

Reprinted from Danninger T, Stundner O, Rasul R, et al. Factors associated with hospital admission after rotator cuff repair: the role of peripheral nerve blockade. *J Clin Anesth*. 2015;27:566-573, with permission from Elsevier.

associated with a reduction in the need for postoperative hospital admission after ambulatory surgery. Although the reason for this finding has to remain speculative, better pain control may play a role (Table 4).

▶ This careful study offers the potential for incremental improvement in the care of the patient having rotator cuff surgery. Assessing more than 27 000 procedures, the authors were able to provide several important insights. The addition of a peripheral nerve block to a general anesthetic statistically decreases the potential for an overnight, or longer, admission. The authors then further address the next 2 logical questions.

Is the block associated with an increased complication rate? Not statistically. Is the addition of the block more costly? No, not when considering the avoidance of the cost of admission (Table 4). This is a useful and well-done study.

B. F. Morrey, MD

Arthroscopic Repair for Chronic Massive Rotator Cuff Tears: A Systematic Review

Henry P, Wasserstein D, Park S, et al (Univ of Toronto, Ontario, Canada; et al)
Arthroscopy 31:2472-2480, 2015

Purpose.—To systematically review the available evidence for arthroscopic repair of chronic massive rotator cuff tears and identify patient demographics, pre- and post-operative functional limitations, reparability and repair techniques, and retear rates.

Methods.—Medline, Embase, the Cochrane Database of Systematic Reviews, and the Cochrane Central Register of Controlled Trials were searched to identify all clinical papers describing arthroscopic repair of chronic massive rotator cuff tears. Papers were excluded if a definition of "massive" was not provided, if the definition of "massive" was considered inappropriate by agreement between the 2 reviewers, or if patients with smaller tears were also included in the study population. Study quality and clinical outcome data were pooled and summarized.

Results.—There were 18 papers that met the eligibility criteria; they involved 954 patients with a mean age of 63 (range, 37 to 87), 48% of whom were female. There were 5 prospective and 13 retrospective study designs. The overall study quality was poor according to the Modified Coleman Methodology Score. Of the 954 repairs, 81% were complete repairs and 19% were partial repairs. The follow-up range was between 33 and 52 months, and the mean duration between symptom onset and surgery was 24 months. Single-row repairs were performed in 56% or patients, and double-row repairs were performed in 44%. A pooled analysis demonstrated an improvement in visual analog scale from 5.9 to 1.7, active range of motion from 125° to 169°, and the Constant-Murley score from 49 to 74. The pooled retear rate was 79%.

Conclusions.—Arthroscopic repair of chronic massive rotator cuff tears is associated with complete repair in the majority of cases and consistently improves pain, range of motion, and functional outcome scores; however, the retear rate is high. Existing research on massive rotator cuff repair is limited to poor- to fair-quality studies.

Level of Evidence.—Level IV, systematic review including Level IV studies.

▶ One of the values of this study is to demonstrate the progression of the practice to treat massive rotator cuff tears arthroscopically. The combined results from 18 studies with almost 1000 patients report both objective and subjective improvement. However, despite functional improvement, the imaging studies suggest a retear rate of almost 80%. However, on the basis of the Coleman manuscript quality scoring system, the quality of the papers to arrive at this conclusion is consider poor to fair. Regardless, this is helpful information for the reasons stated.

B. F. Morrey, MD

Alterations of the Deltoid Muscle After Open Versus Arthroscopic Rotator Cuff Repair

Cho NS, Cha SW, Rhee YG (Kyung Hee Univ, Seoul, Korea)
Am J Sports Med 43:2927-2934, 2015

Background.—Open repair can be more useful than arthroscopic repair for immobile and severely retracted, large to massive rotator cuff tears. However, it is not known whether the deltoid muscle is altered after open repair or to what extent the deltoid origin remains detached after surgery.

Purpose.—To compare postoperative alterations of the deltoid muscle in open versus arthroscopic repair for severely retracted, large to massive rotator cuff tears.

Study Design.—Case-control study; Level of evidence, 3.

Methods.—Enrolled in this study were 135 patients who underwent surgical repair for severely retracted, large to massive rotator cuff tears and who had routine follow-up MRIs at least 6 months after surgery. Open repairs were performed in 56 cases and arthroscopic repairs in 79 cases. The detachment and thickness of the deltoid muscle at its proximal origin were recorded in 5 zones on MRI. The alterations of the deltoid muscle and postoperative integrity of the repaired rotator cuff were evaluated.

Results.—Partial detachment of the deltoid occurred in 1 patient (1.8%) in the open group and in 2 patients (2.5%) in the arthroscopic group ($P = .80$). All the partial detachments occurred in zones 2 and 3. Attenuation of the proximal origin of the deltoid was found in 3 patients (5.4%) in the open group and in 4 patients (5.1%) in the arthroscopic group ($P = .87$). Atrophy of the deltoid muscle was shown in 3 patients (5.4%)

in the open group and 4 patients (5.1%) in the arthroscopic group (P =.61). The retear rate of the repaired cuff was 30.4% (17/56) in the open group and 38.0% (30/79) in the arthroscopic group (P =.74).

Conclusion.—Between open and arthroscopic repair for severely retracted, large to massive rotator cuff tears, there was no significant difference in detachment of the deltoid origin and alterations of the deltoid muscle after repair. Postoperative alterations of the deltoid occurred in arthroscopic surgery as well as in open surgery. For immobile massive rotator cuff tear, open repair is an acceptable technique as long as the deltoid muscle is meticulously reattached after surgery.

▶ I could not help but think of the literature regarding modular tibial knee components as I read this article. The commonality was to test the proposed value of the specific point in question. At the knee, the modular feature of the tibial component has proven to be of no or limited value to increase motion by downsizing, or simply replacing a worn insert. So, too, these authors provide a reasonable sample of open and arthroscopic procedures for a specific clinical entity: the repair of a large cuff tear. They provide carefully attained and studied data that support their conclusion. There is no functional advantage to the arthroscopic repair, and there is no disadvantage of excessive deltoid damage with the open procedure. The message? Do what works best in your hands.

B. F. Morrey, MD

Functional Outcomes and Health-Related Quality of Life After Surgical Repair of Full-Thickness Rotator Cuff Tears Using a Mini-Open Technique: A Concise 10-Year Follow-up of a Previous Report

Saraswat MK, Styles-Tripp F, Beaupre LA, et al (Univ of Alberta, Edmonton, Canada; Covenant Health-Grey Nuns Community Hosp, Edmonton, Alberta, Canada; et al)

Am J Sports Med 43:2794-2799, 2015

Background.—Although good short-term and midterm outcomes are reported for mini-open rotator cuff repair, few prospective studies have investigated long-term results.

Hypothesis.—Function and health-related quality of life (HRQL) outcomes would be maintained 10 years after mini-open rotator cuff repair.

Study Design.—Cohort study; Level of evidence, 2.

Methods.—Patients with a confirmed full-thickness rotator cuff tear who underwent mini-open repair between April 1997 and July 2000 were evaluated preoperatively as well as 1 year and 10 years postoperatively for (1) pain, function, and HRQL using the American Shoulder and Elbow Surgeons (ASES) score and Western Ontario Rotator Cuff Index (WORC) score; (2) active shoulder range of motion (ROM) using goniometry; and (3) satisfaction by an independent evaluator. Changes in function, HRQL, and ROM over time were analyzed using repeated-measures analysis of variance.

Results.—A total of 84 patients were enrolled, of which 61 (73%) were men; the mean (±SD) age was 53.0 ± 9.9 years. At 10 years, 4 (5%) patients were deceased, and 4 (5%) had symptomatic retears. Fifty-nine (74%) patients were evaluated, composed of 43 (73%) men; 26 (44%) were younger than 60 years. Function and HRQL significantly improved over the course of follow-up ($P < .001$), primarily within the first postoperative year. At 10 years, the mean ASES score was 90.4 ± 19.4, similar to the 1-year score of 91.1 ± 12.0 ($P = .83$). The mean WORC score at 10 years was 88.7 ± 17.8, with no change from the 1-year score of 88.4 ± 13.6 ($P = .93$). This relationship did not change after adjusting for age and tear size. Shoulder ROM was also maintained over 10 years. Flexion ROM improved in the first postoperative year, and this improvement was sustained at 10 years after surgery ($P \geq .30$). External rotation ROM was slower to improve postoperatively, and significant improvements were seen between 1 and 10 years ($P < .01$). Fifty-three patients (90%) were satisfied or very satisfied with their results. Tear size, workers' compensation board claimant status, sex, and smoking status did not influence HRQL or shoulder ROM ($P > .06$).

Conclusion.—Postoperative improvements in function and HRQL after mini-open rotator cuff repair were retained at 10 years.

▶ In the past, this topic would simply be entitled the long-term outcomes of the mini-open cuff repair. Today we must define the nature of the surveillance as health-related quality of life. Oh well, this is the way it is. Importantly, these investigators reveal a 90% 10-year satisfaction rate with cuff repair using this technique. This does not surprise me. What I do not understand is the contrary finding of what is well established: worker's compensation, size of tear, and smoking are adverse predictors of outcome. This was not observed in this experience.

B. F. Morrey, MD

Age-related differences in the use of total shoulder arthroplasty over time: use and outcomes

Singh JA, Ramachandran R (Univ of Alabama at Birmingham)

Bone Joint J 97-B:1385-1389, 2015

We assessed the age-related differences in the use of total shoulder arthroplasty (TSA) and outcomes, and associated time-trends using the United States Nationwide Inpatient Sample (NIS) between 1998 and 2010. Age was categorised as < 50, 50 to 64, 65 to 79 and ≥ 80 years. Time-trends in the use of TSA were compared using logistic regression or the Cochran Armitage test.

The overall use of TSA increased from 2.96/100 000 in 1998 to 12.68/100 000 in 2010. Significantly lower rates were noted between 2009 and 2010, compared with between 1998 and 2000, for: mortality, 0.1% *versus* 0.2% ($p = 0.004$); discharge to an inpatient facility, 13.3% *versus* 14.5% ($p = 0.039$), and hospital stay > median, 29.4% *versus* 51.2% ($p < 0.001$).

The rates of use of TSA/100 000 by age groups, < 50, 50 to 64, 65 to 79 and ≥ 80 years were: 0.32, 4.62, 17.82 and 12.56, respectively in 1998 ($p < 0.001$); and 0.65, 17.49, 75.27 and 49.05, respectively in 2010 ($p < 0.001$) with an increasing age-related difference over time ($p < 0.001$). Across the age categories, there were significant differences in the proportion: discharged to an inpatient facility, 3.2% *versus* 4.2% *versus* 14.7% *versus* 36.5%, respectively in 1998 ($p < 0.001$) and 1.8% *versus* 4.3% *versus* 12.5% *versus* 35.5%, respectively in 2010 ($p < 0.001$) and the proportion with hospital stay > median, 39.7% *versus* 40.2% *versus* 53% *versus* 69%, respectively in 1998 ($p < 0.001$) and 17.2% *versus* 20.6% *versus* 28.7% *versus* 50.7%, respectively in 2010 ($p < 0.001$).

In a nationally representative sample, we noted a time-related increase in the use of TSA and increasing age-related differences in outcomes indicating a changing epidemiology of the use of TSA. Age-related differences in outcomes suggest that attention should focus on groups with the worst outcomes.

▶ With the ever-increasing awareness of the impact of the aging population on the consumption of medical resources, studies such as this are worthwhile. Using a large national database with a representative sample of 20%, the methodology is considered adequate to draw the conclusions discussed in the article. The 4-fold increase in total shoulder arthroplasty from 1998 to 2010 is in line with the growth of arthroplasty in general. The unique feature is the stratification by age group, which demonstrates the faster growth in the 65- to 79-year age group. The key is to determine whether the increased utilization effects a prolonged independence in this age group and hence an improved quality of life. Trends in shorter hospital stay and fewer dismissals to rehabilitation units are encouraging and aligned with overall trends in orthopedics.

B. F. Morrey, MD

CORR Insights®: Obesity is Not Associated with Increased Short-term Complications After Primary Total Shoulder Arthroplasty

Gross RM (GIKK Ortho Specialists, Omaha, NE)

Clin Orthop Relat Res 474:796-798, 2016

Background.—Since the Food and Drug Administration (FDA) approved the reverse total shoulder, shoulder arthroplasty has been used considerably more often than in the past. However, this procedure is generally more suitable for older individuals, who may also be obese. The status of obesity as a risk factor for complications after shoulder replacement has been unclear.

Methods for Calculating Obesity.—The body mass index (BMI) is calculated by dividing weight in kilograms by height in meters and is the standard index used by the National Institutes of Health (NIH). Twenty-five is the upper limit of normal for men and women. Criticisms of the BMI include (1) men and women are seen as having the same body physique; (2) height adds 10% to the BMI for tall persons and subtracts 10% for short individuals, which makes it overly important; (3) and heavily muscled individuals can be deemed obese. However, it is a simple method with a high degree of sensitivity, especially at the higher end of the range. Although other methods have been proposed to overcome the concerns, none have evidence to support their use as essential.

Relevance.—The risk profile for shoulder replacement in patients with moderate to severe obesity indicates that the procedure is relatively safe up to a BMI of 40. Even surgical experts will have difficulty avoiding complications in patients whose BMI exceeds 40. Thus the determination of BMI is an essential step in evaluating risks for patients having shoulder replacement.

Another essential step is the consideration of alternative procedures. Patients with painful arthritic shoulders but a strong glenoid and rotator cuff and balanced wear pattern can successfully undergo hemiarthoplasty, especially a subscapularis sparing approach, and achieve excellent results. The procedure is simpler and may address the patient's problem without a high degree of risk.

A third essential is the surgeon's truthful appraisal of his or her own skill in performing shoulder arthroplasty and in helping the specific patient being considered. Not all patients with a BMI over 40 are alike, with some having reasonable surgical risk profiles and others presenting an unacceptable likelihood of complications. Therefore the surgeon must evaluate the facts of each case and his or her skill level to determine the best course of action.

Conclusions.—Considering the aging population, the fact that obesity is common, and the high expectations of patients, it is not unusual that arthroplasties will be requested. Surgeons need to assess each situation and determine not only the patient's BMI but also the alternative procedures that could be done and their own degree of skill in performing the demanding shoulder arthroplasty procedure.

▶ This contribution is a little unusual because it is a comment on a recently published article on the subject. It was selected here because the topic is growing in relevance. The discussion itself is accurate. My additional comments are to reinforce the "threshold" body mass index (BMI) not just for shoulder but for hip, knee, and probably elbow is a BMI of 40—gross obesity. However, it should also be considered that the considerable literature on this subject consistently indicated that the extent of improvement of the grossly obese patient is as good if not better than those with a lower BMI. So to operate on this category of patient will see increasing pressure in our society: patients will benefit, but at an increased cost to the patient, surgeon, and society.

B. F. Morrey, MD

Conversion of Stemmed Hemi- or Total to Reverse Total Shoulder Arthroplasty: Advantages of a Modular Stem Design

Wieser K, Borbas P, Ek ET, et al (Univ of Zurich, Switzerland)

Clin Orthop Relat Res 473:651-660, 2014

Background.—If revision of a failed anatomic hemiarthroplasty or total shoulder arthroplasty is uncertain to preserve or restore satisfactory rotator cuff function, conversion to a reverse total shoulder arthroplasty has become the preferred treatment, at least for elderly patients. However, revision of a well-fixed humeral stem has the potential risk of loss of humeral bone stock, nerve injury, periprosthetic fracture, and malunion or nonunion of a humeral osteotomy with later humeral component loosening.

Questions/Purposes.—The purposes of this study were to determine whether preservation of a modular stem is associated with (1) less blood loss and operative time (2) fewer perioperative and postoperative complications, including reoperations and revisions and/or (3) improved Constant and Murley scores and subjective shoulder values for conversion to a reverse total shoulder arthroplasty compared with stem revision.

Methods.—Between 2005 and 2011, 48 hemiarthroplasties and eight total shoulder arthroplasties (total = 56 shoulders 54 patients) were converted to an Anatomical™ reverse total shoulder arthroplasty system without (n = 13) or with (n = 43) stem exchange. Complications and revisions for all patients were tallied through review of medical and surgical records. The outcomes scores included the Constant and Murley score and the subjective shoulder value. Complete clinical followup was available on 80% of shoulders (43 patients 45 of 56 procedures, 32 with and 13 without stem exchange) at a minimum of 12 months (mean, 37 months range, 12–83 months).

Results.—Blood loss averaged 485 mL (range, 300–700 mL SD, 151 mL) and surgical time averaged 118 minutes (range, 90–160 minutes SD, 21 minutes) without stem exchange and 831 mL (range, 350–2000 mL SD, 400 mL) and 176 minutes (range, 120–300 minutes SD, 42 minutes) with stem exchange ($p = 0.001$). Intraoperative complications (8% versus 30% odds ratio [OR], 5.2) and reinterventions (8% versus 14% OR, 1.9) were substantially fewer in patients without stem exchange. The complication rate leading to dropout from the study was substantial in the stem revision group (six patients 43 shoulders [14%]), but there were no complication-related dropouts in the stem-retaining group. If, however, such complications could be avoided, with the numbers available we detected no difference in the functional outcome between the two groups.

Conclusions.—Patients undergoing revision of stemmed hemiarthroplasty or total to reverse total shoulder arthroplasty without stem exchange had less intraoperative blood loss and operative time, fewer intraoperative complications, and fewer revisions than did patients whose index revision procedures included a full stem exchange. Therefore modularity of a shoulder arthroplasty system has substantial advantages if

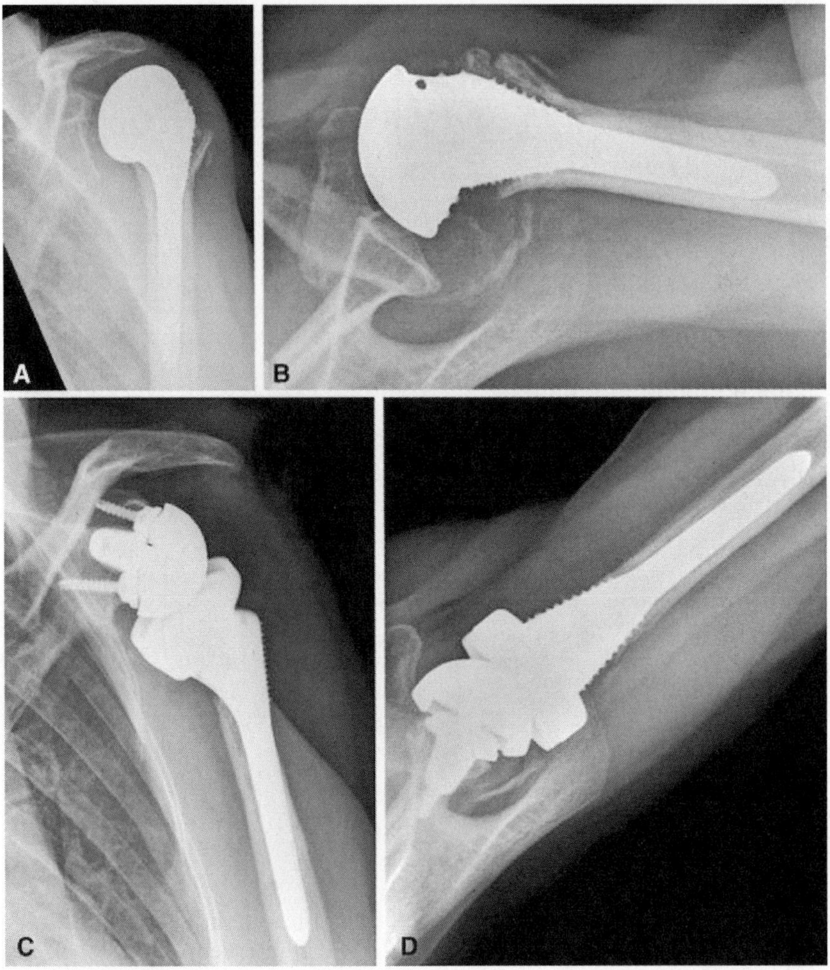

FIGURE 2.—A 55-year old woman presented with severe a pseudoparalysis of her left arm 7 months after a hemiarthroplasty as a result of a four-part humeral head fracture. Her (**A**) AP and (**B**) axial radiographs show a well-fixed humeral stem with anterosuperior instability resulting from rotator cuff insufficiency. Two years after conversion to a reverse total shoulder arthroplasty, the patient had a pain-free overhead function with good component positioning without any signs of loosening observed on the (**C**) AP and (**D**) axial radiographs. (Reprinted from Wieser K, Borbas P, Ek ET, et al. Conversion of stemmed hemi- or total to reverse total shoulder arthroplasty: advantages of a modular stem design. *Clin Orthop Relat Res.* 2014;473:651-660, with permission from The Association of Bone and Joint Surgeons.)

conversion to reverse total shoulder arthroplasty becomes necessary and should be considered as prerequisite for stemmed shoulder arthroplasty systems.

Level of Evidence.—Level III, therapeutic study (Fig 2).

▶ In the world of shoulder reconstructive surgery, it's all about the reverse.

Although we do not know where this path will take us, data are emerging that help us to understand our way forward. Modular implants, although attractive conceptually, have not necessarily demonstrated their clinical value. This study is of a small sample, but with modest surveillance, the findings are relevant. A modular design that allows conversion from a conventional to a reverse prosthesis is of significant value (Fig 2). The demonstration of the utility of this strategy will clearly increase with time.

B. F. Morrey, MD

6 Spine

Introduction

This year's Spine section in the YEAR BOOK of Orthopedics has marked a changing of the guard. As I settle in as the new editor for this section, I tried to sample hot topics in a variety of spine surgical aspects. In years to come, one or a few themes will be selected. This year's selections span the gambit from screw-fix cage implants in the cervical and lumbar spine and their early clinical outcomes to a systematic review of the use of BMP-2 in spine surgery. The primary goal of these reviews will be to distill the dense portions of original research articles into concise summary points and commentary regarding the quality of the work and its importance with respect to other literature on the topic. Screw fixed cages are becoming commonplace in anterior spinal fusion surgery. The reports reviewed this year support the equivalence to standard techniques. The impact on long term outcomes is still unknown. BMP-2 does not appear to be carcinogenic and it clearly increases the rate of fusion compared to other bone graft options. Osteoporotic medications may impact spinal fusion according to early animal testing, but the actual clinical implication is currently being evaluated and likely something we will cover next year. Articles defining surgical complications are very important additions to the literature. This year, complications like graft extrusion, neurological deterioration and implant malposition with minimally invasive techniques were reviewed. I hope you appreciate this year's diversity in topics and I look forward to a more thematic approach in the years to come.

Brett A. Freedman, MD

Comparative analysis of clinical outcomes between zero-profile implant and cages with plate fixation in treating multilevel cervical spondilotic myelopathy: A three-year follow-up

Chen Y, Chen H, Wu X, et al (Second Military Med Univ, Shanghai, China)
Clin Neurol Neurosurg 146:72-76, 2016

Objectives.—This study aimed to figure out three-year clinical outcomes and complications of ACDF with Zero-p in treating multilevel cervical spondylotic myelopathy (MCSM) by comparing with plate fixation.

Clinical Materials and Methods.—Patients with MCSM caused by degenerative disc herniation only were recruited from April 2010 to December 2010. According to the surgical procedures, the patients were divided into two groups at random, the plate group and Zero-P group. The data was collected before surgery and at three-year follow-up. Clinical parameters, including Japanese orthopedic association (JOA) score, neck disabled index (NDI) were evaluated. Cervical segmental lordosis was calculated and fusion in each level was assessed on lateral radiographs. The Bazaz's criterion and the short Swallowing and Quality of Life (SQOL) questionnaires were used to evaluate the dysphagia incidence and severity respectively. The presence of ALOD was observed and recorded on lateral radiographs.

Results.—A total of 72 patients (46 men and 26 women) were recruited. The mean age at operation was 52.9 ± 7.9 years, ranged from 43 to 69 years. There was no significant difference between two groups preoperatively in age, sex, operative levels, JOA, NDI, cervical lordosis, dysphagia incidence, SQOL and ALOD incidence. JOA, NDI and cervical lordosis improved postoperatively and postoperative SQOL got restitution in both groups. However, no difference was detected. There were 7 patients with ALOD in the plate group after surgeries while there was only 1 patient in Zero-P group. The difference of AOLD incidence between them was significant. Of the 7 patients with ALOD in the plate group, 4 patients developed ALOD in cranial level, 2 in caudal level and 1 in both levels. The patient in Zero-P group developed ALOD in caudal level.

Conclusion.—Based on the three-year follow-up, we could not conclude that Zero-P was superior to plate fixation in clinical outcomes such as neurological results, cervical lordosis, fusion rate and the incidence and severity of dysphagia in treating MCSM. However, it had the advantage of reducing ALOD incidence which tended to happen in ACDF with plate fixation.

▶ The impact of plate encroachment on adjacent levels following anterior cervical discectomy and fusion (ACDF) has gained significant attention since Park's original report.[1] It is clear that when plates encroach on adjacent segments (< 5 mm plate to disc), the incidence of ossification of the tissues anterior to the disc (ALOD) increases. Whether this has clinical impact is less certain. However, most agree that it would be advantageous to avoid this phenomenon. In this article, the authors have evaluated in what appears to be a prospective randomized trial with 3-year follow-up, the impact of using a screw-fixed cage (Synthes Zero-P) versus a standard anterior plate and cage (Medtronic Atlantis plate and Stryker Solis PEEK cage) to stabilize ACDFs of various lengths conducted between April and December 2010 at their institution. Milled autograft was used in all patients. Seventy-two patients (38 Plate, 34 Zero-P) were enrolled. All patients in each group went onto solid fusion (assessed by flexion-extension films) by 3 years. It is always difficult to accept reports of a 0% nonunion rate after multilevel ACDF, but this does not distract too much from the primary finding, which is that there was significantly more ALOD in the plate group versus the Zero-P group (18% vs 3%; most commonly at the cephalad adjacent level). Interestingly, the incidence of dysphagia was not significantly different between the 2 groups (nor was JOA or NDI change), suggesting that the dysphagia that is frequently encountered following ACDF is more related to the surgical exposure than to the plate.

B. Freedman, MD

Reference

1. Park JB, Cho YS, Riew KD. Development of adjacent-level ossification in patients with an anterior cervical plate. *J Bone Joint Surg Am.* 2005;87:558-563.

Application of a stand-alone anchored spacer in noncontiguous anterior cervical arthrodesis with radiologic analysis of the intermediate segment

Shi S, Liu Z-D, You W-J, et al (Shanghai Jiaotong Univ, PR China; Second Military Med Univ, Shanghai, PR China)

J Clin Neurosci 25:69-74, 2016

The purpose of this study was to describe the clinical features of noncontiguous cervical degenerative disc disease (cDDD), investigate the efficacy and complications of a stand-alone anchored spacer (SAAS) for patients with noncontiguous cDDD, and present radiologic analysis of the intermediate segment (IS) after skip-level fusion. Nineteen consecutive patients with noncontiguous cDDD who underwent skip-level anterior cervical discectomy and fusion (ACDF) with SAAS from January 2010 to December 2012 were enrolled in this study. Clinical outcomes were assessed preoperatively and at 24 months postoperatively using the Japanese Orthopaedic Association score, Neck Disability Index, and Visual Analog Scale. Overall cervical alignment (OCA) of the cervical spine, and the range of motion (ROM), intervertebral disc height (IDH), disc signal intensity and disc protrusion of IS were measured and compared before and after surgery. Clinical outcomes significantly improved compared to preoperative scores. The OCA was corrected and maintained at 24 months postoperatively compared with preoperative values ($p < 0.05$). There were no significant differences in the ROM and IDH of the IS at each follow-up ($p > 0.05$). However, decreased signal intensity on T2-weighted MRI was evidenced in three mobile IS at final follow-up (20.0%). Skip-level ACDF with SAAS may be an efficacious option for the treatment of noncontiguous cDDD.

▶ Noncontiguous cervical degenerative disc disease is a challenging problem. The authors have done a good job framing this issue and selecting a research topic that is impactful. Their approach is to avoid surgery at the intervening normal segment and to use low-profile implants. They evaluated the efficacy of this approach in a prospective clinical study evaluating the 24-month outcome following anterior cervical discectomy and fusion (ACDF) performed using a stand-alone anchored spacer (Synthes Zero-P - PEEK) filled with excised local bone fragments for graft by a single spine surgeon. The low-profile implants may reduce dysphagia and are easier to work around if the intervening segment goes on to degenerate and require subsequent surgery. Overall, cervical lordosis was significantly improved, and there was no change in range of motion, disc height, or degeneration of the intervening segment at 24 months. All patients went onto fusion as documented on flexion-extension radiographs. Unfortunately, this report only contains the outcomes of 19 patients who underwent this procedure during the period of their study. In addition, this was an observational study with no comparison cohort. But in terms of proof of concept, the evidence generated supports consideration of this technique for this challenging situation.

B. Freedman, MD

Anterior lumbar interbody fusion with integrated fixation and adjunctive posterior stabilization: A comparative biomechanical analysis

Yeager MS, Dupre DA, Cook DJ, et al (Allegheny General Hosp, Pittsburgh, PA; et al)

Clin Biomech (Bristol, Avon) 30:769-774, 2015

Background.—Interbody fusion cages with integrated fixation components have become of interest due to their ability to provide enhanced post-operative stability and mitigate device migration. A recently approved anterior lumbar interbody fusion cage with integrated fixation anchors has yet to be compared *in vitro* to a standard polyetheretherketone cage when used in combination with an interspinous process clamp.

Methods.—Twelve human cadaveric lumbar segments were implanted at L4–L5 with a Solus interbody cage (n = 6) or standard polyetheretherketone cage (n = 6) following Intact testing and discectomy. Each cage was subsequently evaluated in all primary modes of loading after supplementation with the following posterior constructs: interspinous process clamp, bilateral transfacet screws, unilateral transfacet screw with contralateral pedicle screws, and bilateral pedicle screws. Range of motion results were normalized to Intact, and a two-way mixed analysis of variance was utilized to detect statistical differences.

Findings.—The Solus cage in combination with all posterior constructs provided significant fixation compared to Intact in all loading conditions. The polyetheretherketone cage also provided significant fixation when combined with all screw based treatments, however when used with the interspinous process clamp a significant reduction was not observed in lateral bending or axial torsion.

Interpretation.—Interbody cages with integrated fixation components enhance post-operative stability within the intervertebral space, thus affording clinicians the potential to utilize less invasive methods of posterior stabilization when seeking circumferential fusion. Interspinous process clamps, in particular, may reduce peri-operative and post-operative comorbidities compared to screw based constructs. Further study is necessary to corroborate their effectiveness *in vivo*.

▶ Yeager et al have reported a simple biomechanical study that highlights a few things that are worthwhile to know. First stand-alone anterior lumbar interbody cages that do not possess integrated fixation (ie, screws or other fixation features) do not significantly reduce range of motion (ROM) over the intact or even destabilized state, especially when loaded in axial torsion or lateral bending. These devices require the addition of supplemental posterior fixation. However, this is not posterior instrumentation of a native spine but rather one in which the anterior cage inherently limits flexion-extension ROM; thus, the robustness of the posterior portion of the construct may be minimized. In this study, if the anterior cage had integrated fixation, any posterior supplemental fixation was enough to significantly reduce ROM from the intact state in all modes of loading. The authors conclude that of the 3 types (interspinous clamp, facet screws, pedicle screws) of supplemental posterior fixation test, that the simplest and the one that required the least soft tissue disruption, may be clinically best, namely, a interspinous clamp. However, in the absence of integrated fixation, an interspinous clamp was not sufficient to control against torsion and lateral bending. A significant limitation is that anterior plate testing of the simple anterior cage was not included, and the 12 cadaveric samples were likely very degenerative at baseline because radical discectomy did not significantly change the ROM. Despite the limitations, this article and those cited in the Discussion provide a good evidence base for surgeons to consider when selecting best means for reconstruction after anterior discectomy.

B. Freedman, MD

Effect of Zoledronic Acid on Spinal Fusion Outcomes in an Ovariectomized Rat Model of Osteoporosis

Yasen M, Li X, Jiang L, et al (Fudan Univ, Shanghai, China)
J Orthop Res 33:1297-1304, 2015

To evaluate the effect of zoledronic acid (ZA) on spinal fusion in ovariectomized (OVX) rats. Female SD rats ($n = 50$) were OVX or sham-operated and randomized into five groups: Sham, OVX control, ZOL-20 (20 μg/kg), ZOL-100 (100 μg/kg), and ZOL-500 (500 μg/kg). Eight weeks after OVX, bilateral lumbar spinal fusion was performed using autologous iliac bone with ZA or saline according to the grouping. The lumbar spines were harvested at 8 weeks and subjected to radiographic, manual palpation, micro-computed tomographic (micro-CT), and histological analysis. The manual palpation result differed significantly only between the ZOL-500 (fused: partially fused: not fused, 9:0:0) and OVX control (4:2:3) ($p < 0.05$). The radiographic scales were also differed significantly only between these two groups. According to the micro-CT results, the bone volume fraction (BV/TV) were significantly higher in all ZA-treated groups

(54.2%, 65.9%, and 73.6%) than OVX control (43.7%) ($p < 0.01$). At clinical dose or lower, ZA didn't alter the spinal fusion, but a higher dose increased the spinal fusion rate significantly. This study suggests ZA may have a positive effect on spinal fusion in the presence of osteoporosis, and spinal fusion surgery outcome is not likely to be altered by ZA at clinical dose.

▶ Yasen et al. report their results from an animal experimentation study evaluating the impact zoledronic acid (ZA) has on spinal fusion in ovariectomized rats. The model is well validated and well performed. Fifty rats either had ovaries removed (to induce osteoporosis) or not (sham) 8 weeks before an L4-5 posterolateral spinal fusion using autologous iliac crest bone. Immediately after spinal fusion surgery rats were injected 1 time with no, 20 μg/kg, 100 μg/kg (equivalent to 5-mg human dose) or 500 μg/kg ZA. Eight weeks later, the animals were euthanized. At that point x-ray, micro—CT, manual palpation and histology were used to quantify fusion rate. Interestingly, sham (ie, normal bone quality) and ovariectomy-induced osteoporosis did not significantly affect fusion. At clinically relevant doses ZA had no significant impact on fusion status, but at higher doses (500 μg/kg), it led to 100% solid fusion rate versus 44% in the control group, and it was a more robust and dense fusion mass. This finding is important because animal work to date has provided conflicting results as to whether osteoclast inhibition due to bisphosphonates (BP) has an inhibitory, neutral, or beneficial impact on spinal fusion. In a rabbit model without surgically induced osteoporosis, we found that alendronate administration delayed and reduced bone fusion mass development.[1] The beneficial effect of ZA (a high-potency, high-affinitiy BP, which exerts a clinical effect for 1 year from dosing) demonstrated in this study needs to be reconfirmed in larger animals, and assuming this is successful, clinical studies should be performed, similar to that mentioned in the Introduction, to validate this approach, because the use of active osteoporosis medications in the perioperative period of spinal fusion is a research topic ripe for yielding significant clinical impact.

B. Freedman, MD

Reference

1. Lehman RA Jr, Kuklo TR, Freedman BA, Cowart JR, Mense MG, Riew KD. The effect of alendronate sodium on spinal fusion: a rabbit model. *Spine J*. 2004;4:36-43.

Effect of a selective estrogen receptor modulator on bone formation in osteoporotic spine fusion using an ovariectomized rat model

Park SB, Kim CH, Hong M, et al (Seoul Natl Univ Boramae Med Ctr, South Korea; Seoul Natl Univ College of Medicine, South Korea; et al)
Spine J 16:72-81, 2016

Background Context.—Selective estrogen receptor modulators (SERMs) are drugs used to treat osteoporosis. Selective estrogen receptor modulators improve bone mineral density and bone mechanical strength. However, there is a lack of data on the effect of SERMs on osteoporotic spinal fusion.

Purpose.—This study aimed to investigate whether treatment with a SERM enhances spinal fusion in an ovariectomized (OVX) rat model.

Study Design.—An in vivo animal study was carried out.

Methods.—Female Sprague Dawley rats (n = 90) were OVX or sham-operated, and randomized into three groups: control (sham-operated+ fusion procedure+saline administration), OVX (OVX+fusion procedure+saline administration), and SERM (OVX+fusion procedure+administration of SERM). Eight weeks after OVX, a bilateral lumbar spinal fusion procedure was performed using autologous iliac bone. In each group, gene expression was evaluated at 2, 4, and 8 weeks after the fusion procedure, histologic analysis was performed at 4 and 8 weeks after the procedure, and bone parameters were measured by micro-computed tomography at 2 days, 4 weeks, and 8 weeks after the procedure.

Results.—Bone mineral density and trabecular quality of the vertebral body were significantly higher in the SERM group compared with the OVX group 16 weeks after OVX. The fusion rate and bone volume ratio were higher in the fusion bed of the SERM group compared with the OVX group 8 weeks after the fusion procedure. Real-time reverse transcription polymerase chain reaction at 4 and 8 weeks after the fusion procedure showed increased expression of the genes for osteoblast-related markers (alkaline phosphatase, osteocalcin, runt-related transcription factor 2, and transforming growth factor) in the SERM group compared with the OVX group. The OVX group showed sparse bone mass between transverse processes. By contrast, the SERM group exhibited a compact bridging fusion mass within the fusion bed at 8 weeks after the fusion procedure.

Conclusions.—Selective estrogen receptor modulator treatment improved the trabecular quality of the vertebral body, enhanced spinal fusion, and increased the amount of compact bone mass within the fusion bed in rats that had received an ovariectomy. Therapeutic SERM treatment may be recommended to improve the fusion rate in osteoporotic patients who undergo spinal fusion.

▶ Park et al. have performed a rigorous, well-designed animal testing protocol to evaluate the effect of 8-week exposure to raloxifene (Evista), a selective estrogen receptor modulator (SERM), has on bone quality and fusion mass after intertransverse posterolateral fusion at the L4-5 level in 90 Sprague-Dawley rats, divided into 3 groups of 30 each. To their credit, they not only included 2 cohorts of rats that had been ovarectomized to induce an osteopenic state, they also included a control cohort that underwent a sham-procedure to ensure blinding at the time of data analysis. As expected, removal of the ovaries resulted in a significant reduction in bone mineral density (BMD) compared with the sham-control group at 8 weeks after the procedure. After this, a posterior spinal fusion procedure was performed in all 90 rats, in which a standardized surgical technique was employed, which included weighing the amount of autogenous iliac bone graft placed into the bilateral L4-5 intertransverse plane. These animals were then either provided raloxifene (n = 30 of the ovarectomized rats; dose = 3 mg/kg/day) or normal saline gavage starting on postoperative day 2 and continued for up to 8 weeks. Fourteen animals in each group were sacrificed early (7 at 2 weeks and 7 and 4 weeks) to allow for real-time polymerase chain reaction (PCR) testing and interval histological assessment. All animals underwent micro–CT to assess areal BMD (g/mm^2) as well as fusion status. Fusion status was also determined by manual palpation (i.e., no bending). Interestingly, the raloxifene group demonstrated significantly higher BMD than the ovarectomized rats that received normal saline, but this effect on BMD was stabilizing, as opposed to anabolic. The BMD in the normal saline cohort continued to diminish following removal of ovaries, while it remained the same, but still significantly lower than the sham controls, in the raloxifene group. Although there was no improvement in BMD (g/mm^2), PCR testing did show increased expression of osteoblastic-related markers, indicating some molecular level of anabolic effect. Likewise, all fusion indices were higher in the raloxifene group compared with the positive controls, but both of the ovarectomized cohorts had less fusion mass than the sham control rats. Thus, this study helps to reiterate the negative impact osteoporosis has in general on spinal fusion, while demonstrating that specific antiosteoporosis medications may have a beneficial effect that mitigates, but does not eliminate, this issue. As populations across the developed world age and remain active, osteoporosis will continue to be a growing challenge for spine surgeons internationally. At the Mayo Clinic we have turned to teriparatide (Forteo), for its anabolic effects, to prepare osteoporotic patients for instrumented spinal fusion; however, this drug has been associated with the development of osteosarcoma in rare cases. Work like that reported in this article needs to continue as we seek an ideal method to optimize bone quality and augment fusion potential in older patients with diminished bone quality undergoing major spine surgery.

B. Freedman, MD

Defining Spino-Pelvic Alignment Thresholds: Should Operative Goals in Adult Spinal Deformity Surgery Account for Age?

Lafage R, International Spine Study Group (NYU Langone Med Ctr; et al)

Spine 41:62-68, 2016

Study Design.—Retrospective review of prospective, multicenter database.

Objective.—The aim of the study was to determine age-specific spinopelvic parameters, to extrapolate age-specific Oswestry Disability Index (ODI) values from published Short Form (SF)-36 Physical Component Score (PCS) data, and to propose age-specific realignment thresholds for adult spinal deformity (ASD).

Summary of Background Data.—The Scoliosis Research Society-Schwab classification offers a framework for defining alignment in patients with ASD. Although age-specific changes in spinal alignment and patient-reported outcomes have been established in the literature, their relationship in the setting of ASD operative realignment has not been reported.

Methods.—ASD patients who received operative or nonoperative treatment were consecutively enrolled. Patients were stratified by age, consistent with published US-normative values (Norms) of the SF-36 PCS (<35, 35–44, 45–54, 55–64, 65–74, >75 y old). At baseline, relationships between between radiographic spino-pelvic parameters (lumbar-pelvic mismatch [PILL], pelvic tilt [PT], sagittal vertical axis [SVA], and T1 pelvic angle [TPA]), age, and PCS were established using linear regression analysis; normative PCS values were then used to establish age-specific targets. Correlation analysis with ODI and PCS was used to determine age-specific ideal alignment.

Results.—Baseline analysis included 773 patients (53.7 y old, 54% operative, 83% female). There was a strong correlation between ODI and PCS ($r = 0.814$, $P < 0.001$), allowing for the extrapolation of US-normative ODI by age group. Linear regression analysis (all with $r > 0.510$, $P < 0.001$) combined with US-normative PCS values demonstrated that ideal spino-pelvic values increased with age, ranging from PT = 10.9 degrees, PI–LL = 10.5 degrees, and SVA = 4.1 mm for patients under 35 years to PT = 28.5 degrees, PI–LL = 16.7 degrees, and SVA = 78.1 mm for patients over 75 years. Clinically, older patients had greater compensation, more degenerative loss of lordosis, and were more pitched forward.

Conclusion.—This study demonstrated that sagittal spino-pelvic alignment varies with age. Thus, operative realignment targets should account for age, with younger patients requiring more rigorous alignment objectives.

▶ Members of the International Spine Study Group have analyzed their prospectively collected outcome data and reported radiographic measures for consecutively enrolled patients in a multicenter registry for adult spinal deformity (n = 773, average age 54, 54% surgically treated). The aim was to assess whether spinopelvic parameters have an age-specific impact on outcome. This was a unique and important research question because adult spinal deformity surgeons have tended to correct patients of all age to the same set of idealized sagittal parameter values (i.e., lumbar-pelvic mismatch [PI–LL] < 10 degrees, pelvic tilt [PT] < 25 degrees, sagittal vertical axis [SVA] < 4-5 cm). Smith et al.'s recent work, highlights the need to assess whether ideal sagittal parameters and compensation are age-dependant.[1] When looking at a sample of 173 adult spinal deformity (ASD) patient (average age 63) undergoing surgery, correcting SVA to < 5 cm resulted in a significantly increased risk of proximal junctional kyphosis.[1] Life is a kyphosing event, and the current study has empirically demonstrated this. The average PI–LL, PT, and SVA were −11 degrees (indicating lumbar lordosis greater than pelvic incidence), 11 degrees and 4 cm, respectively, in young patients (< 35 years old), whereas these sagittal parameters increased in all successive age cohorts, until they peaked at 13.7 degrees, 28.8 degrees and 8 cm in the oldest cohort (> 74 years old). Furthermore, life is a degenerative event, the sum of which leads to progressive dysfunction as assessed by the Physical Component Score of the Short Form—36 and the Oswestry Disability Index (ODI). The normative ODI score increased more than 3 times over adult life from 9.5% in people younger than 35 years to 32.5% in people older than 74 years. Exposing older patients to the substantial risk of ASD surgery demands that we understand what is the age-appropriate geometric goal. This work is an important step in that direction. It is akin to that of Boden et al., who demonstrated in 1990 that not all degenerative findings on MRI of the spine are pathologic.[2] Likewise, not all forward leans and flattened lumbar spines need to be surgically corrected or result in a disability greater than that expected for an age-matched normal peer.

B. Freedman, MD

References

1. Smith MW, Annis P, Lawrence BD, Daubs MD, Brodke DS. Acute proximal junctional failure in patients with preoperative sagittal imbalance. *Spine J.* 2015;15:2142-2148.
2. Boden SD, Davis DO, Dina TS, Patronas NJ, Wiesel SW. Abnormal magnetic-resonance scans of the lumbar spine in asymptomatic subjects. A prospective investigation. *J Bone Joint Surg Am.* 1990;72:403-408.

Appropriate Use of Limited Interventions vs Extensive Surgery in the Elderly Patient With Spinal Disorders

Gussous Y, Than K, Mummaneni P, et al (Univ of California, San Francisco; et al)

Neurosurgery 77:S142-S163, 2015

Surgical management of spinal deformity is elderly patients is characterized by significant variability. In a value-based health care economy, minimization of risks and maximization of benefit and durability of surgery are a priority. The choice of a surgical approach is a significant determinant of risk, cost, and outcome. Informed choice regarding a surgical approach requires participation of the patient and surgeon. Limited interventions may be appropriate for patients with radicular symptoms and focal pain. More extensive surgery may be required for patients with global imbalance of the spine. The role of minimally invasive approaches in limiting complications and improving outcome remains in evolution. An optimal choice of surgical approach requires consideration of patient preferences, values, comorbidities, and goals of care.

▶ Gussous et al provide an interesting commentary on a very relevant event that is occurring in health care systems across the world—the "silver tsunami" and the impact spinal disease in this population will have on the economics of our health care system. Starting in 2011, the oldest baby boomers (born between 1946 and 1964) reached >65 years of age. Currently this accounts for more than 40 million people in the United States, and it is projected to be 72 million or 20% of the US population by 2030. Others have shown that

60% of adults in this age range have some degree of spinal deformity, and this seems to be more commonly a degenerative de novo process as opposed to persistent idiopathic deformity. The combination of these 2 factors is that more and more elderly people with spinal deformity will develop spinal disease and present for surgical consideration in the coming decades. When considering this magnitude of disease, societal factors, namely, cost-effectiveness and utility, are becoming ever more important in the decision process. As the increased rate of complex spinal fusion surgeries outpaces population growth and the costs associated per case have risen 76% in recent time, surgeons, and by proxy patients, will need to empirically demonstrate health outcome benefits to account for these rapidly elevating health care expenditures. Studies have shown mixed results in terms of patient complications, outcomes and satisfaction related to decompression alone, limited decompression-fusion (ie, L4-L5 or L4-S1 fusion for degenerative (dynamic) spondylolisthesis, while ignoring the balanced coronal and/or sagittal deformity above) and long segment decompression-fusion. As expected, more complex surgery leads to higher complication rates, but oddly it also seems to breed higher patient satisfaction. Economic decisions need to be couched in the long run, "an approach that is more expensive for the index surgery may be cost-saving over time." If decompression alone in the setting of spinal deformity, which is far cheaper than fusion surgery, results in equivalent short-term results, but at long-term produces far more complicated deformity-related spinal disease, then is it really cost-effective? The middle option may become the most cost-effective and durable of the 3 options. Limited fusions localized to 1 to 3 levels that ignore adjacent (preferably well-balanced) spinal deformity, offer the ability to widely decompress the focal compressive disease, control the segmental deformity, provide some local deformity correction, and, in the case of lumbosacral disease (fractional curves and spondylolisthesis), set a stable base, if long-segment deformity becomes necessary. This is an excellent review article on the topic for those who are interested. As with most things in medicine, the simplest and the most complex are rarely the best generic solution. Something in the middle will likely be the best option for the masses, and the masses are coming.

B. Freedman, MD

Adult Spinal Deformity Patients Recall Fewer Than 50% of the Risks Discussed in the Informed Consent Process Preoperatively and the Recall Rate Worsens Significantly in the Postoperative Period

Saigal R, Clark AJ, Scheer JK, et al (Univ of California San Francisco; Univ of California San Diego; et al)
Spine 40:1079-1085, 2015

Study Design.—Recall of the informed consent process in patients undergoing adult spinal deformity surgery and their family members was investigated prospectively.

Objective.—To quantify the percentage recall of the most common complications discussed during the informed consent process in adult spinal deformity surgery, assess for differences between patients and family members, and correlate with mental status.

Summary of Background Data.—Given high rates of complications in adult spinal deformity surgery, it is critical to shared decision making that patients are adequately informed about risks and are able to recall preoperative discussion of possible complications to mitigate medical legal risk.

Methods.—Patients undergoing adult spinal deformity surgery underwent an augmented informed consent process involving both verbal and video explanations. Recall of the 11 most common complications was scored. Mental status was assessed with the mini-mental status examination-brief version. Patients subjectively scored the informed consent process and video. After surgery, the recall test and mini-mental status examination-brief version were readministered at 5 additional time points: hospital discharge, 6 to 8 weeks, 3 months, 6 months, and 1 year postoperatively. Family members were assessed at the first 3 time points for comparison.

Results.—Fifty-six patients enrolled. Despite ranking the consent process as important (median overall score: 10/10; video score: 9/10), median patient recall was only 45% immediately after discussion and video reenforcement and subsequently declined to 18% at 6 to 8 weeks and 1 year postoperatively. Median family recall trended higher at 55% immediately and 36% at 6 to 8 weeks postoperatively. The perception of the severity of complications significantly differs between patient and surgeon. Mental status scores showed a transient, significant decrease from preoperation to discharge but were significantly higher at 1 year.

Conclusion.—Despite being well-informed in an optimized informed consent process, patients cannot recall most surgical risks discussed and recall declines over time. Significant progress remains to improve informed consent retention.

Level of Evidence.—3.

▶ Saigal et al have provided great insight into a new area of concern for the spine surgeon, in their prospective assessment of recall bias in 56 patients following a thorough informed consent process (verbal + 20 min video) before adult spinal deformity surgery. Immediately after completing the process, patients only recalled 45% of the 11 complications discussed, family members, when present, were able to recall 55%. This recall plummeted to <27% (18% at 1 year) at all postoperative time points for patients and about 36% for family members. Mini-Mental Exam showed that poor cognition was not to blame. Lessons learned are as follows: (1) complicated surgery demands a thorough consent strategy; (2) regardless of thoroughness, patient recall is poor so surgeon documentation should be robust; (3) having family present increases recall, but prior spine surgery or experiencing 1 of the discussed complications after surgery does not; and (4) patient and surgeon's prioritize complication severity differently. Patients were most concerned about blood transfusion and cerebrospinal fluid leak, whereas surgeons felt that weakness, blindness, and death were the most severe risks. In the era of shared decision making, studies like this are needed to inform all parties of the limitations of complex information transfer. This is clearly an area for future work.

B. Freedman, MD

Clinical Depression Is a Strong Predictor of Poor Lumbar Fusion Outcomes Among Workers' Compensation Subjects

Anderson JT, Haas AR, Percy R, et al (Case Western Reserve Univ School of Medicine, Cleveland, OH; Ohio Bureau of Workers' Compensation, Columbus; et al)
Spine 40:748-756, 2015

Study Design.—Retrospective cohort study.

Objective.—Determine how psychosocial factors, particularly depression, impact lumbar fusion outcomes in a workers' compensation (WC) setting.

Summary of Background Data.—WC patients are less likely to return to work (RTW) after fusion. Few studies evaluate risk factors within this clinically distinct population.

Methods.—A total of 2799 Ohio WC subjects were identified who underwent lumbar fusion between 1993 and 2013 using *Current Procedural Terminology (CPT)* procedural and *International Classification of Diseases, Ninth Revision (ICD-9)* diagnosis codes. A total of 123 subjects were diagnosed with depression before fusion. Subjects with a smoking history, prior lumbar surgery, permanent disability, and failed back syndrome were excluded. The primary outcome was whether subjects returned to work within 2 years of fusion and sustained this RTW for more than 6 months of the following year. To determine the impact depression had on RTW status, we performed a multivariate logistic regression analysis. We also compared time absent from work and other secondary outcomes using χ^2 and t tests.

Results.—Subjects with preoperative depression had significantly higher rates of legal representation, degenerative lumbar disease, and higher medical costs, and used opioid analgesics for considerably longer before and after fusion ($P < 0.001$). Depression group (10.6% [13/123]) and controls (33.0% [884/2676]) met our RTW criteria ($P < 0.001$). Preoperative depression was a negative predictor of RTW status ($P < 0.001$; odds ratio [OR]: 0.38). Additional predictors included working during same week as fusion (OR: 2.15), age more than 50 years (OR: 0.58), chronic preoperative opioid analgesia (OR: 0.58), and legal representation (OR: 0.64). After surgery, depression subjects were absent from work 184 more days compared with controls ($P < 0.001$).

Conclusion.—Overall, RTW rates after fusion were low, which was especially true for those with pre-existing depression. Depression was a strong negative predictor of postoperative RTW status. Psychological screening and treatment may be beneficial in these subjects. The poor outcomes in this study may highlight a more limited role for fusion among WC subjects with chronic low back pain where RTW is the treatment goal.

Level of Evidence.—3.

▶ Anderson et al report the retrospectively observed rates of return to work (RTW) within 2 years of spinal fusion surgery, with at least 6 months sustained work after the return, in 2676 patients without preoperatively diagnosed depression versus 123 depressed patients from the Ohio worker's compensation (WC) administrative database. As expected, those with depression did very poorly, with only 10.6% RTW rate versus 33% for those who were not diagnosed with depression before surgery. The authors dug deep in the database, which generated several interesting findings. Almost 3 times more patients were diagnosed with depression in the 3 years after fusion surgery (n = 430 of the 2676; 16%), than before surgery. Based on preoperative psychological testing completed, it appears this more likely indicates failure to diagnose preexisting disease than new onset. Adjusting for this did not significantly change the differences in RTW. Clinically depressed patients were 2.6 times less likely to RTW. Those who were able to continue work up until surgery were 2.5 times more likely to RTW after surgery, however, which meant that 51% of patients who were working before surgery were able to return. Age > 50, use of narcotic pain medications for more than 1 year before surgery, and legal representation were all negative prognosticators for RTW. The overall RTW for WC patients is only 32%, whereas 41% of WC patients with or without depression were declared permanently disabled within 3 years of undergoing spinal fusion surgery. Furthermore, 1 in 5 WC patients underwent another lumbar spine surgery within 3 years of the index procedure. This study identifies significant negative predictors for RTW in WC patients. This and similar studies are needed to define optimal predictors of successful occupational outcomes in WC patients.

B. Freedman, MD

Patient-Reported Outcome Instruments in Spine Surgery

Guzman JZ, Cutler HS, Connolly J, et al (Icahn School of Medicine at Mount Sinai, NY; et al)

Spine 41:429-437, 2016

Study Design.—A critical review of the current literature.

Objective.—The purpose of this study was to determine frequency, trends, and methods of utilization of spine-related PROIs over the last 10 years.

Summary of Background Data.—Patient-reported outcome instruments (PROIs) have become the gold standard to assess the efficacy of various medical and surgical treatments. Currently, however, there is an expansive range of PROIs without a clear consensus or guideline addressing which PROIs should be used for a particular diagnosis or surgical intervention.

Methods.—A PubMed search was conducted from 2004 to 2013 of 5 orthopedic journals (*The Journal of Bone and Joint Surgery, The Bone and Joint Journal, The Spine Journal, The European Spine Journal, and Spine*) that publish spine articles, chosen on the basis of readership and impact factor. Journal abstracts were inspected for spine surgery and inclusion of at least 1 PROI. All articles containing PROIs and investigating a surgical intervention with a level of evidence (LOE) 1 to 4 were included for analysis. Article title, LOE, journal, and chosen PROI were recorded for selected articles.

Results.—Out of 19,736 articles published in our selected time frame, 1,079 utilized PROIs. Most studies were LOE 4 (32.7%). Nearly half (48.9%) of all articles addressed degenerative thoracolumbar conditions. In total, there were 206 unique PROIs in the studies chosen for inclusion. The top 6 instruments utilized were the (1) visual analog scale, (2) Oswestry disability index, (3) Short Form-36, (4) Japanese Orthopaedic Association Outcome Questionnaire, (5) Neck Disability Index, and (6) Scoliosis Research Society-22.

Conclusion.—The breadth of PROIs in spine surgery is extensive. Although there are preferred patient-reported outcome measures, a consensus or guideline addressing which instruments should be used for a particular diagnosis or procedure may be warranted.

▶ Guzman et al. have provided a concise demonstration of the need for better and more consistent use of patient-reported outcome instruments (PROIs) related to spinal disease. In their literature review of 19 736 articles reporting clinical results from spine surgery between 2004 and 2013, only 1079 (5.5%) reported the results of at least 1 PROI and a total of 206 unique PROIs were used in these studies. There was a proclivity toward 6 particular PROIs (visual analog scale, used in 48% of included studies; Oswestry Disability Index, 38%; Short Form-36 (SF-36), 21%; Japanese Orthopaedic Association Outcome Questionnaire, 15%; Neck Disability Index, 8%; and Scoliosis Research Society-22, 6%). With a pivot toward performance-based reimbursement, we must be more proactive in defining results of our surgical interventions, using a consistent set of validated outcome measures to provide the empiric support for our anecdotal understanding that spine surgery in well-selected patients provides meaningful clinical benefit. Unfortunately, of the 6 commonly used PROIs, only SF-36 can be readily converted into quality-adjusted life years for health utility assessment. The authors saw an early favorable trend toward annually increased use of PROIs from 2004 to 2008, but in 2009, use dropped to 2005 levels and then started an upward trend again. Another interesting finding in this study is that about 15% of clinical reports regarding spine surgery were Level 1 evidence, while most commonly the level of evidence was 4 (33%). The authors have hit the head on the nail in their conclusion: the leadership in spinal medical literature (ie, established authors and editors) needs to select a specific set of PROIs that become the standard outcome assessment tools so that meaningful comparisons between studies can be drawn and our medical literature can inform cumulatively as opposed to independently.

B. Freedman, MD

A Cost-Utility Analysis of Lumbar Decompression With and Without Fusion for Degenerative Spine Disease in the Elderly

Devin CJ, Chotai S, Parker SL, et al (Univ Med Ctr, Nashville, TN; et al)
Neurosurgery 77:S116-S124, 2015

Background.—Value-based purchasing is rapidly being implemented to rein in the unsustainably rising costs of the US healthcare system. With a growing elderly population, it is vital to understand the value of spinal surgery in this group of individuals.

Objective.—To compare the cost-effectiveness of lumbar decompression with and without fusion for degenerative spine disease in elderly vs non-elderly patients.

Methods.—A total of 221 patients undergoing elective primary surgery for degenerative lumbar pathology who were enrolled in a prospective longitudinal registry were analyzed. Patient-reported outcomes of Oswestry Disability Index, numeric rating scale for back and leg pain, and quality-of-life scores (EuroQol-5D) were recorded. Two-year back-related medical resource use, missed work, and health-state values (quality-adjusted life-years [QALYs]) were assessed. Two-year resource use was multiplied by unit costs based on Medicare national allowable payment amounts (direct cost). Patient and caregiver workday losses were multiplied by gross-of-tax wage rate (indirect cost). Patients were divided into age groups <70 and ≥70 years.

Results.—Mean cumulative 2-year QALYs gained were statistically similar between younger and older patients for both decompression alone (0.67 ± 0.65 vs 0.56 ± 0.65; $P = .47$) and decompression with fusion (0.56 ± 0.55 vs 0.59 ± 0.55; $P = .26$). Mean 2-year cost per QALY gained between younger and older patients was similar for both decompression alone ($24 365 vs $31 750 per QALY; $P = .11$) and decompression with fusion ($64 228 vs $60 183 per QALY; $P = .09$).

Conclusion.—Surgical treatment provided significant improvements in pain, disability, and quality of life for elderly patients with degenerative lumbar disease. Observed costs per QALY gained for lumbar decompression with and without fusion were similar for younger and older patients, demonstrating that lumbar spine surgery in the elderly is an equally cost-effective and valuable intervention.

▶ Devin et al continue a dialogue that is lacking in our literature in their attempt to define the value we know to be present for spine surgery in well-selected patients of all ages. The strength of this article is that they conducted this work using the metrics and terminology of the health economist (quality-adjusted life-years—QALY), who will become ever more intrusive in the sacred bond between patient and surgeon. This article determines the cost per QALY for lumbar decompression with or without fusion in patients younger and older than 70 years of age by retrospectively analyzing their prospectively collected patient-reported outcome's (Oswestry Disability Index being the primary outcome for determining minimal clinically important difference (>14.9% improvement) in 221 patients (>18 with degenerative lumbar spinal disease undergoing decompression with or without fusion over a 4-year period). Although an enrollment stratification chart is sorely lacking, because the Vanderbilt group has certainly performed >221 such lumbar spinal surgeries between 2010 and 2014, this does not fatally corrupt the conclusions. Lumbar spine surgery performed on adult patients with disc herniation, stenosis, and/or spondylolisthesis who present with back and leg pain and fail at least 3 months of nonoperative care, provides clinically significant and cost-effective benefit.

B. Freedman, MD

Cadaveric Analysis of Posterior Pharyngoesophageal Wall Thickness: Implications for Anterior Cervical Spine Surgery

Nam KH, Kim DH, Kim HS, et al (Pusan Natl Univ Hosp, Busan, Korea)
Spine 41:E262-E267, 2016

Study Design.—A cadaveric study

Objective.—To investigate possible variations of posterior pharyngoesophageal (PE) wall thickness in the horizontal plane and their implications for anterior spine surgery.

Summary of Background Data.—Lower cervical levels (C5–7) are most commonly involved in cases of PE injury, and PE wall thickness could be one of the proposed reasons for the high incidence of PE injuries at these levels. The purpose of this study was to document thickness variations of the posterior PE wall at different cervical spine levels, because the study could provide valuable anatomical information that could reduce iatrogenic injuries caused by retractors or instrumentation.

Methods.—Thirteen formaldehyde-fixed cadaveric specimens were included in current study. PE specimens were harvested from epiglottis to suprasternal notch within 2 months of formaldehyde fixation and sectioned axially. Four slices corresponding to the superior and inferior borders of thyroid cartilage, cricoid cartilage, and 2 cm below cricoid cartilage were sectioned. Posterior PE wall thickness was measured at three zones as follows: median, lateral, and paramedian. Posterior PE wall thicknesses were measured by a pathologist.

Results.—Based on one-way ANOVA, posterior PE wall thickness showed several significantly different variations depending on cervical level and horizontal plane. PE walls were thinnest at the level of cricoid cartilage ($P < 0.05$). This difference was more pronounced in the median zone, because of thickness variations in the muscular layer ($P < 0.001$).

Conclusion.—The posterior PE wall was thinnest in the median zone at the cricoid cartilage level. Variations in muscle layer thickness caused PE wall thickness differences. The smaller wall thickness at the level of the cricoids cartilage and in the midline zone may place it at higher risk of injury, and special care should be taken during dissection, retraction, and instrument placement.

▶ Nam et al. in a simple but relevant cadaveric study (n = 13, formaldehyde-fixed, all males; aged 42-56) have identified that the pharyngoesophageal posterior wall is thinnest (1.41-1.57 mm) at and 2 cm below the cricoid level as opposed to the thyroid cartilage levels, especially in the midline. This is important in the contest of anterior cervical spine surgery, where damage to the pharynx/esophagus is rare (0.02%-1.62%) but catastrophic (mortality is up to 20%-50% or higher). Unfortunately, the area of the cervical spine that is most commonly addressed by anterior cervical spine surgery C5-C7 is the area where the pharyngoesophageal wall is thinnest. Not only does this have implications during surgical exposure, it also means that anterior plate and screws will most commonly be in contact with this vulnerable section. Adding further insult is that this is a section with the highest amplitude peristaltic waves. The additive effects of these factors probably explain why esophageal perforation after anterior cervical spine surgery is most common in the subaxial spine after placement of a plate. The pharyngoesophageal wall is composed of mucosa, submucosa, and muscularis propria without serosa. The absence of a serosal layer amplifies the consequence of events that pierce or thin the wall.

B. Freedman, MD

Incidence of graft extrusion following minimally invasive transforaminal lumbar interbody fusion

Bakhsheshian J, Khanna R, Choy W, et al (Univ of Southern California Keck School of Medicine, Los Angeles; Northwestern Feinberg School of Medicine, Chicago, IL; et al)

J Clin Neurosci 24:88-93, 2016

Minimally invasive transforaminal lumbar interbody fusion (MI-TLIF) has been scrutinized for having a complex learning curve. Careful assessment of MI-TLIF complications and critical analyses of prevention may aid a safe adoption of this technique. The current report focuses on the incidence of interbody cage extrusions following MI-TLIF in a series of 513 patients. The authors discuss their experience with graft extrusions and provide methods to minimize this complication. This study retrospectively reviewed 513 prospectively followed patients who underwent MI-TLIF over a 10 year period. The inclusion criteria consisted of all patients who underwent one to three level MI-TLIF, from whom the incidence of cage extrusion was analyzed. Cage extrusion was defined as an interbody graft migrating outside the cephalad and caudal vertebral body posterior margin. Cage extrusions were diagnosed by comparing the intraoperative radiographs to the postoperative radiographs. Patients with >10° coronal curves, significant sagittal malalignment, infection, and preoperative instrumentation failure were excluded. Of 513 patients undergoing MI-TLIF, five patients (0.97%) were diagnosed with cage migrations. The mean follow-up duration was 13.6 ± standard deviation of 8.8 months. Complications included asymptomatic cage migration alone (two patients) neurological decline (two patients) and epidural hematoma (one patient). On average, cage migrations cost a university hospital an additional $US17,217 for revision treatment. While the incidence of cage migrations is low (0.97%), it can lead to postoperative complications that require revision surgery and increased hospital costs. The risk for this significant complication can be minimized with proper technique and patient selection.

▶ Bakhsheshian et al. reported the incidence of cage extrusion in the first post-operative year is about 1% following minimally invasive transforaminal lumbar interbody fusion in the largest series to date to evaluate this risk, which has been previously reported to occur 1% to 6% of the time. This is a retrospective review of 513 consecutive patients who underwent a nonstandardized (i.e., surgeon-dependant technique regarding: 1, 2 or 3 level fusion, polyetherether-ketone (PEEK) cage vs other type, bone graft vs bone morphogenetic protein (BMP) and bilateral vs unilateral screw fixation, but the vast majority received 12 mg of BMP-2 mixed with local autograft (94%), in a PEEK cage (86%) with bilateral pedicle screws (99%) for a 1-level fusion (84%)) minimally invasive transforaminal lumbar interbody fusion over a 10-year period. Five cases of cage extrusion were detected in their medical record review. Two of 5 (40%) were asymptomatic. All cases had posterior migration (this was an inclusion criteria in the Methods). Thus, the rate of lateral or anterior migration or misplacement is not assessed in this cohort. Although this is a rather simple study and has methodological flaws inherent to a Level 3 study, it does provide a reasonably valid assessment of the rare but real chance of cage extrusion occurring when interbody fusion devices are placed by any of the described posterior approaches in the lumbar spine. Further, this risk appears to be no more common when the technique is minimally invasive.

B. Freedman, MD

Early complications after instrumentation of the lumbar spine using cortical bone trajectory technique

Patel SS, Cheng WK, Danisa OA (Loma Linda Univ Med Ctr, CA)
J Clin Neurosci 24:63-67, 2016

This retrospective chart review aimed to identify and report on a series of early complications that resulted from instrumentation of the lumbar spine using the cortical bone trajectory (CBT) technique. CBT technique is a novel method for fixation of the lumbar spine. Since it was first described in 2009 this technique has gained significant popularity. Here we report a series of early complications that have developed in patients who had lumbar spine fusion using the CBT technique. A retrospective chart review was performed in which all cases utilizing the CBT technique for instrumentation of the lumbar spine by two fellowship trained spine surgeons at our institution between July 2012 and May 2014 were reviewed. Medical records were reviewed to determine the number of patients who went on to develop an early complication after instrumentation with this technique. An early complication was defined as any of the following occurring within 3 months of surgery: (1) early screw loosening confirmed by post-operative CT scan, (2) evidence of fracture development confirmed by post-operative CT scan, (3) intra-operatively identified durotomy, (4) superficial or deep post-operative infection and (5) neurological injury. A total of 22 cases using the CBT technique were performed in our department. Of these cases two patients went onto develop early screw loosening, one developed an intra-operative pars fracture, one developed a dural tear and lastly, one patient developed both a pedicle fracture and early screw loosening. At our institution a total of five patients thus far have developed early complications after undergoing instrumentation of the lumbar spine using the CBT technique between 2012–2014.

▶ Patel et al have provided one of the earliest reports of complications related to the use of the cortical bone trajectory (CBT) for the placement of screws into the lumbar spine. Although this technique, as an officially named and defined method, is relatively new (2009), most spine surgeons have (unintentionally) employed this trajectory at some point in their career for decades, we just called them laterally malpositioned screws. Joking aside, the theory is reasonable. A screw that is aimed in a caudal to cephalad and medial to lateral trajectory can reach upwards of 30 mm and engage cortical bone for most of the length of the screw, as opposed to trabecular bone in the setting of the traditional pedicle screw technique. In this consecutive case series of 22 patients operated on between July 2012 and May 2014, 5 experienced an early (< 3 months postoperative) screw-related complication (23% complication rate). Sixty percent of complications were related to screw loosening, and 1 went on to early revision surgery for pedicle fracture and screw loosening (via anterior lumbar interbody fusion), and the other 2 are scheduled for revision surgery. This brings up another point in the learning curve for this technique, which is, what is the ideal revision method in the setting of a loose CBT screw—anterior or posterior? In a cadaveric study, we have previously shown that immediately redirecting a lateral breached pedicle screw into an ideal center-center trajectory results in an approximately 25% reduction in fixation strength.[1] Another purported benefit of the CBT technique is that the lateral trajectory is aimed away from the canal; as such, it should reduce durotomy and/or neural injury, but 1 of the 5 complications in this series was a screw preparation–related durotomy with a resultant 3 months of left foot numbness. Lastly, this is not the first group to report that the CBT trajectory can weaken the caudal pars. If this leads to pars fracture (as it did in 1 case in this series), it would jeopardize the stability of the caudal adjacent segment. Because there is nothing new under the sun, attempts to reinvent the wheel should always be challenged before accepted. This article and this group's honest description of their experience is 1 step in the pathway of validating the virtue of this technique in comparison to traditional pedicle screw fixation.

B. Freedman, MD

Reference

1. Stauff MP, Freedman BA, Kim JH, Hamasaki T, Yoon ST, Hutton WC. The effect of pedicle screw redirection after lateral wall breach—a biomechanical study using human lumbar vertebrae. *Spine J*. 2014;14:98-103.

Value of intraoperative neurophysiological monitoring to reduce neurological complications in patients undergoing anterior cervical spine procedures for cervical spondylotic myelopathy

Thirumala PD, Muralidharan A, Loke YK, et al (Univ of Pittsburgh, PA; Univ of Michigan, Ann Arbor; Univ of East Anglia, Norwich, UK)
J Clin Neurosci 25:27-35, 2016

The primary aim of this study was to conduct a systematic review of reports of patients with cervical spondylotic myelopathy and to assess the value of intraoperative monitoring (IOM), including somatosensory evoked potentials, transcranial motor evoked potentials and electromyography, in anterior cervical procedures. A search was conducted to collect a small database of relevant papers using key words describing disorders and procedures of interest. The database was then shortlisted using selection criteria and data was extracted to identify complications as a result of anterior cervical procedures for cervical spondylotic myelopathy and outcome analysis on a continuous scale. In the 22 studies that matched the screening criteria, only two involved the use of IOM. The average sample size was 173 patients. In procedures done without IOM a mean change in Japanese Orthopaedic Association score of 3.94 points and Nurick score by 1.20 points (both less severe post-operatively) was observed. Within our sub-group analysis, worsening myelopathy and/or quadriplegia was seen in 2.71% of patients for studies without IOM and 0.91% of patients for studies with IOM. Variations persist in the existing literature in the evaluation of complications associated with anterior cervical spinal procedures. Based on the review of published studies, sufficient evidence does not exist to make recommendations regarding the use of different IOM modalities to reduce neurological complications during anterior cervical procedures. However, future studies with objective measures of neurological deficits using a specific IOM modality may establish it as an effective and reliable indicator of injury during such surgeries.

▶ Thirumala et al have performed a systematic review of the literature describing neurological outcomes after the use or lack of use of intraoperative neuromonitoring (IOM) during anterior cervical spine surgery in the setting of cervical myelopathy. Although there appears to be a benefit in protecting against all adverse neurological events (ie, palsies, dysphagia, dysphonia, and myelopathic progression; 9.3% total (range 0%–54.3%) versus 1.3% total (range 0.14%–2.5%), without and with IOM use), the data published to date does not refute or support the impact IOM has on specifically preventing myelopathic progression. This limitation is due to inconsistent means used to measure myelopathy in prior studies. The administrative database survey by Ney et al reviewed in this years YEAR BOOK also found that evidential support for IOM in anterior cervical fusion surgery was lacking. The results of this study and that of Ney et al are in conflict with standard practice, where anterior cervical spine surgery, especially in the setting of myelopathy, is one of the most common indications for use of IOM in those who use this technology. I think that the current article gets at the matter, which is to say the prior research has not adequately addressed this question. Only 2 studies reported neurological outcomes after IOM use with anterior cervical spine surgery cases and neither measured preoperative and postoperative Japanese Orthopaedic Association (JOA) or Nurick scores. Given that the rate of significant myelopathic progression after anterior cervical surgery was low (2.71% vs 0.91%) in this study, it would be challenging to generate sufficient power in a single-center prospective study, but a multicenter study employing a standardized array of tests and neurological assessment tools (ie, preoperative and postoperative graded manual muscle testing as well as documented Nurick and JOA scores) seems feasible, and it could once and for all answer the question of whether IOM is protective against all types of neurological events related to anterior cervical spine surgery. Short of that, we are left with surgeon discretion as the gold standard for the use of IOM as a means to improve outcomes associated with spine surgery.

B. Freedman, MD

Does intraoperative neurophysiologic monitoring matter in noncomplex spine surgeries?

Ney JP, van der Goes DN, Nuwer MR (Univ of Washington, Seattle; Univ of New Mexico, Albuquerque; Univ of California, Los Angeles)
Neurology 85:2151-2158, 2015

Objectives.—To determine associations between intraoperative neurophysiologic monitoring (IOM) for spinal decompressions and simple fusions with neurologic complications, length of stay, and hospitalization charges.

Methods.—Adult discharges in the Nationwide/National Inpatient Sample (NIS) (2007–2012) with spinal decompressions and simple spinal fusions were included. Revision surgeries, instrumentations, complicated approaches, and tumor- and trauma-related surgeries were excluded. Extracted data included patient demographics, medical comorbidities, primary spinal surgery type, and hospital characteristics. Bivariate and multiple regression analyses using NIS survey design variables correlated IOM use with neurologic complications, hospital charges, and length of stay.

Results.—IOM was reported in 4.9% of an estimated 1.1 million discharges in the weighted sample. Discharges reporting IOM were more often privately insured (61% vs 57%, $p < 0.001$) and had slightly more comorbidities (25% vs 24% with 3+ comorbidities, $p = 0.01$). Spinal fusions more often reported IOM than decompressions. The IOM group had fewer neurologic complications (0.8% vs 1.4% of controls) with no difference in length of stay (3.0 days for each group), but increased hospital charges (39% greater). Multiple regression adjustment showed significant associations of IOM with fewer neurologic complications (odds ratio 0.60, 95% confidence interval [CI] 0.47, 0.76, $p < 0.001$), while the estimated percentage of hospital charges was sizably diminished from the unadjusted analysis (IOM effect +9%, 95% CI +4%, +13%, $p < 0.001$), and length of stay was reduced (IOM effect −0.26 days, 95% CI −0.42, −0.11, $p < 0.001$).

Conclusions.—IOM was associated with better clinical outcomes and some increased hospital charges among discharges of simple spinal fusions and laminectomies in a large, multiyear, nationally representative dataset.

▶ Ney et al. have abstracted a very large sample size (1.1 million discharges from 2007 to 2012) from the Nationwide Inpatient Survey administrative database to yield the power to detect real differences in clinical and cost-associated outcomes (total cost and LOS) following "low-risk" spinal surgeries that mainly included laminectomy and uninstrumented anterior cervical fusion procedures, in which intraoperative monitoring (IOM) was used or not used. Although this article is clearly written from the perspective a true believer in the benefit of IOM, the empirical data support the cause. Neurological complications, which occur in about 1% of all types of spinal surgeries,[1-3] were reported to have occurred almost 50% less commonly in the 4.9% cases that were monitored versus those case in which unmonitored (0.8% vs 1.4%; $P < .001$). Use of IOM was associated with a front-end 9% adjusted increased cost per hospitalization; however, this statistic fails to factor in the health care and societal cost savings inherent to preventing this dreaded complication. Oddly, because the rate of neurological complication was so low after anterior cervical fusion surgery (<0.2%), this surgery type was the only that showed no benefit with IOM use, yet it is a simple surgery compared with IOM, and its use is more commonly accepted. Conversely, simple laminectomy in which the routine use of IOM is generally less common, showed the greatest clinical benefit, significantly reducing the reported neurological complication rate from 2.7% to 1.7%. Although the use of such a high sample size all but guarantees the identification of statistically significant findings, the magnitude of the differences were clinically relevant. Summarizing this relevance is the determination that a neurological complication is averted in every 167 cases that are monitored as opposed to being unmonitored. Although the granularity of data abstracted from administrative databases prevents clear understanding of this burden of disease because the magnitude of neurological injury nor its transience cannot be determined, these data, along with the large observational studies that consistently demonstrate a rare but real risk of neurological injury associated with complex and simple spine surgery, provide foundational support for the concept. Although the rarity of these events may make prospective confirmation of these findings cost-prohibitive, there does appear to be sufficient information presented in this study to defend its current use. Based on these data, at a minimum, selection of IOM should be an option left to surgeons so that they may do all they can to fulfill their primum *nocere* promise to their patients.

B. Freedman, MD

References

1. Williams BJ, Smith JS, Saulle D, et al. Complications associated with surgical treatment of traumatic spinal fractures: a review of the scoliosis research society morbidity and mortality database. *World Neurosurg*. 2014;81:818-824.
2. Reames D, Smith JS, Fu KM, et al. Scoliosis Research Society Morbidity and Mortality Committee. Complications in the surgical treatment of 19,360 cases of pediatric scoliosis: a review of the Scoliosis Research Society Morbidity and Mortality database. *Spine (Phila Pa 1976)*. 2011;36:1484-1491.
3. Cramer DE, Maher PC, Pettigrew DB, Kuntz C 4th. Major neurologic deficit immediately after adult spinal surgery: incidence and etiology over 10 years at a single training institution. *J Spinal Disord Tech*. 2009;22:565-570.

Early Secondary Neurologic Deterioration After Blunt Spinal Trauma: A Review of the Literature

Oto B, Corey DJ II, Oswald J, et al (Univ of New England, Portland, ME; Northeastern Univ, Boston, MA; Ambulance Victoria, Australia; et al)
Acad Emerg Med 22:1200-1212, 2015

Objectives.—The objectives were to review published reports of secondary neurologic deterioration in the early stages of care after blunt spinal trauma and describe its nature, context, and associated risk factors.

Methods.—The authors searched the MEDLINE, EMBASE, and CINAHL databases for English-language studies. Cases were included meeting the criteria age 16 years or older, nonpenetrating trauma, and experiencing neurologic deterioration during prehospital or emergency department (ED) care prior to definitive management (e.g., discharge, spinal clearance by computed tomography, admission to an inpatient service, or surgical intervention). Results were qualitatively analyzed for characteristics and themes.

Results.—Forty-one qualifying cases were identified from 12 papers. In 30 cases, the new deficits were apparently spontaneous and were not detected until routine reassessment. In 12 cases the authors did attribute deterioration to temporally associated precipitants, seven of which were possibly iatrogenic; these included removal of a cervical collar, placement of a halo device, patient agitation, performance of flexion/extension films, "unintentional manipulation," falling in or near the ED, and forced collar application in patients with ankylosing spondylitis. Thirteen cases occurred during prehospital care, none of them sudden and movement-provoked, and all reported by a single study.

Conclusions.—Published reports of early secondary neurologic deterioration after blunt spinal trauma are exceptionally rare and generally poorly documented. High-risk features may include altered mental status and ankylosing spondylitis. It is unclear how often events are linked with spontaneous patient movement and whether such events are preventable.

▶ Oto et al have added an interesting bit of knowledge to the medical literature, with their structured literature review of all identified cases of secondary neurological decline in patients sustaining blunt injury to any aspect of the spinal column. Although I think their work is a worthwhile read for its novelty and clinical import, their math and/or attention to detail is sometimes lacking in their reporting of results. For case inclusion, the deterioration (from normal to some degree of deficit or from an incomplete deficit to a more severe one) had to occur in the time between which the patient received prehospital care through the time in which the definitive spinal treatment was performed. The purpose of this work was to assess whether the anecdotal concern for patients under medical care of emergency providers are at risk of new or worsened neurological deficits related to care received. They were able to identify only 41 cases in the published literature from 12 papers. One-third of deteriorations occurred before reaching the emergency department. Two-thirds of deteriorations were unwitnessed, not directly attributable to a specific treatment event but rather detected on serial examination. Thirty-two percent were intact before decline, and 34% each had incomplete deficits or insufficient documentation to determine baseline neurological status. About half of the declines that were felt to be temporally related to a precipitating factor were considered iatrogenic. Alternatively, <17% of secondary neurological injury was considered iatrogenic. Neurological decline in spine-injured patients under medical supervision is extremely rare. Ankylosing spondylitis and altered mental status seem to be the only identifiable risk factors for this rare event.

B. Freedman, MD

Provider volume and short-term outcomes following surgery for spinal metastases

De la Garza-Ramos R, Abt NB, Kerezoudis P, et al (Johns Hopkins Univ School of Medicine, Baltimore, MD; Mayo Clinic, Rochester, MN)

J Clin Neurosci 24:43-46, 2016

This study aimed to analyze the impact of surgeon and hospital volume on short-term outcomes following surgery for spinal metastases. Data from the Nationwide Inpatient Sample (NIS; 2003–2009) were extracted. Patients who underwent decompression and/or fusion for metastatic spinal tumors were identified via *International Classification of Diseases, Ninth Revision* codes. Surgeon and hospital volume were evaluated as a continuous variable. Multivariable logistic regression analyses were performed to calculate the adjusted odds ratios (OR) of in-hospital mortality, post-operative complication development, non-routine discharges, prolonged length of stay, and high hospital charges with increasing surgeon and hospital volume. In total 3,069 admissions were examined. The overall in-hospital mortality rate was 4.4% and in-hospital complication rate 29.7%; non-routine discharges occurred in 63.3% of patients. Increasing provider volume was not associated with lower odds of in-hospital mortality. However, increasing surgeon volume was associated with significantly lower odds of developing an in-hospital complication (OR 0.70; 95% confidence interval [CI], 0.58–0.85) and having a non-routine discharge (OR 0.76; 95% CI, 0.66–0.87). Increasing hospital volume was not associated with lower odds of developing a post-operative complication (OR 1.17; 95% CI, 1.00–1.37), but was associated with lower odds of having a non-routine discharge (OR 0.83; 95% CI, 0.73–0.95). Patients operated on by higher volume surgeons were less likely to have a prolonged length of stay (over 14 days); higher hospital volume was associated with increased odds of high hospital charges (over $295,511 USD). In this study utilizing the NIS administrative database, patients with metastatic spinal tumors treated by higher volume surgeons had significantly lower complication rates, were more likely to be discharged home following surgery, and were less likely to have a prolonged length of stay. Increasing hospital volume was associated with lower non-routine discharge rates, but with higher hospital charges. Better outcomes with higher volume surgeons may be a reflection of patient selection, and further research is needed to corroborate our findings.

▶ De la Garza Ramos et al. have reviewed the Nationwide Inpatient Sample (NIS) between 2003 and 2009, to identify 3069 patients who underwent spine surgery for spinal metastasis (average age 60 years old; on average, each had 5.5 medical comorbidities). Analysis of this large sample demonstrated what has been demonstrated for just about all complex surgical procedures, which is surgeons and hospitals with greater experience (measured in case volume) have better clinical outcomes. This is known as the volume-outcome relationship (VOR). In surgery (decompression and/or fusion) for spinal metastasis, high-volume surgeons have lower complications (average 30% reduction), shorter length of stay, and are more likely to discharge the patient to home. Conversely, when it comes to being identified a high-volume hospital for the treatment of spinal metastasis, experience breeds more efficient disposition (i.e., more likely to discharge home), but it also breeds (tertiary) referral of complicated patients who more frequently go on to consume the most health care dollars. Lastly, spine surgery for metastatic disease is fraught with adversity, with an overall 4.4% inpatient mortality and 30% complication rate, regardless of surgeon and hospital experience. Given our population is aging, spinal metastasis complicates 5% to 14% of all cancer cases, and health care dollars especially for government-insured patients are becoming evermore scarce, as a health care system we need to evaluate the most efficient and effective strategy for dealing with this disease.

B. Freedman, MD

A Systematic Review of Lumbar Fusion Rates With and Without the Use of rhBMP-2

Galimberti F, Lubelski D, Healy AT, et al (Cleveland Clinic Lerner College of Medicine, OH; Cleveland Clinic, OH; et al)
Spine 40:1132-1139, 2015

Study Design.—Systematic review.

Objective.—To evaluate literature comparing fusion rates in anterior lumbar interbody fusion (ALIF), posterior lumbar interbody/transforaminal lumbar interbody fusion (PLIF/TLIF), and posterolateral lumbar fusion (PLF) with and without recombinant human bone morphogenetic protein-2 (rhBMP-2).

Summary of Background Data.—rhBMP-2 is used for the FDA approved indication of single-level ALIF with LT-Cage and off-label for PLIF/TLIF, and PLF. Due to recent controversies, it is essential to evaluate the literature for its effects on fusion rates to evaluate whether benefits outweigh potential complications.

Methods.—A Medline search was performed of clinical studies published between May 2000 and May 2012 comparing fusion rates after ALIF, PLIF/TLIF, and PLF surgery with versus without rhBMP-2. Only studies with a control arm were reviewed.

Results.—16 studies were reviewed (1794 patients, 995 treated with rhBMP-2 and 799 without). 5 of 5 studies for PLIF/TLIF (including 301 of 301 patients), 1 of 4 for ALIF (including 279 of 589 patients), and 3 of 7 for PLF (including 272 of 904 patients) reported no significant improvement in fusion rates with rhBMP-2 compared with those without rhBMP-2 at longest follow-up investigated. Average fusion rate 24 months after surgery was 97.8% for ALIF (n = 316), 95.7% for PLIF/TLIF (n = 141), and 93.6% for PLF (n = 422) with rhBMP-2 and 88.2% (n = 228), 89.5% (n = 86), and 83.1% (n = 372) without rhBMP-2, for ALIF, PLIF/TLIF, and PLF, respectively. Odds ratio of fusion were calculated as 7.08 (95% CI: 1.54–32.7) in ALIF, 1.98 (95% CI: 0.39–10.1) in PLIF/TLIF, and 3.06 (95% CI: 1.61–5.80) in PLF with rhBMP-2 as compared with without rhBMP-2.

Conclusion.—Although numerous studies did not show statistically significant improvement in fusion rates with rhBMP-2 use, analysis of combined studies revealed significant improvement in fusion rate with rhBMP-2 in ALIF and PLF patients. Notably, even when pooling data from several studies, rhBMP-2 did not result in statistically significantly improved fusion rates in PLIF/TLIF. However, heterogeneity of rhBMP-2 dosing, surgical techniques, and quality of papers reviewed may limit the validity of conclusions drawn.

Level of Evidence.—4.

▶ Galimberti et al (Cleveland Clinic group) present a review of the literature regarding the fusion rate with and without bone morphogenetic protein (BMP) in on-label (anterior lumbar interbody fusion [ALIF] in LT cage or perimeter cage) and mostly off-label use. The primary intention of BMP (specifically BMP-2, commercially marketed at InFuse, Medtronic, Inc) is to serve as a bone graft substitute in support of fusion, so the primary outcome should come from this perspective.

This study took on the challenge of reviewing the published literature to date to specifically define the effect of BMP on fusion rate. Key lessons learned from this review of 16 clinical studies reporting the outcomes for 1794 patients was that although essentially all studies showed a trend toward higher fusion rates with BMP, only 6 of 15 studies found the difference to be significant, but when the results are pooled across procedure (broken down into ALIF [single-level], posterior lumbar interbody/transforaminal lumbar interbody fusion [PLIF/TLIF], or PSF), the trends are clearly significant for ALIF and PSF with odds ratios showing an average 2 to 7 times fusion advantage with BMP use in PSF and ALIF, respectively. In the 5 studies that reported on BMP use with PLIF/TLIF, which contained 301 total patients, 0 of 5 showed a significant difference within the study and pooling results also showed no significant difference. Of note, the PLIF/TLIF articles have the lowest level of evidence (1 randomized controlled trial, 1 prospective study, and 3 retrospective studies). Sixty percent of the retrospective studies in this review were from this procedural cohort. The single study that looked at multilevel PLIF/TLIF fusion found a statistically significant difference in fusion rate.

With regard to the PSF group, it is important to note that the largest studies used substantially higher doses of BMP per level (40 mg vs 4.3-12 mg in the ALIF and PLIF/TLIF cohorts). It was the results of these studies and a US Food and Drug Administration review for a new indicated use of BMP in posterior lumbar spinal fusion surgery that generated concern for BMP carcinogenicity because there was a trend toward higher incidence of newly diagnosed cancer in the BMP-treated cohort. These were older patients, the distribution of new cancers identified essentially mirrored Surveillance, Epidemiology, and End Results data, and 1 cancer was a pancreatic cancer that was diagnosed at high grade shortly after spinal fusion surgery. This work prompted the YODA analyses, which included the review of case report forms for all industry-sponsored clinical trials using BMP.

In demonstration of the ambiguity of the data surrounding BMP adverse events and their interpretation, 2 respected research groups from 2 sides of the planet reviewed the same base data and came up with 2 different opinions on whether BMP posed a significant cancer risk.[1,2] More productively, the YODA studies drew attention to other complications that are now well-established BMP-related adverse events that had hitherto been underreported in the primary publications for the industry-sponsored trials.[1-3] The failure to report these complications in the initial articles has come under scrutiny of late. Although we still have things to learn about the risk profile of BMP in spinal fusion surgery, this article helps confirm in an apparently nonbiased fashion that there appears to be at a minimum a fusion advantage of BMP over autogenous bone graft in lumbar fusion surgery. This advantage, which was also noted by Simmonds et al (increased fusion rate 12%; confidence interval 2%-23%), was demonstrated reviewing mostly single-level fusion surgery trials; thus, it can be extrapolated, and the studies that included multiple levels showed, that in the more challenging situation of multilevel fusion, where the limitations of the total volume of harvestable iliac crest bone graft are real, BMP would demonstrate a definite fusion advantage over autogenous bone graft.[2]

Lastly, although I appreciate the authors' opinion regarding the use of BMP in PLIF/TLIF stated in their conclusion paragraph, as they have pointed out, the existing data on which they based this conclusion is low-quality and heterogeneous. As such, this incomplete data set does not support a conclusion one way or the other about the fusion advantage of BMP in PLIF/TLIF procedures, especially in multilevel cases. Rather, it most strongly supports the need for continued clinical research on the topic. On the basis of currently available data, use of BMP as a bone graft substitute demands an informed counseling process that discusses and weighs demonstrated risks and benefits of this technique over more traditional bone graft sources.

B. Freedman, MD

References

1. Fu R, Selph S, McDonagh M, et al. Effectiveness and harms of recombinant human bone morphogenetic protein-2 in spine fusion: a systematic review and meta-analysis. *Ann Intern Med.* 2013;158:890-902.
2. Simmonds MC, Brown JV, Heirs MK, et al. Safety and effectiveness of recombinant human bone morphogenetic protein-2 for spinal fusion: a meta-analysis of individual-participant data. *Ann Intern Med.* 2013;158:877-889.
3. Rodgers MA, Brown JV, Heirs MK, et al. Reporting of industry funded study outcome data: comparison of confidential and published data on the safety and effectiveness of rhBMP-2 for spinal fusion. *BMJ.* 2013;346:f3981.

Epidural Corticosteroid Injections for Radiculopathy and Spinal Stenosis: A Systematic Review and Meta-analysis

Chou R, Hashimoto R, Friedly J, et al (Oregon Health & Science Univ, Portland; Spectrum Res, Tacoma, WA; Univ of Washington, Seattle; et al)
Ann Intern Med 163:373-381, 2015

Background.—Use of epidural corticosteroid injections is increasing.

Purpose.—To review evidence on the benefits and harms of epidural corticosteroid injections in adults with radicular low back pain or spinal stenosis of any duration.

Data Sources.—Ovid MEDLINE (through May 2015), Cochrane Central Register of Controlled Trials, Cochrane Database of Systematic Reviews, prior systematic reviews, and reference lists.

Study Selection.—Randomized trials of epidural corticosteroid injections versus placebo interventions, or that compared epidural injection techniques, corticosteroids, or doses.

Data Extraction.—Dual extraction and quality assessment of individual studies, which were used to determine the overall strength of evidence (SOE).

Data Synthesis.—30 placebo-controlled trials evaluated epidural corticosteroid injections for radiculopathy, and 8 trials were done for spinal stenosis. For radiculopathy, epidural corticosteroids were associated with greater immediate-term reduction in pain (weighted mean difference on a scale of 0 to 100, −7.55 [95% CI, −11.4 to −3.74]; SOE, moderate), function (standardized mean difference after exclusion of an outlier trial, −0.33 [CI, −0.56 to −0.09]; SOE, low), and short-term surgery risk (relative risk, 0.62 [CI, 0.41 to 0.92]; SOE, low). Effects were below predefined minimum clinically important difference thresholds, and there were no longer-term benefits. Limited evidence showed no clear effects of technical factors, patient characteristics, or comparator interventions on estimates. There were no clear effects of epidural corticosteroid injections for spinal stenosis (SOE, low to moderate). Serious harms were rare, but harms reporting was suboptimal (SOE, low).

Limitations.—The review was restricted to English-language studies. Some meta-analyses were based on small numbers of trials (particularly for spinal stenosis), and most trials had methodological shortcomings.

Conclusion.—Epidural corticosteroid injections for radiculopathy were associated with immediate reductions in pain and function. However, benefits were small and not sustained, and there was no effect on long-term surgery risk. Limited evidence suggested no effectiveness for spinal stenosis.

▶ Chou et al, with funding from Agency for Healthcare Research and Quality at the request of the Centers for Medicare & Medicaid Services, have performed a systematic review of the available literature from randomized clinical trials to determine whether there is evidence to support a clinical benefit for epidural steroid injection (ESI), by any method, including intralaminar, transforaminal, and caudal, with or without radio-guidance, in the treatment of radiculopathy, sciatica, and/or symptoms related to spinal stenosis. Fifty-nine trials that included randomized comparison between epidural steroid and placebo, local anesthetic alone, and/or another steroid were selected for review. Five of 59 (8%) were rated as good quality trials, and 24% were poor quality; the remainder were fair, exposing conclusions from this analysis to the bad-in, bad-out phenomenon. The only statistically significant benefits across all time points (out to >1 year follow-up) were detected in the immediate term (5 days—less than 2 weeks), and none of these differences reached minimal clinically important differences (15 points on 100-point pain scale, 10-point Oswestry Low Back Pain Disability Index change, 3 point Roland—Morris Disability Questionnaire [RDQ] change). On average epidural corticosteroid injections (ESIs) provided a 7.6-point reduction in pain score in the first 2 weeks after injections performed for radiculopathy in 30 trials where radiculopathy was the primary disease state. As a result of these immediate effects, ESIs did significantly reduce the conversion to surgical decompression on average by 38% in the 3-month period after injection, but this ability to prevent surgery did not persist at longer durations. The literature was even more sparse for ESI use in spinal stenosis, in which there was only 1 good quality study (n = 386). This showed a statistically, but not clinically, significant improvement in RDQ (1.8-point reduction on 24-point scale) at 3 weeks, which was lost by 6 weeks.

There was significant heterogeneity between studies included in this systematic review, and this effects the summary statistics regardless of pooling methods. This cannot be discounted, nor should the immediate beneficial effect for this intervention, which carries almost no risk for serious harm, be dismissed. Ameliorating disabling symptoms and/or expediting the resolution of a neurological condition that results in substantial time off from work and diminished quality of life has benefit to society and the patient. Also overlooked in this study's utilitarian assessment of the impact ESIs have on patients, is the diagnostic effect they provide. Although nonoperative care, including injections, to treat an episode of radiculopathy or sciatica will be successful in upward of 50% of patients, those who fail to receive a durable therapeutic effect can benefit from the diagnostic information gleaned during the immediate response to the injection. Patients who receive excellent but nonlasting pain relief from an injection placed in the area of neurological compression related to a disc herniation, and less reliably, degenerative spinal stenosis, will often respond favorably and in a more lasting fashion to surgical decompression. The utility of optimizing treatment for a physically debilitating condition that most commonly affects working-age adults cannot be accurately distilled to a signal metric. Research to date consistently fails to evaluate the totality of effect treatment has on a problem of this magnitude.

B. Freedman, MD

Conus Medullaris Level in Vertebral Columns With Lumbosacral Transitional Vertebra

Kershenovich A, Macias OM, Syed F, et al (Geisinger Health System, Danville, PA; ISSSTE, Mexico; et al)

Neurosurgery 78:62-70, 2016

Background.—The estimated prevalence of lumbar or sacral transitional vertebrae (LSTV) in the population is 4% to 30%. Few small patient series have studied the normal level of the conus medullaris (CM) in individuals with LSTV.

Objective.—To determine, by using a large cohort of patients, whether individuals of all ages with LSTV have different CM positions in the spinal canal in comparison with the rest of the population with normal vertebral columns.

Methods.—We performed an institutional retrospective analysis of spinal magnetic resonance images on individuals with LSTV of all ages, sexes, and pathologies during a 10-year period. Fifty-seven percent of patients (n = 467) had a lumbarized vertebra and 43% had sacralized vertebra (n = 355). Mean age at the time of the study was 55 ± 19 years (range 1-97 years). Fifty-two percent were male and 48% were female. Sixty percent of subjects with a sacralized vertebra were female, and 54.5% of those with a lumbarized vertebra were male ($P = .001$).

Results.—The CM in individuals with a lumbarized vertebra was seen to be lower at L1-2 to L2s, than un those with a sacralized vertebra where most conuses were at T12-L1 to L1s ($P \leq 0.001$). The CM level was similarly distributed among sexes and ages.

Conclusion.—In our series, the CM level, when lumbarization occurred, was lower, with a mean level at L1-L2, whereas a more superior mean level at T12-L1 was seen when sacralization occurred. CM level was not influenced by sex, age, or pathology other than tethered cords.

▶ Transitional lumbosacral anatomy is an interesting phenomenon, which is more common than we expect, with a reported prevalence of 4% to 30%. Kershenovich et al. reviewed MRI scans of the lumbar spine for consecutive patients (n = 821) identified as having transitional lumbosacral anatomy over a 10-year period at their single institution to detect the impact this has on the level of the conus medullaris. Transitional anatomy was relatively evenly distributed between the sexes and between lumbarization (57%) and sacralization (43%). Men more commonly had a lumbarized S1, whereas females more commonly had a sacralized L5. The defining characteristic for a lumbarized vertebra is a rectangular shape versus that of a parallelogram for sacralized vertebrae. Among the entire cohort, 4.6% had a low-lying conus (below the L2 level), but only 13% of these had a tethered cord syndrome. The take-home message is that when lumbarization is seen, the conus tends to be located lower in the spinal canal, at the L1-L2 level, whereas when sacralization is present, the conus tends to be higher at the T12-L1 level.

B. Freedman, MD

7 Total Hip Arthroplasty

Introduction

The main themes that run through the literature regarding hip replacement have not changed much. The issue of metal on metal bearings continues to be investigated both from a clinical efficacy perspective as well as investigations into the potential for adverse reactions. In the near future, emphasis on clinical efficacy will lessen somewhat since the use has progressively been abandoned. However, the information regarding adverse reaction will continue for some time. We have also relied on systemic literature reviews and national registry data base studies to address several of the more relevant and ongoing questions regarding hip replacement surgery. This section was difficult to develop due to the large number of really good papers from which to select.

Bernard F. Morrey, MD

High Rates of Interest in Sex in Patients With Hip Arthritis

Lavernia CJ, Villa JM (The Ctr for Advanced Orthopedics at Larkin Hosp, South Miami, FL)
Clin Orthop Relat Res 474:293-299, 2016

Background.—Being sexually active has been associated with a high quality of life. Unfortunately, the topic of sexual limitations in patients undergoing total hip arthroplasty (THA) has not been well studied.

Question/Purposes.—(1) What proportion of patients experience sexual limitations because of hip arthritis before THA; (2) whether patient reports of sexual limitations would be associated with poorer results on general health and hip-specific instruments; and (3) whether patient reports of sexual limitations would be associated with poorer preoperative range of motion.

Methods.—Between May 19, 2003, and August 17, 2009, 403 patients (423 hips) underwent primary THA; of those, 237 patients/hips (59% [237 of 403]) had addressed the new patient questionnaire within 1 year before surgery and had it available for review; and of those, 192 (48% [192 of 403]) had answered the question about sexual function on their questionnaire. This group included 159 patients who were sexually active (82% [159 of 192]). These patients were defined as our study cohort. Among them, 131 patients (82% [131 of 159]) reported some degree of sexual limitations and 28 patients (18% [28 of 159]) did not report limitations. Patient characteristics evaluated included baseline demographics, body mass index, American Society of Anesthesiologists, Charlson in addition to preoperative/postoperative pain intensity/frequency (visual analog scale, 0–10), SF-36, WOMAC, and baseline hip range of motion measures. Outcomes of interest were compared between both groups. Mean age was 65 years. Chi-square, t-tests, and multivariate analysis of variance were used. Alpha was set at 0.05.

Results.—Hip arthritis interfered with the sexual life of 82% (131 of 159) of sexually active patients, more so in women than men (96% [68 of 71], versus 72% [63 of 88]; odds ratio, 8.99; 95% confidence interval, 2.588–31.258; $p = 0.001$). Preoperatively, patients with sexual limitations had a mean pain intensity of 8 ± 1.84 points on the visual analog scale, whereas patients without limitations had 6 ± 1.99 points ($p < 0.001$). Differences were also found in WOMAC pain (11 ± 3.9 versus 8 ± 3.5; $p = 0.004$) and WOMAC stiffness (3.4 ± 2.3 versus 1.4 ± 1.7; $p = 0.001$). Baseline hip flexion (84° ± 22.4° versus 93° ± 16.5°, respectively; $p = 0.04$) and external rotation (23° ± 14.5° versus 30° ± 11.6°; $p = 0.02$) were also different.

Conclusions.—Our data suggest that many patients getting a hip arthroplasty are sexually active but most patients who are sexually active have sexual limitations before surgery as a result of hip arthritis. Women are more affected than men. Patients with these limitations experience more pain and have less flexion and external rotation before surgery. Preoperatively, counseling on sexual activities should be routinely discussed with all patients undergoing THA.

Level of Evidence.—Level III, prognostic study.

▶ It is of course impossible to see this title without assessing it for suitability in the YEAR BOOK. It reminded me of an interaction with a female patient when I was a resident, and my mentor, Dr Mark Coventry, point-blank asked the patient, who was being considered for hip replacement, "What about sex?" I remember the answer: "It's a problem." So now we have a little science applied to the issue. It is not surprising that loss of flexion and external rotation are associated with discomfort with sexual activity. The important point, which frankly I never quite incorporated into my interview, is that it is reasonable to inquire regarding this considerable functional deficiency. I'm not sure it is the ultimate discriminator of whether to offer replacement, but it is certainly useful to appreciate this "quiet" implication of our intervention.

B. F. Morrey, MD

Association between changes in global femoral offset after total hip arthroplasty and function, quality of life, and abductor muscle strength: a prospective cohort study of 222 patients

Mahmood SS, Mukka SS, Crnalic S, et al (Umeå Univ, Sweden; et al)

Acta Orthop 87:36-41, 2016

Background and Purpose.—There is no consensus on the association between global femoral offset (FO) and outcome after total hip arthroplasty (THA). We assessed the association between FO and patients' reported hip function, quality of life, and abductor muscle strength.

Patients and Methods.—We included 250 patients with unilateral hip osteoarthritis who underwent a THA. Before the operation, the patient's reported hip function was evaluated with the Western Ontario and McMaster Universities Osteoarthritis (WOMAC) index and quality of life was evaluated with EQ-5D. At 1-year follow-up, the same scores and also hip abductor muscle strength were measured. 222 patients were available for follow-up. These patients were divided into 3 groups according to the postoperative global FO of the operated hip compared to the contralateral hip, as measured on plain radiographs: the decreased FO group (more than 5 mm reduction), the restored FO group (within 5 mm restoration), and the increased FO group (more than 5 mm increment).

Results.—All 3 groups improved ($p < 0.001$). The crude results showed that the decreased FO group had a worse WOMAC index, less abductor muscle strength, and more use of walking aids. When we adjusted these results with possible confounding factors, only global FO reduction was statistically significantly associated with reduced abductor muscle strength. The incidence of residual hip pain and analgesics use was similar in the 3 groups.

Interpretation.—A reduction in global FO of more than 5 mm after THA appears to have a negative association with abductor muscle strength of the operated hip, and should therefore be avoided.

▶ This is an interesting study that addresses a commonly discussed issue in hip replacement surgery. There is no question that femoral offset is an important variable for at least 2 reasons, which are probably related: hip abductor strength and stability. The value of this study is that in a prospective model with specific objective outcome parameters, the threshold of inadequate offset is quantified. To know that decreasing the nominal offset by more than 5 mm is associated with measurable weakness is an important finding that is useful in the clinical setting.

B. F. Morrey, MD

Hemiarthroplasty *versus* internal fixation for displaced intracapsular fractures of the hip in elderly men: a pilot randomised trial

Parker MJ (Peterborough City Hosp, UK)
Bone Joint J 97-B:992-996, 2015

A total of 56 male patients with a displaced intracapsular fracture of the hip and a mean age of 81 years (62 to 94), were randomised to be treated with either a cemented hemiarthroplasty (the Exeter Trauma Stem) or reduction and internal fixation using the Targon Femoral Plate. All surviving patients were reviewed one year after the injury, at which time restoration of function and pain in the hip was assessed. There was no statistically significant difference in mortality between the two groups (7/26; 26.9% for hemiarthroplasty *vs* 10/30; 33.3% for internal fixation). No patient treated with a hemiarthroplasty required further surgery, but eight patients treated by internal fixation did ($p = 0.005$), five requiring hemiarthroplasty and three requiring total hip arthroplasty. Those treated by internal fixation had significantly more pain ($p = 0.02$). The restoration of mobility and independence were similar in the two groups.

These results indicate that cemented hemiarthroplasty gives better results than internal fixation in elderly men with a displaced intracapsular fracture of the hip (Table 3).

▶ Despite the volume of literature on the topic, there is still lack of consensus in the orthopedic community regarding the best management of the patient with a displaced femoral neck fracture. There shouldn't be. This study, although rather limited in numbers, did randomize the patients into either open reduction internal fixation (ORIF) or cemented monoblock hemireplacement. The study is a

TABLE 3.—Operative Details and Post-operative Complications by Implant

	Hemiarthroplasty	Internal Fixation	*p*-Value
Mean operating time (mins) (SD)	53.3 (19.2)	36.7 (16.9)	0.001
Number of patients transfused (n, %)	2 *(7.7)*	0	0.2
Pneumonia (n, %)	1 *(3.8)*	0	0.5
Atrial fibrillation (n, %)	0	1 *(3.3)*	1.0
Myocardial infarction	0	1	1.0
Acute renal injury (n, %)	1 *(3.8)*	0	0.5
Urinary retention (n, %)	5 *(19.2)*	2 *(6.7)*	0.2
Deep vein thrombosis (n, %)	1 *(3.8)*	0	0.5
Pressure sores (n, %)	1 *(3.8)*	0	0.5
Re-operations (n, %)	0 *(0.0)*	8 *(26.7)*	0.005
Mean hospital stay (days) (SD)	24.2 *(22.5)*	15.9 *(12.1)*	0.09
Mean total hospital stay (days) (SD)	25.1 (23.8)	19.4 (18.2)	0.3
Mortality 30 days (n, %)	1 *(3.8)*	3 *(10.0)*	0.6
Mortality one year (n, %)	7 *(26.9)*	10 *(33.3)*	0.8

SD, standard deviation.

single center, so confounding variables regarding technique and postoperative care are standardized. The key is the statistically fewer reoperations in the hemireplacement. I was surprised to see the operative time so much shorter for the ORIF patient. The cultural difference in management is noted with the length of stay being several weeks (Table 3).

The bottom line is that there should no longer be any uncertainty regarding this question.

B. F. Morrey, MD

Cemented Bipolar Hemiarthroplasty Provides Definitive Treatment for Femoral Neck Fractures at 20 Years and Beyond

von Roth P, Abdel MP, Harmsen WS, et al (Charité Universitätsmedizin Berlin, Germany; Mayo Clinic, Rochester, MN)

Clin Orthop Relat Res 473:3595-3599, 2015

Background.—Displaced femoral neck fractures frequently are treated with bipolar hemiarthroplasties. Despite the frequency with which bipolar hemiarthroplasty is used to treat these fractures, there are few long-term data.

Questions/Purposes.—We sought to evaluate (1) the cumulative incidence of revision for any reason of bipolar hemiarthroplasties at 20 years, and the proportion of patients who lived more than 20 years who still have the prosthesis in situ from the index arthroplasty, (2) the cumulative incidence of aseptic loosening at 20 years, and (3) the Harris hip score of the surviving patients at long term.

Methods.—We performed 376 cemented bipolar hemiarthroplasties for displaced femoral neck fractures in 359 patients between 1976 and 1985. At a minimum of followup of 20 years (mean, 24 years; range, 20–31 years), 339 of 359 patients (94%) were deceased, leaving 20 patients in the study group. Of those, one patient was confirmed to be lost to followup and two others had radiographic followup only. Three hundred fifty-nine patients (99.2%) (376 of the original 379 hips) were followed until death, revision of the hemiarthroplasty, or for at least 20 years (of clinical followup). Bipolar hemiarthroplasty was performed for displaced femoral neck fractures. Cemented fixation was the standard of care between 1976 and 1985 at our institution. The mean age of the patients at the time of surgery was 79 years (range, 60–99 years). The cumulative incidence of revision, estimated with death as a competing risk, and radiographs were evaluated for signs of aseptic loosening by a surgeon not involved in the clinical care of the patients. Clinical function was evaluated with the Harris hip score. The mean age of the patients at the time of surgery was 79 years.

Results.—The 20-year cumulative incidence of revision for any reason was 3.5% (95% CI, 1.6%–5.3%). Of the 20 patients who survived more than 20 years, seven had the implant intact. The 20-year cumulative incidence of revision for aseptic loosening was 1.4% (95% CI, 0.2%–

2.6%). The mean Harris hip score in patients who were still living and patient who did not have revision surgery was 63 ± 22, however 13 of the 20 patients had undergone revision surgery.

Conclusions.—The long-term survivorship of bipolar hemiarthroplasty prostheses used to treat displaced femoral neck fractures in the elderly was high, and the procedure can be considered definitive for the majority of elderly patients with a femoral neck fracture. In this series, 6% (20 patients, 339 of 359) of the patients survived more than 20 years after treatment of a femoral neck fracture with a bipolar hemiarthroplasty. Of those, 35% (seven of 20) survived with their index prosthesis in situ.

Level of Evidence.—Level IV, therapeutic study.

▶ This is an attractive study because it asks a focused and important clinical question and answers it definitively. We had a discussion in the surgeons lounge just this week on this very topic, and the comment was made that there is no good study to direct our decision making. It would seem this report with a large sample with careful long-term surveillance would answer the question. Although a cemented bipolar implant may not be the only solution for a displaced femoral neck fracture in the older patient, it is a viable solution. The expectation on the part of the surgeon and patient is that it will not need to be revised in approximately 95% of cases.

B. F. Morrey, MD

CORR Insights®: Primary Ceramic-on-ceramic Total Hip Arthroplasty Using a 32-mm Ceramic Head with a Titanium-alloy Sleeve

D'Antonio JA (Greater Pittsburgh Orthopaedic Associates, Moon Township, PA)

Clin Orthop Relat Res 473:3788-3789, 2015

Background.—Ceramic-on-ceramic bearings are replacing conventional polyethylene in total hip arthroplasty (THA). These bearings offer the advantages of scratch resistance, a low coefficient of friction, less-reactive particulate debris, and superior wear resistance. Having higher-quality alumina ceramic bearings with greater burst strength mated with implants with excellent fixation records and high taper tolerances represents another improvement, but ceramic fracture, neck socket impingement, and squeaking remain concerns. Smaller-diameter femoral heads, malpositioned sockets, and trunnion debris and/or damage are associated with a higher risk of fracture. Implant position, design, and material properties can affect impingement and squeaking. Larger-diameter femoral heads have an increased risk of fretting corrosion and adverse local tissue responses (ALTRs). When retrieved from in vivo settings and during in vitro studies, there appears to be less fretting corrosion at the head-neck junction when ceramic rather than metal is used. Adding a titanium (Ti) sleeve has been proposed to diminish fracture risks from trunnion debris and/or damage. Metal sleeves, however, can contribute to fretting corrosion and ALTRs. A review of one investigation of ceramic heads with Ti sleeves and suggestions for improvement were offered.

Study Results.—A review by Lim and colleagues of alumina ceramic bearings with a Ti sleeve in the modular ceramic femoral head evaluated their performance for a minimum of 5 years. Most clinical studies of alumina ceramic bearings not protected by Ti sleeves have at least a 10-year follow-up. Comparison of the bearings included survivorship for revision for any reason, ceramic fracture, and the incidence of osteolysis. Lim and colleagues reported 97% survivorship for revision of any reason, which is comparable to the findings of other studies. The added Ti sleeve did not prevent fracture of the femoral head within 6 years of placement for 0.36% of the cases. The fracture risk has been estimated to be about 2%. Osteolysis also developed, which is uncommon in most other studies with a follow-up period of at least 10 years.

Recommendations.—This group of patients should be followed up for more than 10 years to determine if longer-term survivorship, fracture risk, and osteolysis incidence are sufficient to justify the addition of the Ti sleeve in the ceramic femoral head. Any retrievals of these implants should add important information about fretting corrosion as well.

Conclusions.—Improvements or even new materials may be developed to help minimize or eliminate the problems seen with alumina ceramic hips. Surgeons should also be careful to properly position implants and restore biomechanics to avoid fractures. Fracture risk is increased when there is edge loading, trunnion debris and/or damage, and ceramic components secured to either femoral or acetabular implants. Surgical assist devices to accurately position implants and restore biomechanics can also improve survivorship. Highly cross-linked polyethylene (HXLPE)–mounted metal and/or ceramic prostheses also offer lower wear and higher survivorship profiles.

▶ This review of the status of the 32-mm ceramic head remains relevant as the search for the ideal articulation for the young person continues. In addition to the concern about sqeeking and the requirement for precise acetabular placement, head fracture remains a major factor that has affected the acceptance of this solution. This review places the incidence of head fracture as considerably higher than the .02% quoted by the manufacturer. In fact, fracture may occur as frequently as 2%. The justified concern regarding the difficulty of managing the fractured head will continue to influence the acceptance of the ceramic head, at least in North America.

B. F. Morrey, MD

CORR Insights®: Otto Aufranc Award: Large Heads Do Not Increase Damage at the Head-neck Taper of Metal-on-polyethylene Total Hip Arthroplasties

Noble PC (Baylor College of Medicine, Houston, TX)
Clin Orthop Relat Res 474:339-341, 2016

Background.—Large femoral heads are associated with a lower risk of dislocation for total hip arthroplasties (THAs). However, metal-on-metal (MoM) THAs fail at a higher rate with larger head sizes—even greater than that of hip resurfacing cases using the same articulation design. The cause appears to be increased corrosion products produced in the modular head-neck junction area. Whether larger heads, specifically those larger than 32 mm, implanted with metal-on-polyethylene (MoP) articulations are associated with a higher risk for inflammatory reactions secondary to trunnion wear and corrosion remains a question and studies have returned divergent findings. A study was undertaken to determine the combination of implant materials, design features, and surgical practices that will eliminate tissue reactions at modular junctions without having a major impact on current procedures.

Study Results.—The study by Triantafyllopoulos and colleagues used data taken from a long-term retrieval collection. Authors examined 154 MoP components with six taper designs and head sizes ranging from 22 to 44 mm, 80% of which were 32 mm or smaller. Implantation period ranged from a few months to more than 20 years. The study revealed no association between fretting or corrosion of the head and trunion and differences in head size, although fretting and corrosion were common occurrences.

Analysis.—The wide range of components and conditions analyzed will likely include situations reflective of today's THA practices. However, the wide range also indicates how impossible it is to have large numbers of components of a single alloy composition and a single design of modular connection that have been followed up for 5 to 10 years.

Unfortunately, the conclusions related to components or materials no longer in service are not helpful to today's practitioners. In addition, the conclusions of the study assume that there are no clustering effects related to specific implant designs and head sizes for specific modes of fixation and types of patients. These issues should be addressed in future studies to determine if the conclusions can indeed be generalized to today's practice and what variables may alter the findings.

Additional issues must also be addressed in appropriate studies. These include whether head diameters similar to natural femoral head size are useful for MoP joints and will not jeopardize the modular junction; whether large heads increase the incidence of outlier results; whether highly wear-resistant polyethylenes alter the effect of head size on bearing friction; what effect various factors have on frictional forces; if ceramic or ceramicized heads will minimize problems; and whether head size makes it more difficult to assemble the modular junction in the body, especially with the small incisions used today.

Conclusions.—Researchers should ensure that all analyses of data from retrieval and registry sources include all the variables identified as having an influence on the fretting and corrosion of components. The conditions present at the joint above the modular junction also affect the loads and torques imposed on the trunnion-head interface and must be considered. Once all the variables have been either quantified or held constant, the number of cases evaluated must be sufficiently large to permit the drawing of valid conclusions that are relevant to future patients having THAs.

▶ The original article and this analysis represent the next generation of investigation and, hopefully, improvement in hip prosthetic design. The basis for the analysis is the increasing acceptance of the large prosthetic femoral head to improve stability. I would point out that increasing head diameter has a secondary effect on stability. That is, the impact is minimal if an anterior approach is used. Regardless, the larger heads will be used because the improvements in cross-linked polyethylene would seem to allow thinner liners without the previously described adverse effects of polyethylene less than 6 mm thick. The fact that larger heads do not create increased adverse debris generation at the trunnion is good to know. However, as we continue to drive toward an anatomic-sized head and as the polyethylene becomes thinner—beware.

B. F. Morrey, MD

CORR Insights®: Metal-on-conventional Total Hip Arthroplasty Bearing Surfaces Have a Higher Risk of Revision Than Metal-on-highly Crosslinked Polyethylene: Results From a US Registry

McCalden RW (Univ of Western Ontario, London, Canada)

Clin Orthop Relat Res 473:1449-1450, 2015

Background.—Conventional polyethylene has been largely replaced by highly cross-linked polyethylene (XLPE) for total hip arthroplasty (THA). Good evidence shows femoral head penetration, plus presumably polyethylene wear, and periprosthetic osteolysis are associated with XLPE used for THA, an improvement over conventional polyethylene. A clear reduction in revision rates related to XLPE in mid- or long-term follow-up has not yet been shown.

Current Evidence.—The clinical benefits of using XLPE rather than conventional polyethylene were revealed in an observational study of a large database of US patients. This effort focused on two specific implant designs and found that revision rates were significantly decreased for XLPE compared to conventional polyethylene. However, longer-term follow-up is needed to confirm these benefits. In addition, the effects of a range of variables on XLPE performance remain to be determined. These variables include surgical approach, surgeon experience, implant design, XLPE properties, femoral head size, and patient gender, race, and activity level.

Analysis.—To demonstrate long-term clinical benefits related to XLPE will require ongoing surveillance and reports of long-term results from current databases. In addition, national and/or large population-based registries, especially from North America, should be established that will include validated patient outcome scores, functional scores, and survivorship data. These new sources should be supplemented by the findings of ongoing randomized controlled trials (RCTs) comparing XLPE and conventional polyethylene.

Conclusions.—Currently it is unethical to begin new RCTs comparing XLPE and conventional polyethylene because the evidence in support of XLPE for THA strongly indicates it is the best choice. However, long-term follow-up, extending for 15 to 20 years or more, is needed, as are cross-sectional imaging (computed tomography scans) to quantify any periarticular osteolysis that develops, which is a precursor to implant failure.

▶ I feel there are a few points to be made with this review. Despite the widespread adoption of the highly cross-linked polyethylene cup, some intermediate-term studies show no definite advantage. The larger studies with longer surveillance clearly reveal the true advantage of this polyethylene. So the old adage holds: absence of evidence is not evidence of absence. The earlier, smaller studies were simply inadequate to demonstrate reality. It is also important to know that not all highly cross-linked polyethylenes are created equal. Hence, there is merit in reviewing the data on the specific brand when making a design selection.

B. F. Morrey, MD

Highly cross-linked polyethylene decreases the rate of revision of total hip arthroplasty compared with conventional polyethylene at 13 years' follow-up

Hanna SA, Somerville L, McCalden RW, et al (Univ of Western Ontario, London, Canada)

Bone Joint J 98-B:28-32, 2016

Aims.—The purpose of this study was to compare the long-term results of primary total hip arthroplasty (THA) in young patients using either a conventional (CPE) or a highly cross-linked (HXLPE) polyethylene liner in terms of functional outcome, incidence of osteolysis, radiological wear and rate of revision.

Methods.—We included all patients between the ages of 45 and 65 years who, between January 2000 and December 2001, had undergone a primary THA for osteoarthritis at our hospital using a CPE or HXLPE acetabular liner and a 28 mm cobalt-chrome femoral head.

From a total of 160 patients, 158 (177 hips) were available for review (CPE 89; XLPE 88). The mean age, body mass index (BMI) and follow-up in each group were: CPE: 56.8 years (46 to 65); 30.7 kg/m^2 (19 to 58); 13.2 years (2.1 to 14.7) and HXLPE: 55.6 years (45 to 65); BMI: 30 kg/m^2 (18 to 51); 13.1 years (5.7 to 14.4).

Results.—The mean Harris hip score (HHS) at final follow-up was 89.3 for the CPE group and 90.9 for the HXLPE group ($p = 0.078$). Osteolysis was present around 15 acetabular (17%) and 16 femoral (18%) components in the CPE hips compared with none (0%) in the HXLPE hips. The mean radiological linear wear of the CPE liners was 0.11 mm/year compared with 0.035 mm/year for the HXLPE liners ($p = 0.006$). The cumulative implant survival, with revision for polyethylene wear as the endpoint, was 86% (95% confidence interval 78 to 94) in the CPE group and 100% in the HXLPE group at 13 years (numbers at risk at 13 years - CPE: 65, XLPE: 61).

Discussion.—This study shows that HXLPE liners are associated with significantly less osteolysis and a lower rate of revision THA than CPE liners at long-term follow-up.

Take home message: The findings of this study highlight the clinical benefits of using HXLPE liners in THA and support the routine use of the material in order to improve implant longevity and to decrease the number of patients needing revision for aseptic osteolysis.

Low Wear Rates Seen in THAs With Highly Crosslinked Polyethylene at 9 to 14 Years in Patients Younger Than Age 50 Years

Garvin KL, White TC, Dusad A, et al (Univ of Nebraska Med Ctr, Omaha; et al)
Clin Orthop Relat Res 473:3829-3835, 2015

Background.—Patients 50 years or younger are at high risk for wear-related complications of their total hip arthroplasty (THA) because of their generally higher levels of activity. Highly crosslinked polyethylene (HXLPE) is believed to be more durable for this population than conventional polyethylene because of its improved wear; however, limited information is available on the wear of HXLPE in this population, particularly the wear of HXLPE when it articulates with alternative bearings like Oxinium (Smith & Nephew, Memphis, TN, USA).

Questions/Purposes.—The purpose of this study was to evaluate two questions relative to this population of patients undergoing THA. First, what was the linear and volumetric wear rate of HXLPE in patients 50 years or younger at a minimum followup of 9 years and was osteolysis observed in any of these hips? Given the potential for damage to the Oxinium femoral head surface, was the wear of HXLPE in the patients with this material similar to the other bearings or was there accelerated or runaway wear that was visible in any of the patients?

Methods.—From November 1999 to April 2005, 105 THAs were performed in 95 patients 50 years of age or younger (mean, 42 years;

range, 20–50 years). The mean body mass index was 30 kg/m^2 (range, 17–51 kg/m^2).The mean followup was 12 years (range, 9–14 years). Two patients died, five patients (one bilateral) were lost to followup, and one hip was revised elsewhere for pain. The patients' information was not included in the study, which left 87 patients with 96 hips for analysis. Highly crosslinked polyethylene was the acetabular bearing for all of the hips. We analyzed the linear and volumetric wear of all of the hips using the Martell method. Eighty hips had the same diameter head (28 mm) allowing us to more accurately compare the different bearing materials. The type of femoral head used was related to our sequential use of materials beginning with cobalt chrome (14), ceramic (23) followed by Oxinium (43) in the hips with 28-mm heads. Although cobalt-chrome was used early in this study, our previous experience with ceramic on polyethylene encouraged us to use it as an alternative bearing. The Oxinium was used consecutively for the remaining hips.

Results.—The mean wear of the HXLPE after 1 year of bedding-in (true linear wear) was 0.022 mm/year (95% confidence interval [CI], 0.015–0.030 mm/year). The mean volumetric wear of HXLPE after 1 year of bedding-in (true volumetric wear) was 9 mm^3/year (95% CI,

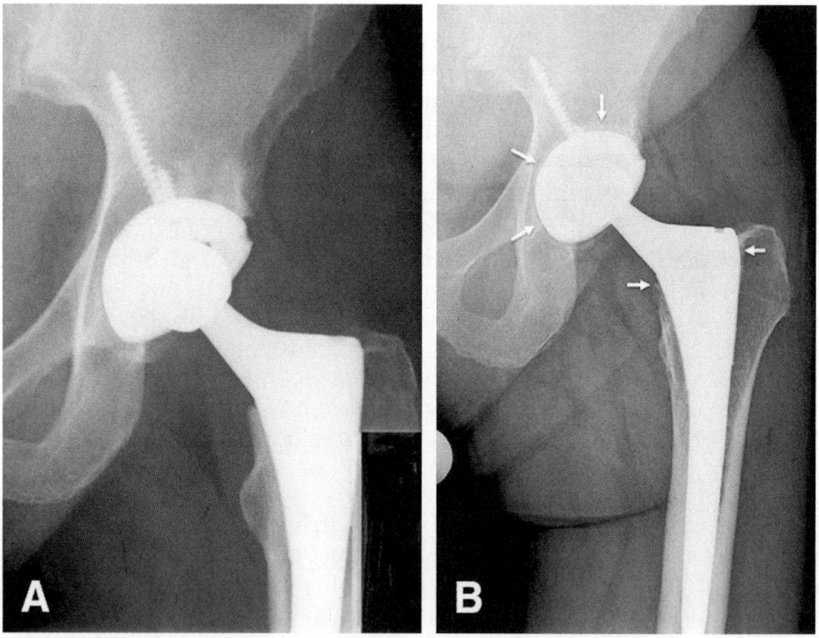

FIGURE 1.—(A) The figure is an AP pelvis radiograph obtained 6 weeks after THA in a 47-year-old woman. (B) The figure is an AP pelvis radiograph obtained 12 years after THA. The radiolucencies are evident (arrows) around the acetabular component and the proximal femoral component in Zone 1 and Zone 7. (Reprinted from Garvin KL, White TC, Dusad A, et al. Low wear rates seen in THAs with highly crosslinked polyethylene at 9 to 14 years in patients younger than age 50 years. *Clin Orthop Relat Res.* 2015;473:3829-3835, with permission from The Association of Bone and Joint Surgeons.)

4–14 mm^3/year). None of the hip radiographs had evidence of loosening or osteolysis. Wear was not associated with femoral head material ($p = 0.58$ for linear wear/year versus head material and $p = 0.52$ for volumetric wear/year versus head material).

Conclusions.—In our study of patients 50 years of age or younger undergoing THA, the linear and volumetric wear rates of HXLPE were very low regardless of the bearing surface material. The laboratory concerns of Oxinium surface damage are serious but at this time we have not seen high wear of the HXLPE or osteolysis in this population.

Level of Evidence.—Level III, therapeutic study (Fig 1).

► The articles by Hanna et al and Garvin et al continue to contribute to the body evidence that highly cross-linked polyethylene is the solution our profession has been looking for. Both studies are what we can considered long-term averaging over 10 years with a minimum surveillance of 9 years. Both use a 28-mm CoCr head.

The study by Hanna from Canada is a prospective controlled but not strictly randomized study of about 90 patients with conventional and 90 with highly cross-linked poly all with 28-mm femoral heads. The survival for poly wear of the conventional poly is good at 86%, but not as good as the crossed-linked product of 100% survival for poly wear at 13 years ($P = .006$; Fig 1, Hanna et al). The calculated linear wear rate was .035 mm/year by Hanna and .022 mm/year by Garvin. These and other similar positive findings from these 2 reports prompts me, a math major in college, to summarize: Q.E.D.

B. F. Morrey, MD

Five-year comparison of wear using oxidised zirconium and cobalt–chrome femoral heads in total hip arthroplasty: a multicentre randomised controlled trial

Jassim SS, Patel S, Wardle N, et al (Univ College London Hosps, London, UK; et al)

Bone Joint J 97-B:883-889, 2015

Oxidised zirconium (OxZi) has been developed as an alternative bearing surface for femoral heads in total hip arthroplasty (THA). This study has investigated polyethylene wear, functional outcomes and complications, comparing OxZi and cobalt–chrome (CoCr) as part of a three-arm, multicentre randomised controlled trial. Patients undergoing THA from four institutions were prospectively randomised into three groups. Group A received a CoCr femoral head and highly cross-linked polyethylene (XLPE) liner; Group B received an OxZi femoral head and XLPE liner; Group C received an OxZi femoral head and ultra-high molecular weight polyethylene (UHMWPE) liner. At five years, 368 patients had no statistically significant differences in short-form-36 ($p = 0.176$ mental, $p = 0.756$ physical), Western Ontario and McMaster Universities Osteoarthritis

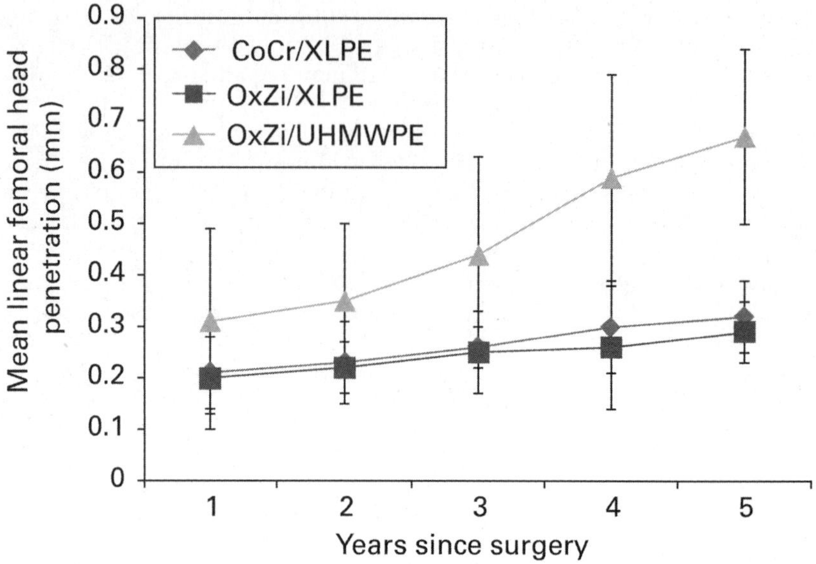

FIGURE 2.—Line graph demonstrating mean five-year linear wear of acetabular liner for groups of Cobalt-chrome (CoCr)/cross-linked polyethylene (XLPE), Oxidised zirconium (OxZi)/XLPE and OxZi/ultra-high molecular weight polyethylene (UHMWPE) (standard deviation in error bars). (Reprinted from Jassim SS, Patel S, Wardle N, et al. Five-year comparison of wear using Oxidised zirconium and cobalt-chrome femoral heads in total hip arthroplasty: a multicentre randomised controlled trial. *Bone Joint J.* 2015;97-B:883-889, with permission from The British Editorial Society of Bone & Joint Surgery.)

Index ($p = 0.847$), pain scores ($p = 0.458$) or complications. The mean rate of linear wear was 0.028 mm/year (standard deviation (SD) 0.010) for Group A, 0.023 mm/year (SD 0.010) for Group B, and 0.09 mm/year (SD 0.045) for Group C. Penetration was significantly higher in the UHMWPE liner group compared with both XLPE liner groups ($p < 0.001$) but no significant difference was noted between CoCr and OxZi when articulating with XLPE ($p = 0.153$). In this, the largest randomised study of this bearing surface, it appears that using a XLPE acetabular liner is more important in reducing THA component wear than the choice of femoral head bearing, at mid-term follow-up. There is a non-significant trend towards lower wear, coupling OxZi rather than CoCr with XLPE but long-term analysis is required to see if this observation changes with time and becomes significant (Fig 2).

▶ This is a very valuable contribution. The strength of the science is strong because this is a prospective randomized study. The follow-up period is adequate for the initial conclusion.

Whether there is added value in a ceramic compared with a cobalt chromium head is relevant, especially when one considers the expense and the potential for fracture with the ceramic head. Further, it provides added information regarding the clinical performance of highly cross-linked polyethylene. Fig 2 says it all. With the use of the highly crossed-linked product, the ceramic head offers little additional value. In both instances, the reduction in wear is dramatic.

B. F. Morrey, MD

No association between pseudotumors, high serum metal-ion levels and metal hypersensitivity in large-head metal-on-metal total hip arthroplasty at 5–7-year follow-up

Hjorth MH, Stilling M, Soballe K, et al (Aarhus Univ Hosp, Aarhus C, Denmark; et al)

Skeletal Radiol 45:115-125, 2016

Objective.—The relationship between metal wear debris, pseudotumor formation and metal hypersensitivity is complex and not completely understood. The purpose of this study was to assess the prevalence of pseudotumor formation in a consecutive series of metal-on-metal (MoM) total hip arthroplasty (THA) and to investigate its relationship to serum metal-ion levels and hypersensitivity to metal.

Methods.—Forty-one patients (31 males), mean age 52 (28–68) years, with a total of 49 large-head MoM THA participated in a 5–7-year follow-up study. Patients underwent ultrasonography, serum metal-ion concentrations were measured, metal allergy and atopic dermatitis were evaluated, and the questionnaires of the Oxford Hip Score (OHS), Harris Hip Score (HHS) and the Short-Form Health Survey (SF-36) were completed.

Results.—Pseudotumors were found in eight patients, but they were asymptomatic and their serum metal-ion levels were similar to those observed in patients with no pseudotumors ($p > 0.36$). The capsule-stem distance of mean 8.6 mm (SD 3.82, 95% CI: 5.40–11.79) was wider ($p = 0.02$) in patients with pseudotumours than in patients without pseudotumors of mean 5.6 mm (SD 2.89, 95% CI: 4.68–6.58). Positive patch test reactions were seen in three patients. Higher serum metal-ion levels of chromium and cobalt were significantly correlated with steeper cup inclination and smaller femoral head sizes, and were associated with female gender ($p < 0.04$).

Conclusion.—We found no association between pseudotumor formation, serum metal-ion levels, metal patch test reactivity, and atopic dermatitis. However, clinicians should be aware of asymptomatic pseudotumors, and we advise further exploration into the mechanisms involved in the pathogenesis of pseudotumors.

▶ This study offers more information regarding metal on metal bearings and host concerns. In this small sample, the potential correlation with serum ion concentration and the presence or size of the pseudotumor could not be made. There was also was no correlation to atopy or patch testing. All this is good to know. The finding of the smaller head diameters having higher ion concentrations has been pretty well demonstrated. It is useful to observe the correlation of more vertical cup positioning and offset with metal ion concentration. The real key is how do we identify the hyperreactor, that is, the potential aseptic lymphocyte dominated vasculitis associated lesion—prone patient. Lacking this, the attractiveness of the metal bearing will continue to wane. Finally, note the use of ultrasound to define the size of the lesions.

B. F. Morrey, MD

Adverse Reactions to Metal on Metal Are Not Exclusive to Large Heads in Total Hip Arthroplasty

Lombardi AV Jr, Berend KR, Adams JB, et al (Joint Implant Surgeons, Inc, New Albany, OH; et al)
Clin Orthop Relat Res 474:432-440, 2016

Background.—There is some suggestion that smaller diameter heads in metal-on-metal total hip arthroplasty (MoM THA) may be less prone to the adverse reactions to metal debris (ARMD) seen with large-diameter heads.

Questions/Purposes.—We reviewed our population of patients with small head (≤ 32 mm) MoM THA to determine (1) the frequency of ARMD; (2) potential risk factors for ARMD in this population; and (3) the etiology of revision and Kaplan-Meier survivorship with revision for all causes.

Methods.—Small-diameter head MoM devices were used in 9% (347 of 3753) of primary THAs during the study period (January 1996 to March 2005). We generally used these implants in younger, more active, higher-demand patients. Three hundred hips (258 patients) had MoM THA using a titanium modular acetabular component with a cobalt-chromium tapered insert and were available for review with minimum 2-year followup (mean, 10 years; range, 2–19 years). Complete followup was available in 86% of hips (300 of 347). Clinical records and radiographs were reviewed to determine the frequency and etiology of revision. Kaplan-Meier survivorship analysis was performed.

Results.—ARMD frequency was 5% (14 of 300 hips) and represented 70% (14 of 20) of revisions performed. Using multivariate analysis, no variable tested, including height, weight, body mass index, age, cup diameter, cup angle, use of screws, stem diameter, stem type, head diameter, preoperative clinical score, diagnosis, activity level, or sex, was significant as a risk factor for revision. Twenty hips have been revised: two for infection, four for aseptic loosening, and 14 for ARMD. Kaplan-Meier analysis revealed survival free of component revision for all causes was 95% at 10 years (95% confidence interval [CI], 91%–97%), 92% at 15 years (95% CI, 87%–95%), and 72% at 19 years (95% CI, 43%–90%), and survival free of component revision for aseptic causes was 96% at 10 years (95% CI, 92%–98%), 92% at 15 years (95% CI, 88%–95%), and 73% at 19 years (95% CI, 43%–90%).

Conclusions.—The late onset and devastating nature of metal-related failures is concerning with this small-diameter MoM device. Although

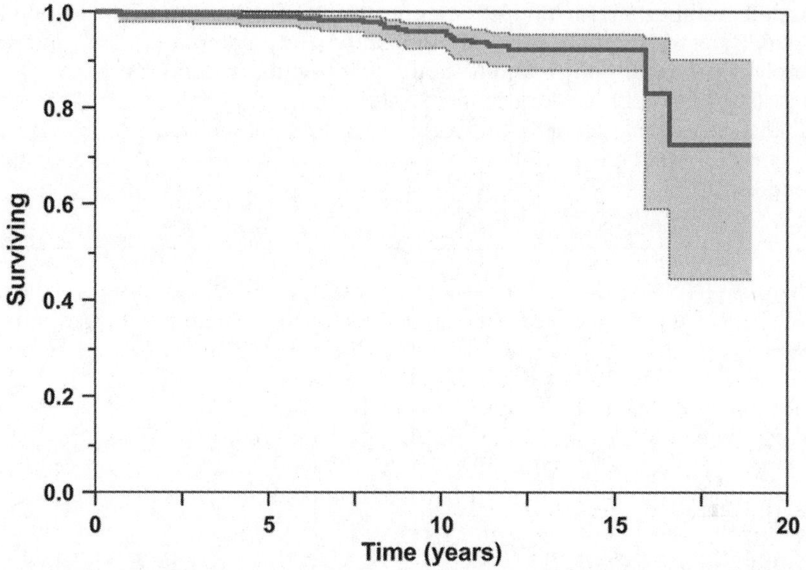

FIGURE 2.—Kaplan-Meier analysis revealed survival free of component revision for all causes was 95% at 10 years (95% CI, 91%–97%), 92% at 15 years (95% CI, 87%–95%), and 72% at 19 years (95% CI, 43%–90%). (Reprinted from Lombardi AV Jr, Berend KR, Adams JB, et al. Adverse reactions to metal on metal are not exclusive to large heads in total hip arthroplasty. *Clin Orthop Relat Res.* 2016;474:432-440, with permission from The Association of Bone and Joint Surgeons.)

the liner is modular, it cannot be exchanged and full acetabular revision is required. Patients with all MoM THA devices should be encouraged to return for clinical and radiographic followup, and clinicians should maintain a low threshold to perform a systematic evaluation. Symptomatic patients should undergo thorough investigation and vigilant observation for ARMD.

Level of Evidence.—Level IV, therapeutic study (Fig 2).

▶ I have included fewer articles regarding the metal-on-metal (MOM) articulation in recent years since the potential adverse effects are well known today. The main focus of the study is the survival and adverse response to the smaller head implant. This question is answered, but the most important finding is that the considerable adverse effects may not be demonstrated until 15 years after insertion (Fig 2). The bottom line is that the adverse effects of the MOM bearing is most significant if implanted in the younger patient. This is exactly the patient who many feel is the ideal candidate. In fact, it is quite the opposite.

B. F. Morrey, MD

Are all metal-on-metal hip revision operations contributing to the National Joint Registry implant survival curves? A study comparing the London Implant Retrieval Centre and National Joint Registry datasets

Sabah SA, Henckel J, Koutsouris S, et al (Great Ormond Street Hosp for Children, London, United Kingdom; Royal Natl Orthopaedic Hosp Trust, Stanmore, Middlesex, United Kingdom; Univ College London, United Kingdom; et al)

Bone Joint J 98-B;33-39, 2016

Aims.—The National Joint Registry for England, Wales and Northern Ireland (NJR) has extended its scope to report on hospital, surgeon and implant performance. Data linkage of the NJR to the London Implant Retrieval Centre (LIRC) has previously evaluated data quality for hip primary procedures, but did not assess revision records.

Methods.—We analysed metal-on-metal hip revision procedures performed between 2003 and 2013. A total of 69 929 revision procedures from the NJR and 929 revised pairs of components from the LIRC were included.

Results.—We were able to link 716 (77.1%) revision procedures on the NJR to the LIRC. This meant that 213 (22.9%) revision procedures at the LIRC could not be identified on the NJR. We found that 349 (37.6%) explants at the LIRC completed the full linkage process to both NJR primary and revision databases. Data completion was excellent (> 99.9%) for revision procedures reported to the NJR.

Discussion.—This study has shown that only approximately one third of retrieved components at the LIRC, contributed to survival curves on the NJR. We recommend prospective registry-retrieval linkage as a tool to feedback missing and erroneous data to the NJR and improve data quality.

Take Home Message.—Prospective Registry – retrieval linkage is a simple tool to evaluate and improve data quality on the NJR.

▶ This is a really interesting and important study because it addresses a question we rarely consider: how accurate are the data from the registry? The related question is: does it impact clinical decision making? This assessment clearly demonstrates a major weakness, at least in the UK registry. That 23% of revisions are not recorded is a major problem because it understates the effectiveness of implant survival requiring revision, but by a magnitude that is variable and not predictable.

B. F. Morrey, MD

Increased risk of revision of cementless stemmed total hip arthroplasty with metal-on-metal bearings

Varnum C, Pedersen AB, Mäkelä K, et al (Vejle Hosp, Denmark; Aarhus Univ Hosp, Denmark; Turku Univ Hosp, Finland; et al)

Acta Orthop 86:491-497, 2015

Background and Purpose.—Data from the national joint registries in Australia and England and Wales have revealed inferior medium-term survivorship for metal-on-metal (MoM) total hip arthroplasty (THA) than for metal-on-polyethylene (MoP) THA. Based on data from the Nordic Arthroplasty Register Association (NARA), we compared the revision risk of cementless stemmed THA with MoM and MoP bearings and we also compared MoM THA to each other.

Patients and Methods.—We identified 32,678 patients who were operated from 2002 through 2010 with cementless stemmed THA with either MoM bearings (11,567 patients, 35%) or MoP bearings (21,111 patients, 65%). The patients were followed until revision, death, emigration, or the end of the study period (December 31, 2011), and median follow-up was 3.6 (interquartile range (IQR): 2.4–4.8) years for MoM bearings and 3.4 (IQR: 2.0–5.8) years for MoP bearings. Multivariable regression in the presence of competing risk of death was used to assess the relative risk (RR) of revision for any reason (with 95% confidence interval (CI)).

Results.—The cumulative incidence of revision at 8 years of follow-up was 7.0% (CI: 6.0–8.1) for MoM bearings and 5.1% (CI: 4.7–5.6) for MoP bearings. At 6 years of follow-up, the RR of revision for any reason was 1.5 (CI: 1.3–1.7) for MoM bearings compared to MoP bearings. The RR of revision for any reason was higher for the ASR (adjusted RR = 6.4, CI: 5.0–8.1), the Conserve Plus (adjusted RR = 1.7, CI: 1.1–2.5) and "other" acetabular components (adjusted RR = 2.4, CI: 1.5–3.9) than for MoP THA at 6 years of follow-up.

Interpretation.—At medium-term follow-up, the survivorship for cementless stemmed MoM THA was inferior to that for MoP THA, and metal-related problems may cause higher revision rates for MoM bearings with longer follow-up.

► It is generally accepted that there is an association between an increased rate of infection in the rheumatoid patient and the use of immunosuppressive medical treatment. Yet there are few hard data to quantify this increased risk. This registry study of almost 400 000 patients does confirm patients with rheumatoid arthritis have experienced an increased infection rate since 2002. Unfortunately, as with many registry studies, the granularity of the data is such that a cause and effect relationship can only be surmised. Adding to the confusion is that the advantage in this study of using antibiotics in the cement appears to be time sensitive and of no value in the first 3 months after surgery.

B. F. Morrey, MD

A longitudinal study of MARS MRI scanning of soft-tissue lesions around metal-on-metal total hip arthroplasties and disease progression

Briant-Evans TW, Lyle N, Barbur S, et al (Hampshire Hosps NHS Foundation Trust, Basingstoke, United Kingdom)

Bone Joint J 97-B:1328-1337, 2015

We investigated the changes seen on serial metal artefact reduction magnetic resonance imaging scans (MARS-MRI) of metal-on-metal total hip arthroplasties (MoM THAs). In total 155 THAs, in 35 male and 100 female patients (mean age 70.4 years, 42 to 91), underwent at least two MRI scans at a mean interval of 14.6 months (2.6 to 57.1), at a mean of 48.2 months (3.5 to 93.3) after primary hip surgery. Scans were graded using a modification of the Oxford classification. Progression of disease was defined as an increase in grade or a minimum 10% increase in fluid lesion volume at second scan. A total of 16 hips (30%) initially classified as 'normal' developed an abnormality on the second scan. Of those with 'isolated trochanteric fluid' 9 (47%) underwent disease progression, as did 7 (58%) of 'effusions'. A total of 54 (77%) of hips initially classified as showing adverse reactions to metal debris (ARMD) progressed, with higher rates of progression in higher grades. Disease progression was associated with high blood cobalt levels or an irregular pseudocapsule lining at the initial scan. There was no association with changes in functional scores. Adverse reactions to metal debris in MoM THAs may not be as benign as previous reports have suggested. Close radiological follow-up is recommended, particularly in high-risk groups.

▶ This study provides important insights into the ongoing concern regarding metal-on-metal hip replacements. Using reliable imaging with a modest-sized cohort, but followed with care and precision, the authors demonstrate progressive adverse MRI changes in the bone around the prosthetic replacement. Of note, these changes correlated with increased concentrations of serum cobalt levels. Because these patients were and largely remain asymptomatic, the conclusion of the authors appears to be spot on: close radiological follow-up is recommended, particularly in high-risk groups.

B. F. Morrey, MD

An evaluation of the role of nuclear medicine imaging in the diagnosis of periprosthetic infections of the hip

Trevail C, Ravindranath-Reddy P, Sulkin T, et al (Royal Cornwall Hosps NHS Trust, Truro, UK)

Clin Radiol 71:211-219, 2016

Aim.—To validate the role of nuclear medicine (NM) imaging in hip periprosthetic joint infection (PJI) of hip arthroplasties.

Materials and Methods.—This was a retrospective study of 235 consecutive patients referred to NM for investigation of a symptomatic hip prosthesis. Imaging comprised Tc-99m bone scintigraphy, In-111 white cell scintigraphy, and bone marrow scintigraphy if required. Imaging findings were compared with intraoperative microbiology and histology, clinical findings and follow up for ≥24 months.

Results.—There were 14 exclusions. Of the 221 remaining patients, there were 16 true positives, one false positive, 200 true negatives, and four false negatives. The algorithm used at this centre demonstrated an accuracy of 97.7% with high specificity of 99.5% and sensitivity of 80%.

Conclusion.—When modern NM techniques and accurate reporting criteria are used, scintigraphy is an effective tool for diagnosing PJI of the hip. NM is only given a marginal role in the recent American Association of Orthopedic Surgeons guidelines, and the orthopaedic community should reconsider their evaluation of this technique (Fig 2).

▶ I found this to be an interesting article because it has political implications. This well-done study demonstrates a nuclear medicine strategy to diagnosis of periprosthetic total hip arthroplasty infections is highly sensitive and specific (Fig 2). The key is the T99 test indicates those with either loosening or infection. The addition of the 111 white cell scan is only of value when indicated by the T99 scan and interpreted in concert with it. The authors refer to American

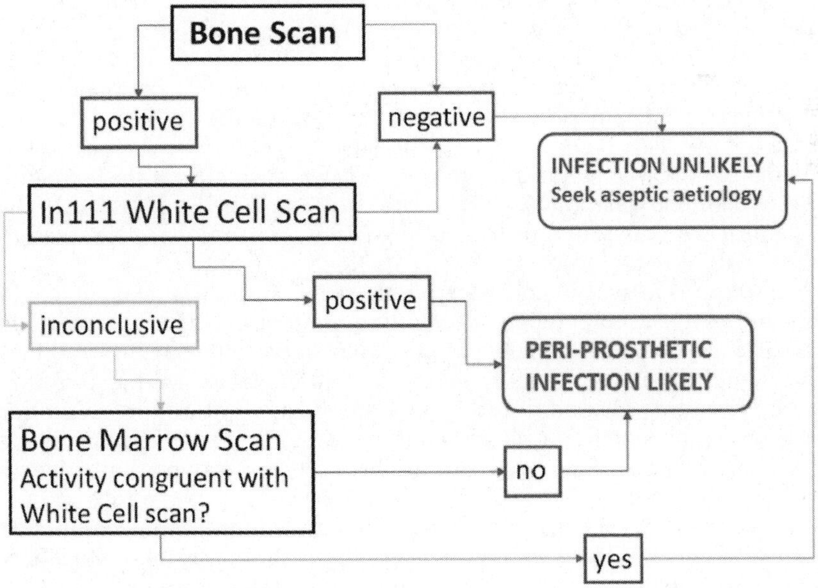

FIGURE 2.—Imaging algorithm for NM investigation of painful hip prostheses. (Reprinted from Trevail C, Ravindranath-Reddy P, Sulkin T, et al. An evaluation of the role of nuclear medicine imaging in the diagnosis of periprosthetic infections of the hip. *Clin Radiol.* 2016;71:211-219, with permission from The Royal College of Radiologists.)

Academy of Orthopedic Surgeons guidelines that indicate there is weak evidence for nuclear medicine studies to diagnose infected hip implants. The authors suggest this position should be reevaluated. Maybe they have a point; these data are pretty compelling. But this protocol must be followed to reach this benefit.

B. F. Morrey, MD

Missed low-grade infection in suspected aseptic loosening has no consequences for the survival of total hip arthroplasty: 173 patients followed for 6 to 9 years

Boot W, Moojen DJF, Visser E, et al (Univ Med Ctr Utrecht, the Netherlands; Onze Lieve Vrouwe Gasthuis, Amsterdam, the Netherlands; et al)
Acta Orthop 86:678-683, 2015

Background and Purpose.—Aseptic loosening and infection are 2 of the most common causes of revision of hip implants. Antibiotic prophylaxis reduces not only the rate of revision due to infection but also the rate of revision due to aseptic loosening. This suggests under-diagnosis of infections in patients with presumed aseptic loosening and indicates that current diagnostic tools are suboptimal. In a previous multicenter study on 176 patients undergoing revision of a total hip arthroplasty due to presumed aseptic loosening, optimized diagnostics revealed that 4–13% of the patients had a low-grade infection. These infections were not treated as such, and in the current follow-up study the effect on mid- to long-term implant survival was investigated.

Patients and Methods.—Patients were sent a 2-part questionnaire. Part A requested information about possible re-revisions of their total hip arthroplasty. Part B consisted of 3 patient-related outcome measure questionnaires (EQ5D, Oxford hip score, and visual analog scale for pain). Additional information was retrieved from the medical records. The group of patients found to have a low-grade infection was compared to those with aseptic loosening.

Results.—173 of 176 patients from the original study were included. In the follow-up time between the revision surgery and the current study (mean 7.5 years), 31 patients had died. No statistically significant difference in the number of re-revisions was found between the infection group (2 out of 21) and the aseptic loosening group (13 out of 152); nor was there any significant difference in the time to re-revision. Quality of life, function, and pain were similar between the groups, but only 99 (57%) of the patients returned part B.

Interpretation.—Under-diagnosis of low-grade infection in conjunction with presumed aseptic revision of total hip arthroplasty may not affect implant survival.

▶ This is a challenging report, in my opinion. It addresses real dilemmas encountered in prosthetic revision surgery: first, how does one diagnose subclinical infection? Second, how is one sure this is an infection? Third, should an unexpected positive culture be treated as an infection? I am not convinced that all 22 patients were in fact infected. The article references the selection criteria but does not list the inclusion criteria but just the phrase "optimized diagnostics." Furthermore, there is no information on the presumed infecting organisms. Regardless, the fact that there was at least a strong possibility of an infection in the study group that was not specifically treated is an important insight. The authors note no prior similar study of any joint. We did in fact study this issue for total elbows and found a similar long-term outcome as reported here—with no treatment.[1] We concluded that an unexpected positive culture at the time of revision was probably a contaminant if isolated in broth only. In this case, no long-term antibiotic was administered with a similar survival, as reported.

B. F. Morrey, MD

Reference

1. Wee AT, Morrey BF, Sanchez-Sotelo J. The fate of elbows with unexpected positive intraoperative cultures during revision elbow arthroplasty. *J Bone Joint Surg Am.* 2013;95:109-116.

Cost-effectiveness of antibiotic prophylaxis for dental patients with prosthetic joints: Comparisons of antibiotic regimens for patients with total hip arthroplasty

Skaar DD, Park T, Swiontkowski MF, et al (Univ of Minnesota, Minneapolis; St. Louis College of Pharmacy, MO; et al)

J Am Dent Assoc 146:830-839, 2015

Background.—Clinician uncertainty concerning the need for antibiotic prophylaxis to prevent prosthetic joint infection (PJI) after undergoing dental procedures persists. Improved understanding of the potential clinical and economic risks and benefits of antibiotic prophylaxis will help inform the debate and facilitate the continuing evolution of clinical management guidelines for dental patients with prosthetic joints.

Methods.—The authors developed a Markov decision model to compare the lifetime cost-effectiveness of alternative antibiotic prophylaxis strategies for dental patients aged 65 years who had undergone total hip arthroplasty (THA). On the basis of the authors' interpretation of previous recommendations from the American Dental Association and American Academy of Orthopaedic Surgeons, they compared the following strategies: no prophylaxis, prophylaxis for the first 2 years after arthroplasty, and lifetime prophylaxis.

Results.—A strategy of foregoing antibiotic prophylaxis before dental visits was cost-effective and resulted in lower lifetime accumulated costs ($11,909) and higher accumulated quality-adjusted life years (QALYs) (12.375) when compared with alternative prophylaxis strategies.

Conclusions.—The results of Markov decision modeling indicated that a no-antibiotic prophylaxis strategy was cost-effective for dental patients who had undergone THA. These results support the findings of case-control studies and the conclusions of an American Dental Association Council on Scientific Affairs report that questioned general recommendations for antibiotic prophylaxis before dental procedures.

Practical Implications.—The results of cost-effectiveness decision modeling support the contention that routine antibiotic prophylaxis for dental patients with total joint arthroplasty should be reconsidered.

▶ This topic is of great importance in that it discusses one of the most commonly asked, and poorly understood, questions in joint replacement surgery. We have long known the science to justify routine prophylaxis before dental procedures after joint replacement is thin. This analysis reinforces the scientifically based recommendation that continues to fly in the face of what we feel is appropriate. I am not sure I will change my practice of one gm before and one gm after dental procedures, but I will continue to be concerned that I have an ever-eroding scientific basis for my practice.

B. F. Morrey, MD

Antibiotic cement was associated with half the risk of re-revision in 1,154 aseptic revision total knee arthroplasties

Bini SA, Chan PH, Inacio MCS, et al (The Permanente Med Group, Oakland, CA; Kaiser Permanente, San Diego, CA; et al)

Acta Orthop 87:55-59, 2016

Background and Purpose.—Aseptic revisions comprise 80% of revision total knee arthroplasties (TKAs). We determined the incidence of re-revision TKA, the reasons for re-revision, and risk factors associated with these procedures.

Patients and Methods.—We conducted a retrospective cohort study of 1,154 patients who underwent aseptic revision TKA between 2002 and 2013 and were followed prospectively by a total joint replacement registry in the USA. Revision was defined as any operation in which an implanted component was replaced. Patient-, surgeon-, and procedure-related risk factors were evaluated. Survival analyses were conducted.

Results.—There were 114 re-revisions (10%) with a median time to reoperation of 3.6 years (interquartile range (IQR): 2.6−5.2). The infection rate was 2.9% (34/1,154) and accounted for 30% of re-revisions (34 of 114). In adjusted models, use of antibiotic- loaded cement was associated with a 50% lower risk of all-cause re-revision surgery (hazard ratio (HR) = 0.5, 95% CI: 0.3−0.9), age with a 20% lower risk for every 10-year increase (HR = 0.8, CI: 0.7−1.0), body mass index (BMI) with a 20% lower risk for every 5-unit increase (HR = 0.8, CI: 0.7−1.0), and a surgeon's greater cumulative experience ($\geq$ 20 cases vs. < 20 cases) with a 3 times higher risk of re-revision (HR = 2.8, CI: 1.5–5).

Interpretation.—Revised TKAs were at high risk of subsequent failure. The use of antibiotic-loaded cement, higher age, and higher BMI were associated with lower risk of further revision whereas a higher degree of surgeon experience was associated with higher risk.

▶ This is a useful contribution in our knowledge from an uncommon source of a US single-practice system database. Every one of the factors contributing to a greater revision failure rate is of interest. The age and body mass index issues have been previously documented. However, the use of antibiotic impregnated cement is a bit controversial. There is some question as whether this practice can lessen the infection rate in primary procedures. However, these data indicate antibiotic-impregnated cement is of measurable value in revision surgery. This has been my practice for 30 years. The finding of the more experienced surgeon as an independent risk factor is interesting. In the past, we assumed these surgeons do the more difficult cases. I can only hope such is the case.

B. F. Morrey, MD

Acetabular revision with impaction bone grafting and a cemented polyethylene acetabular component: comparison of the Kaplan-Meier analysis to the competing risk analysis in 62 revisions with 25 to 30 years follow-up

Te Stroet MAJ, Keurentjes JC, Rijnen WHC, et al (Radboud Univ Med Ctr, Nijmegen, The Netherlands)

Bone Joint J 97-B:1338-1344, 2015

We present the results of 62 consecutive acetabular revisions using impaction bone grafting and a cemented polyethylene acetabular component in 58 patients (13 men and 45 women) after a mean follow-up of 27 years (25 to 30). All patients were prospectively followed. The mean age at revision was 59.2 years (23 to 82).

We performed Kaplan–Meier (KM) analysis and also a Competing Risk (CR) analysis because with long-term follow-up, the presence of a competing event (i.e. death) prevents the occurrence of the endpoint of re-revision.

A total of 48 patients (52 hips) had died or had been re-revised at final review in March 2011. None of the deaths were related to the surgery. The mean Harris hip score of the ten surviving hips in ten patients was 76 points (45 to 99).

The KM survivorship at 25 years for the endpoint 're-revision for any reason' was 58.0% (95% confidence interval (CI) 38 to 73) and for 're-revision for aseptic loosening' 72.1% (95% CI 51 to 85). With the CR analysis we calculated the KM analysis overestimates the failure rate with respectively 74% and 93% for these endpoints. The current study

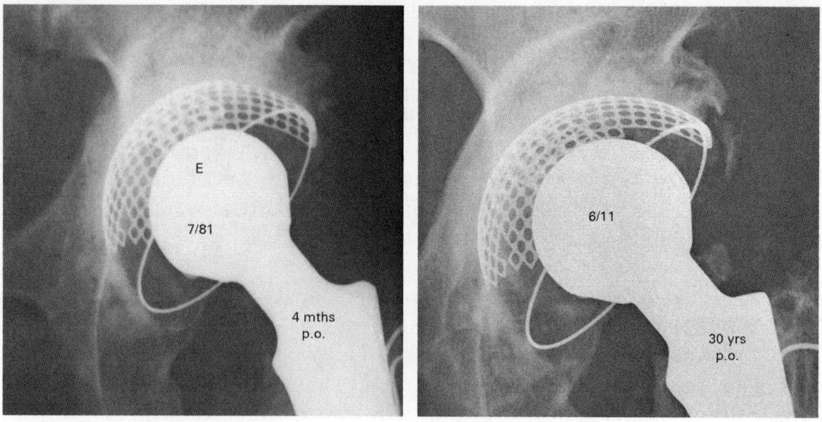

FIGURE 1.—Radiographs of a 21-year-old woman a) four months after revision of a failed resurfacing hip prosthesis with impaction bone grafting and a cemented acetabular component. A metal mesh was placed on top of the graft (a technique no longer recommended); and b) 30 years after the reconstruction showing the position of the acetabular component to be unchanged. There is progressive osteolysis in zone I and at the inferior margin of zone III, but overall, the component is well-fixed. E, code for the patient; 7/81, July 1981; p.o., post-operative; 6/11, June 2011. (Reprinted from Te Stroet MAJ, Keurentjes JC, Rijnen WHC, et al. Acetabular revision with impaction bone grafting and a cemented polyethylene acetabular component: comparison of the kaplan-meier analysis to the competing risk analysis in 62 revisions with 25 to 30 years follow-up. *Bone Joint J.* 2015;97-B:1338-1344, with permission from The British Editorial Society of Bone & Joint Surgery.)

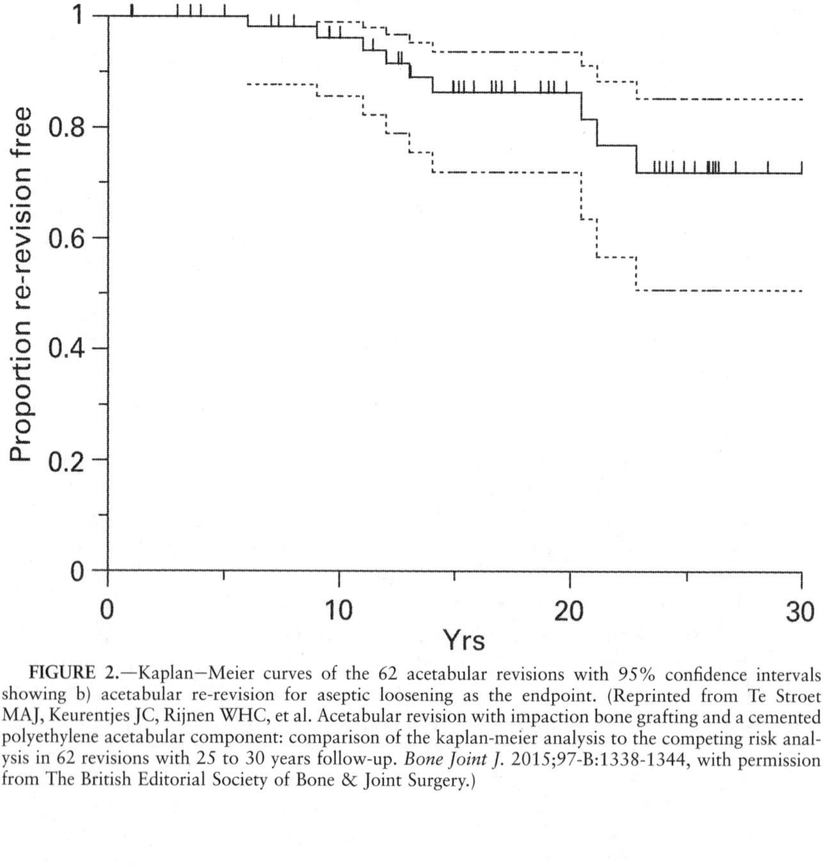

FIGURE 2.—Kaplan–Meier curves of the 62 acetabular revisions with 95% confidence intervals showing b) acetabular re-revision for aseptic loosening as the endpoint. (Reprinted from Te Stroet MAJ, Keurentjes JC, Rijnen WHC, et al. Acetabular revision with impaction bone grafting and a cemented polyethylene acetabular component: comparison of the kaplan-meier analysis to the competing risk analysis in 62 revisions with 25 to 30 years follow-up. *Bone Joint J.* 2015;97-B:1338-1344, with permission from The British Editorial Society of Bone & Joint Surgery.)

shows that acetabular impaction bone grafting revisions provide good clinical results at over 25 years (Figs 1a, b and 2b).

▶ There are few opportunities to document 30-year outcomes. This contribution from the innovator of impaction grafting, Dr T. Slooff, is of great value. This center has been providing long-term surveillance for this technique since it was first introduced. This latest study reveals the long-term outcome of the technique of cancellous impaction grafting for acetabular revision, the indication for which it was first applied (Fig 1a, b). This follow-up period implies an early age of revision, as shown in Fig 1. It is impressive that the revision procedure has a greater than 70% likelihood of survival more than 25 years after revision (Fig 2b). This justifies the use of the concept as described and is the reason we have adapted it for problems at the elbow.

B. F. Morrey, MD

Comparison of the risk of revision in cementless total hip arthroplasty with ceramic-on-ceramic and metal-on-polyethylene bearings: Data on 11,096 patients from the Danish Hip Arthroplasty Registry

Varnum C, Pedersen AB, Kjærsgaard-Andersen P, et al (Odense Univ Hosp, Denmark; Aarhus Univ Hosp, Denmark; et al)

Acta Orthop 86:477-484, 2015

Background and Purpose.—Ceramic-on-ceramic (CoC) bearings were introduced in total hip arthroplasty (THA) to reduce problems related to polyethylene wear. We compared the 9-year revision risk for cementless CoC THA and for cementless metal-on-polyethylene (MoP) THA.

Patients and Methods.—In this prospective, population-based study from the Danish Hip Arthroplasty Registry, we identified all the primary cementless THAs that had been performed from 2002 through 2009 (n = 25,656). Of these, 1,773 THAs with CoC bearings and 9,323 THAs with MoP bearings were included in the study. To estimate the relative risk (RR) of revision, we used regression with the pseudo-value approach and treated death as a competing risk.

Results.—444 revisions were identified: 4.0% for CoC THA (71 of 1,773) and 4.0% for MoP THA (373 of 9,323). No statistically significant difference in the risk of revision for any reason was found for CoC and MoP bearings after 9 years of follow-up (adjusted RR = 1.3, 95% CI: 0.72—2.4). Revision rates due to component failure were 0.5% (n = 8) for CoC bearings and 0.1% (n = 6) for MoP bearings ($p < 0.001$). 6 patients with CoC bearings (0.34%) underwent revision due to ceramic fracture.

Interpretation.—When compared to the "standard" MoP bearings, CoC THA had a 33% higher (though not statistically significantly higher) risk of revision for any reason at 9 years.

▶ Again we turn to the Danish registry to understand the differences, if any exist, between 2 articular options. This analysis does seem to provide the data that support my and many surgeons view of the ceramic-on-ceramic articulation. It reduces wear, but at what cost? The actual complications are similar between the 2 systems. And although the rate of ceramic fracture is low, the implication of managing a fractured ceramic implant are so dire that any fracture would obviate their use, in my opinion. As the authors note, although the overall complication rate is similar, the rate of revision for articular failure is 33% higher in the ceramic-on-ceramic group. QED.

B. F. Morrey, MD

High Survivorship With Cementless Stems and Cortical Strut Allografts for Large Femoral Bone Defects in Revision THA

Kim Y-H, Park J-W, Kim J-S, et al (Ewha Womans Univ School of Medicine, Seoul, Republic of Korea)

Clin Orthop Relat Res 473:2990-3000, 2015

Background.—Numerous studies have investigated the clinical and radiographic results of revision THAs with use of cementless stems and cortical strut allografts. However, to our knowledge, no long-term followup studies have evaluated patients undergoing revision THA with use of cortical strut allografts where the allografts provided the primary stability for extensively coated femoral stems in the presence of extensive femoral diaphyseal bone defects.

Question/Purposes.—We performed this study to determine (1) validated outcomes scores; (2) radiographic signs of fixation and allograft healing; (3) frequency of complications; and (4) survivorship of the components after use of cortical strut onlay allografts in Types IIIB and IV femoral diaphyseal bone defects.

Methods.—Between 1994 and 2003, we performed 140 revision THAs in 130 patients with Paprosky Types IIIB and IV femoral diaphyseal defects. The patients were treated using extensively coated femoral stems and cortical strut allografts because primary axial or rotational stability could not be achieved without grafting. Ten of the patients (10 hips; 7.7%) were lost to followup or died before 10 years; the remaining 120 patients (130 hips) represent the study group in this retrospective study. There were 66 men and 54 women. Their mean age at the time of index surgery was 59 ± 18 years (range, 36–67 years). The primary diagnosis was predominantly osteonecrosis of the femoral head (53%). The most common reason for revision was aseptic loosening (97%), followed by periprosthetic fracture (3%). The mean time from primary to revision

THA was 12 years (range, 8–27 years). The mean duration of followup was 16.1 years (range, 12–20 years).

Results.—The mean Harris hip score was 39 ± 10 points before revision and improved to 86 ± 14 points at 16 years followup ($p = 0.02$). The mean preoperative WOMAC score was 62 ± 29 (41–91) points and improved to 22 ± 19 (11–51) points at 16 years followup ($p = 0.003$). Of the 130 stems, 113 (87%) had bone ingrowth, five (4%) had stable fibrous ingrowth, and 12 (9%) were unstable. All allografts were incorporated. Four hips (3%) had a displaced femoral shaft fracture at the stem tip; four (3%) had a postoperative dislocation; and six (5%) had early postoperative infection. Kaplan-Meier survivorship analysis, with revision or radiographic failure as the endpoint, revealed that the 16-year rate of survival of the components was 91% (95% CI, 0.88%–0.96%).

Conclusion.—Supportive cortical strut onlay allografts provided high survivorship beyond 12 years of followup in revision THAs. Future studies might compare this approach with allograft-prosthesis composites, proximal femoral replacement, or modular fluted, tapered stems.

Level of Evidence.—Level IV, therapeutic study (Fig 2).

▶ As a rule I try to avoid reviewing articles that are highly subspecialized. An exception was made here because I consider the question of long-term incorporation and viability of structural grafts to be relevant to numerous applications in our practice. This is a really good article with an impressive sample of 120 patients followed for a minimum of 12 (mean, 16) years. The findings are really impressive. All grafts incorporated, and the Kaplan-Meier survival

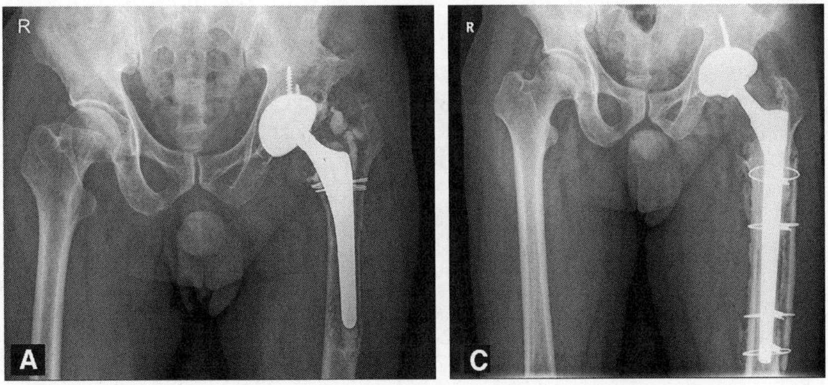

FIGURE 2.—A 65-year-old man had aseptic loosening of the cemented femoral component. (**A**) His prerevision AP radiograph shows a cement fracture, varus shift, and subsidence of the left femoral component. The bone defect of the left femur is Paprosky type IV. (C) The AP radiograph taken 15 years after rerevision surgery shows the Wagner cementless stem is embedded in a satisfactory position with solid bone ongrowth on the entire femoral stem. A two-cortical strut onlay allograft was incorporated in the host bone. The acetabular component is well fixed in a satisfactory position. (Reprinted from Kim Y-H, Park J-W, Kim J-S, et al. High survivorship with cementless stems and cortical strut allografts for large femoral bone defects in revision THA. *Clin Orthop Relat Res.* 2015;473:2990-3000, with permission from The Association of Bone and Joint Surgeons.)

estimate is in excess of 90% at 15 years. This is exceptional, especially when one understands that among the inclusion criteria was that the strut was required for an uncemented stem stability (Fig 2).

B. F. Morrey, MD

Do Rerevision Rates Differ After First-time Revision of Primary THA With a Cemented and Cementless Femoral Component?

Gromov K, Pedersen AB, Overgaard S, et al (Copenhagen Univ Hosp Hvidovre, Denmark; Aarhus Univ Hosp, Denmark; Odense Univ Hosp, Denmark; et al)
Clin Orthop Relat Res 473:3391-3398, 2015

Background.—Worldwide use of cementless fixation for total hip arthroplasty (THA) is on the rise despite some evidence from the world's registries suggesting inferior survivorship compared with cemented techniques. The patterns of bone loss associated with failed cementless and cemented THAs may prejudice the results of future revision procedures; however, this has not been documented.

Questions/Purposes.—The purpose of this study was to compare (1) the risk for rerevision of first revision THA; (2) the patterns of femoral bone loss at the time of first revision of primary THA; (3) the reasons for first revision of primary THA; and (4) the time to first revision of primary THA between primary cementless and cemented femoral components.

Methods.—Primary THAs with cemented (n = 1791) and uncemented (n = 805) femoral components that subsequently sustained first revision of the femoral component were identified from the Danish Hip Arthroplasty Registry (DHR). As of 2012, 120,988 primary THAs and 19,282 revisions were registered in the DHR with completeness of 97% and 90% for primary and revision THA, respectively. Median followup for revisions of primary THA with cemented and cementless femoral component was 4 years (range, 0–17 years) and 2 years (range, 0–16 years), respectively. Survival of first revision THA, with second revision of the femur as outcome, was evaluated using hazard ratios (HRs) with 95% confidence interval (CI) adjusting for potential confounding. All patient- and surgery-related data are collected from Danish medical databases. Recording of bone defects in the DHR is based on surgeons' intraoperative findings.

Results.—With the numbers studied, we found no differences in the risk of second revision between the overall cohort between cementless and cemented techniques (HR, 1.32; 95% CI, 0.97–1.80; $p = 0.076$); however, a second revision for any reason was more likely in patients <70 years old in whom the index arthroplasty was performed using a cementless technique (HR, 1.48; 95% CI, 1.01–2.17; $p = 0.046$). Increasingly severe femoral bone defects of type II (30% [532 of 1791] versus 13% [104 of 805]; $p < 0.001$) type III (11% [200 of 1791] versus 2% [12 of 805]; $p < 0.001$) and type IV (1% [26 of 1791] versus 0.4% [three of 805]; $p = 0.016$) were more frequent at revisions of cemented femoral components compared with cementless femoral components. Indications for first revision differed between primary cemented and uncemented femoral components, because a larger proportion of cemented femoral components was revised as a result of aseptic loosening compared with cementless femoral components (74% [1329 of 1791] versus 25% [197 of 805]; $p < 0.001$), whereas a larger proportion of cementless femoral components was revised as a result of a fracture compared with cemented femoral components (46% [371 of 805] versus 10% [168 of 1791]; $p < 0.001$). Failure before 5 years was more likely in cementless femoral components than cemented femoral components (91% [733 of 805] versus 44% [749 of 1791], $p < 0.001$).

Conclusions.—We found no differences in the risk of second revision in the overall cohort between cementless and cemented techniques; however, we observed an increased risk for rerevision THA performed on patients <70 years whose index THAs were performed using cementless components when looking at all causes for revision, even after adjusting for the most likely confounding factors. Our data suggest that increased use of cementless fixation in primary THA may lead to inferior survivorship of first revision THA.

Level of Evidence.—Level III, therapeutic study.

▶ We need to learn more about the outcome of the efforts to salvage the failed primary implant. The question of the expectation of a successful rerevision has not often been addressed. In the past, it was shown that revision of an uncemented primary was superior to revision of a primary cemented femoral component. This study takes the question to the next level by evaluating the incidence of a second revision based on the original fixation. Surprisingly, the uncemented device had a higher incidence of rerevision than did the cemented option. It is not surprising that neither the cemented primary implants that were revised for loosened nor that the primary uncemented rerevision failures were due to fracture. However, the weakness of registry studies is exemplified here because it is unclear as to whether the fixation used in the first revision was cement. This represents a deficiency of the study.

B. F. Morrey, MD

Hydroxyapatite ceramic-coated femoral components in young patients followed up for 17 to 25 years: an update of a previous report

Syed MA, Hutt NJ, Shah N, et al (Worthing General Hosp, West Sussex, United Kingdom)

Bone Joint J 97-B:749-754, 2015

This study reports the results of 38 total hip arthroplasties (THAs) in 33 patients aged < 50 years, using the JRI Furlong hydroxyapatite ceramic (HAC)-coated femoral component. This represents an update of previous reports of the same cohort at ten and 16 years, which were reported in

2004 and 2009, respectively. We describe the survival, radiological and functional outcomes at a mean follow-up of 21 years (17 to 25). Of the surviving 34 THAs, one underwent femoral revision for peri-prosthetic fracture after 21 years, and one patient (one hip) was lost to follow-up. Using aseptic loosening as the end-point, 12 hips (31.5%) needed acetabular revision but none needed femoral revision, demonstrating 100% survival (95% confidence interval 89 to 100).

In young patients with high demands, the Furlong HAC–coated femoral component gives excellent long-term results.

▶ This case series is of a small cohort but with long-term follow-up. The use of hydroxyapatite (HA) coating is not used extensively in the United States, but it is in Europe. This article should be placed in the historical context of a design period trying to enhance the reliability of the uncemented implant. Simply stated, the HA coating with this design does appear to be effective in ensuring stable long-term fixation. The small sample size should be noted and the similar effectiveness is now available with most systems. So, although this is an effective system, it is probably no more effective than others. For me, the cost would determine which I use.

B. F. Morrey, MD

8 Total Knee Arthroplasty

Introduction

I am aware of the fact that knee replacement is done by most orthopaedic surgeons. Yet, in spite of its prevalence, there is relatively more literature discussing the hip than the knee. I believe this is because it has become such a reliable operation, and so there are fewer controversial issues. One common theme reflected in the reviews this year includes both diagnosis and treating the infected knee replacement. There are emerging data on the effectiveness of blood and culture results to predict the infected joint as well as a trend to consider a single staged revision for the infected joint. As with the hip, analytical reviews of the literature and registry-based analyses have been liberally used in this section to provide insights into the more controversial issues relating to knee replacement. Hence, there are a number of international contributions in this section.

Bernard F. Morrey, MD

Do Patient Race and Sex Change Surgeon Recommendations for TKA?

Dy CJ, Lyman S, Boutin-Foster C, et al (Hosp for Special Surgery, New York; Weill Cornell Med College, New York; et al)
Clin Orthop Relat Res 473:410-417, 2014

Background.—Prior investigations have suggested that physician-related factors may contribute to differential use of TKA among women and ethnic minorities. We sought to evaluate the effect of surgeon bias on recommendations for TKA.

Questions/purpose.—Using an experimental approach with standardized patient scenarios, we sought to evaluate surgeon recommendations regarding TKA, specifically to determine whether recommendations for TKA are influenced by (1) patient race, and (2) patient sex.

Methods.—We developed four computerized scenarios for all combinations of race (white or black) and sex (male or female) for otherwise similar patients with end-stage knee osteoarthritis. Patients gave an orthopaedic history of 2 years worsening pain with decreased functional status and failure of oral antiinflammatory medications and corticosteroid intraarticular injections. Orthopaedic surgeons attending the 2012 annual meetings of the New York State Society of Orthopaedic Surgeons and American Association of Hip and Knee Surgeons were recruited for the study. Surgeons passing an open recruitment table at each meeting were asked to participate. Of the 1111 surgeons in attendance at either meeting, 113 (10.2%) participated in the study. All participants viewed the "control" patient's story (white male) and were randomized to view one of the three "experimental" scenarios (white female, black male, black female). After viewing each scenario, the participants were anonymously asked whether they would recommend TKA. An a priori power analysis showed that 112 participants were needed to detect a 15% difference in the likelihood of recommending surgery for white versus nonwhite patients in the test scenarios evaluated with 90% power at a level of significance of 0.05.

Results.—Of the 39 surgeons who viewed the white male plus black female scenario, there were 33 (85%) concordant responses (TKA offered to both patients) and six discordant responses (TKA offered to only one of the patients), with no effect of patient race and sex ($p = 0.99$). Of the 37 surgeons who viewed the white male plus black male scenario, there were 33 (89%) concordant responses and four discordant responses, with no effect of patient race ($p = 0.32$). Of the 37 surgeons who viewed the white male plus white female scenario, there were 30 (77%) concordant responses and seven discordant responses, with no effect of patient sex ($p = 0.71$).

Conclusion.—After orthopaedic surgeons viewed video scenarios of patients with end-stage knee osteoarthritis, patient race and sex were not associated with a different likelihood of a surgical recommendation. Our findings support the notion that patient race and sex may be less influential on decision making when there are strong clinical data to support a decision. Physician bias may have a greater effect on decision making in situations where the indications for surgery are less clear.

▶ I found this an interesting study because it contradicts prior conclusions regarding race and gender bias in offering joint replacement. The methodology is markedly different from the typical retrospective population-based study. With this methodology, which focuses on patient symptoms and findings, there was no bias demonstrated by these surgeons when presented with the clinical data. This is encouraging, but it does not address the real reason for the documented disparity among race and joint replacement, which is socioeconomically based. Regardless, it is encouraging to see that it appears not to be a direct race or gender bias.

B. F. Morrey, MD

Development of a Prediction Model to Estimate the Risk of Walking Limitations in Patients with Total Knee Arthroplasty

Pua Y-H, Seah FJ-T, Clark RA, et al (Singapore General Hosp; Australian Catholic Univ, Victoria, Australia)

J Rheumatol 43:419-426, 2016

Objective.—Early and accurate risk prediction of walking limitations after total knee arthroplasty (TKA) is important for clinical and economic reasons. However, to our knowledge, no studies have systematically integrated multiple predictors into a single, clinically practical model. Our study aimed to develop a prediction model to estimate the risk of post-TKA walking limitations.

Methods.—We performed a prospective cohort study of 1096 patients who underwent elective, primary TKA between July 2013 and September 2014. Candidate predictors included patient demographics, surgical factors, and pre- and early (1-mo) post-TKA functional measures. The outcome of interest was self-reported walking limitations at 6 months of post-TKA. We used multivariable proportional odds regression with bootstrap internal validation to develop the model.

Results.—In all, 12% of patients reported walking limitations (maximum walk time ≤ 15 min) at 6 months postsurgery. The main predictors of increasing levels of walking limitations were preoperative walking limitations (overall $p < 0.001$), higher levels of body mass index [interquartile range (IQR)-OR 1.3, 95% CI 1.2–1.5], lower values of 1-month post-TKA gait speed (IQR-OR 1.9, 95% CI 1.3–2.6), the presence of contralateral knee pain (OR 1.9, 95% CI 1.2–3.0), and the use of a quadstick preoperatively (OR 3.5, 95% CI 1.7–7.3). The prediction model had an optimism-corrected concordance index of 0.71.

Conclusion.—A small but sizable proportion of patients with TKA had persistent mobility limitations. Our prediction model may help to risk-stratify patients, and external validation is required before the model can be used in clinical practice.

▶ This study provides objective evidence to better discuss post—total knee functional expectations. Distance walked may be the second most important consideration after relief of pain. Walking distance for 15 minutes at 6 months after surgery can be directly correlated to distance walked before surgery, contralateral knee arthritis, and the use of a 4-prong cane. Of course, body mass index (BMI) is also directly correlated with greater impact, observed in patients with BMI in excess of 33. After surgery, gait speed at 1 month also predicted the final outcome. Finally, it is of interest that only 12% had significant walking limitations at 6 months.

B. F. Morrey, MD

Concomitant Methotrexate Protects Against Total Knee Arthroplasty in Patients with Rheumatoid Arthritis Treated with Tumor Necrosis Factor Inhibitors

Asai S, Takahashi N, Funahashi K, et al (Nagoya Univ Graduate School of Medicine, Japan)

J Rheumatol 42:2255-2260, 2015

Objective.—To determine the effects of concomitant methotrexate (MTX) on the incidence of total knee arthroplasty (TKA) resulting from the progression of joint destruction in patients with rheumatoid arthritis (RA) during longterm treatment with tumor necrosis factor (TNF) inhibitors.

Methods.—A total of 155 patients with RA (310 knee joints) received TNF inhibitors at our institute between May 1, 2001, and May 31, 2008. A total of 111 symptomatic (tender and/or swollen) knee joints in 68 patients were retrospectively studied over the course of a minimum of 5 years of followup. The median (interquartile range) followup period was 8.1 (7.0–9.3) years. All data were analyzed using the knee joint as the statistical unit of analysis. TKA during treatment with TNF inhibitors was used as the outcome variable in predictive analyses. The cumulative incidence of TKA was compared by concomitant or no MTX use (MTX ±).

Results.—There were 79 subjects (71%) who received concomitant MTX. According to Kaplan-Meier estimates, the cumulative incidence of TKA for the MTX+ group was significantly lower than that for the MTX− group (24% vs 45% at 5 yrs, respectively, $p = 0.035$). Multivariate analysis using the Cox proportional hazards model revealed that concomitant MTX (HR 0.44, 95% CI 0.22–0.89), Larsen grade (HR 2.93, 95% CI 1.94–4.41), and older age at baseline (HR 1.04, 95% CI 1.01–1.08) were independent predictors of TKA.

Conclusion.—Concomitant MTX reduces the incidence of TKA by 56% in patients with RA during longterm treatment with TNF inhibitors.

▶ I must admit that I did not see this coming. As surgeons, we are sensitive to the various disease-remitting agents our patients are taking as we assess their suitability for surgery.

We are well aware of the adverse effects of tumor necrosis factor and other medications of this type and tend to place methotrexate (MTX) into the same category, at least from the perspective of placing the patient as potentially at greater risk for infection and wound problems. This report from the rheumatology literature is important as a point of reference to reveal the "protective" effect of MTX in preventing a patient with rheumatoid arthritis form ultimately coming to total knee arthroplasty. Worth noting for sure.

B. F. Morrey, MD

Does Tourniquet Use in TKA Affect Recovery of Lower Extremity Strength and Function? A Randomized Trial

Dennis DA, Kittelson AJ, Yang CC, et al (Colorado Joint Replacement, Denver; Univ of Colorado Physical Therapy Program, Aurora, CO; et al)

Clin Orthop Relat Res 474:69-77, 2016

Background.—Tourniquet use during total knee arthroplasty (TKA) improves visibility and reduces intraoperative blood loss. However, tourniquet use may also have a negative impact on early recovery of muscle strength and lower extremity function after TKA.

Questions/Purposes.—The purpose of this study was (1) to determine whether tourniquet use affects recovery of quadriceps strength (primary outcome) during the first 3 postoperative months; and (2) to examine the effects of tourniquet application on secondary outcomes: voluntary quadriceps activation, hamstring strength, unilateral limb balance as well as the effect on operative time and blood loss.

Methods.—Twenty-eight patients (mean age 62 ± 6 years; 16 men) undergoing same-day bilateral TKA (56 lower extremities) were enrolled in a prospective, randomized study. Subjects were randomized to receive a tourniquet-assisted knee arthroplasty on one lower extremity while the contralateral limb underwent knee arthroplasty without extended tourniquet use. In the former group, the tourniquet was inflated just before the incision was made and released after cementation; in the latter group, a tourniquet was not used (10 of 28 [36%]) or inflated only during component cementation (18 of 28 [64%]). The choice of no tourniquet or use just during cementation was based on surgeon choice, because some surgeons felt a tourniquet during cementation was necessary to achieve a dry surgical field to maximize cement fixation. A median parapatellar approach and the identical posterior-stabilized TKA design were used by all four fellowship-trained knee surgeons involved. Isometric quadriceps strength, hamstring strength, voluntary quadriceps activation, and unilateral balance were assessed preoperatively, 3 weeks, and 3 months after bilateral knee arthroplasty. Other factors, including pain, range of motion, and lower extremity girth, were assessed for descriptive purposes at each of these time points as well as on the second postoperative day.

Results.—Quadriceps strength was slightly lower in the tourniquet group compared with the no-tourniquet group (group difference = 11.27 Nm [95% confidence interval {CI}, 2.33–20.20]; $p = 0.01$), and these differences persisted at 3 months after surgery (group difference = 9.48 Nm [95% CI, 0.43–18.54]; $p = 0.03$). Hamstring strength did not differ between groups at any time point nor did measures of quadriceps voluntary activation or measures of unilateral balance ability. There was less estimated intraoperative blood loss in the tourniquet group (84 ± 26 mL) than in the no-tourniquet group (156 ± 63 mL) (group difference = −74 mL [95% CI, −100 to −49]; $p < 0.001$). However, there was no difference in total blood loss between the groups (group difference = −136 mL [95% CI, −318 to 45]; $p = 0.13$).

Conclusions.—Patients who underwent TKA using a tourniquet had diminished quadriceps strength during the first 3 months after TKA, the clinical significance of which is unclear. Future studies may be warranted to examine the effects of tourniquet use on long-term strength and functional outcomes.

Level of Evidence.—Level I, therapeutic study.

▶ This is an uncommon prospective randomized study investigating the effect of different surgical techniques. Not using a tourniquet during a total knee arthroplasty is gaining popularity, primarily driven by the perception of faster rehabilitation and less pain. This study, using a bilateral procedure that allows patients to serve as their own control, is well designed with a reasonable sample size. The short-term weakness in the quadriceps strength is not surprising. That this persists at 3 months is of some concern, even though the clinical function is not obviously affected. It does prompt one to consider the nontourniquet technique.

B. F. Morrey, MD

Intravenous administration of tranexamic acid effectively reduces blood loss in primary total knee arthroplasty in a 610-patient consecutive case series

Pitta M, Zawadsky M, Verstraete R, et al (Medstar Georgetown Univ Hosp, Washington, DC)

Transfusion 56:466-471, 2016

Background.—Tranexamic acid (TXA) has been reported to demonstrate efficacy in reducing blood loss during arthroplasty procedures.

Study Design and Methods.—This study examines the effectiveness of TXA as a central element of a patient blood management program (PBMP) by evaluating blood loss and transfusion of red blood cells in three consecutive groups of patients undergoing routine total knee arthroplasty (TKA). Approximately 200 patients were in each group as follows: Group 1 was a control without TXA, Group 2 was intraarticular administration, and Group 3 was intravenous (IV) administration.

Results.—The IV group demonstrated a small but significant lower blood loss compared to the two other groups measured by hemoglobin (Hb) drift and nadir Hb levels. The routine use of TXA along with the other aspects of our PBMP provided significant cost savings due to the reduction in transfusions as well as a decrease in length of stay and has been an important element of our successful implementation of a PBMP.

Conclusion.—This study demonstrates a significant benefit from the routine use of TXA for total knee arthroplasty and is one of the first studies to demonstrate a small but significant benefit for IV administration in comparison to intraarticular administration. The routine use of TXA as a central element of a PBMP provides a cost savings and can help reduce the rate of transfusions for total knee arthroplasty.

▶ The concept and message in this article are not complicated and require little comment. I have included it here simply to underscore that tranexamic acid use does markedly decrease blood loss after total knee arthroplasty. My sons, surgeons at Mayo and University of Texas Health Science Center—San Antonio, introduced me to this treatment several years ago. I have used it ever since. This modality must be introduced into practice, and this is the reason this article is included here. It is interesting and attractive to note the intravenous administration is as good, and possibly more effective, than direct injection. I am attracted to letting the anesthesiologist administer the drug intravenously, meaning it's one one less thing for me to do and the patient benefits. This must be added to the practice because the trump card: it is also cost-effective. Everyone wins.

B. F. Morrey, MD

Blood Loss and Transfusion After Topical Tranexamic Acid Administration in Primary Total Knee Arthroplasty

Wang H, Shen B, Zeng Y (Sichuan Univ, Chengdu, China)

Orthopedics 38:e1007-e1016, 2015

There has been much debate and controversy about the safety and efficacy of the topical use of tranexamic acid in primary total knee arthroplasty (TKA). The purpose of this study was to perform a meta-analysis to evaluate whether there is less blood loss and lower rates of transfusion after topical tranexamic acid administration in primary TKA. A systematic review of the electronic databases PubMed, CENTRAL, Web of Science, and Embase was undertaken. All randomized, controlled trials and prospective cohort studies evaluating the effectiveness of topical tranexamic acid during primary TKA were included. The focus of the analysis was on the outcomes of blood loss results, transfusion rate, and thromboembolic complications. Subgroup analysis was performed when possible. Of 387 studies identified, 16 comprising 1421 patients (1481 knees) were eligible for data extraction and meta-analysis. This study indicated that when compared with the control group, topical application of tranexamic acid significantly reduced total drain output (mean difference, −227.20; 95% confidence interval, −347.11 to −107.30; $P < .00001$), total blood loss (mean difference, −311.28; 95% confidence interval, −404.94 to −217.62; $P < .00001$), maximum postoperative hemoglobin decrease (mean difference, −0.73; 95% confidence interval, −0.96 to −0.50; $P < .00001$), and blood transfusion requirements (risk ratios, 0.33; 95% confidence interval, 0.24 to 0.43; $P = .14$). The authors found a statistically significant reduction in blood loss and transfusion rates when using topical tranexamic acid in primary TKA. Furthermore, the currently available evidence does not support an increased risk of deep venous thrombosis or pulmonary embolism due to tranexamic acid administration. Topical tranexamic acid was effective for reducing postoperative blood loss and transfusion requirements without increasing the prevalence of thromboembolic complications.

▶ This article is included to reinforce the game-changing effect of tranexa mic acid in reducing blood loss. This may now be well recognized and accepted. Although the data of the advantageous effect of this agent in reducing blood loss is no longer questioned, the efficacy of a topical application is of value. Suffice to say, the topical application of this agent is also measurably effective in reducing blood loss after total knee replacement. Clinical relevance:QED.

B. F. Morrey, MD

The difficult primary total knee arthroplasty: a review

Baldini A, Castellani L, Traverso F, et al (IFCA Inst, Florence, Italy; et al)

Bone Joint J 97-B:30-39, 2015

Primary total knee arthroplasty (TKA) is a reliable procedure with reproducible long-term results. Nevertheless, there are conditions related to the type of patient or local conditions of the knee that can make it a difficult procedure. The most common scenarios that make it difficult are discussed in this review. These include patients with many previous operations and incisions, and those with severe coronal deformities, genu recurvatum, a stiff knee, extra-articular deformities and those who have previously undergone osteotomy around the knee and those with chronic dislocation of the patella.

Each condition is analysed according to the characteristics of the patient, the pre-operative planning and the reported outcomes.

When approaching the difficult primary TKA surgeons should use a systematic approach, which begins with the review of the existing literature for each specific clinical situation (Fig 1).

▶ This comprehensive article is difficult to summarize. Probably the most important point is that a specific review of the literature addressing the problem at hand is the best way to manage the patient. Of note, the authors categorize 7 presenting characteristics that are cause for concern (Fig 1). For me, the key issues are as follows:

1. Wound problems. Solution: Anticipate and always consult a plastic surgeon colleague before the procedure.
2. Varus/valgus alignment. Solution: assess static soft tissue versus osseous contributions. Virtual execution of the procedure before the actual surgery. Beware the valgus knee with >15 degree flexion contracture, which places the peroneal nerve at risk.

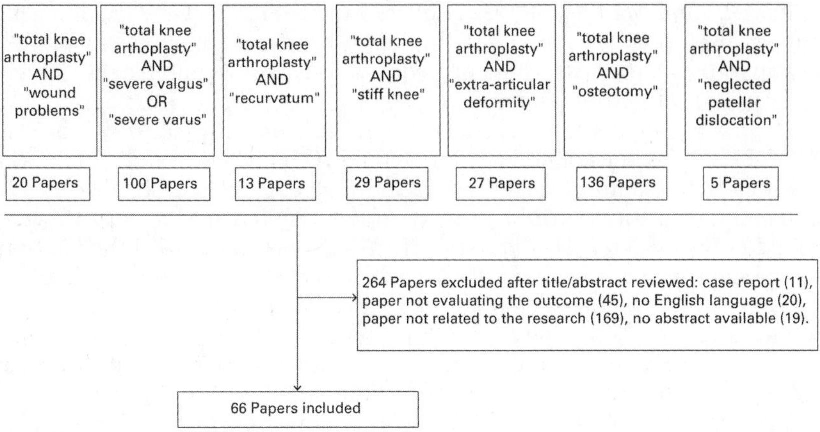

FIGURE 1.—Flow chart of randomised controlled trials and cohort studies identified for the review. (Reprinted from Baldini A, Castellani L, Traverso F, et al. The difficult primary total knee arthroplasty: a review. *Bone Joint J.* 2015;97-B:30-39, with permission from Baldini.)

3. Recurvatum. Solution: assess cause, and adjust cust and soft tissue tension.
4. Stiff/aggressive release as part of the exposure. Solution: be sure the vascular status is understood; often rewires additional osseous resection, thinner poly.
5. Extra-articular deformity. Solution: can it be corrected with the implant, or does it require a staged osteotomy?
6. Prior osteotomy: Solution: beware of posterior scarring of the popliteal artery to the capsule!
7. Patella malalignment: Solution: be prepared to adjust rotatory position of components as well as release and plication.

B. F. Morrey, MD

Effect of rotational alignment on outcome of total knee arthroplasty: a systematic review of the literature and correlation analysis

Valkering KP, Breugem SJ, van den Bekerom MPJ, et al (Amphia Hosp, Breda, the Netherlands; Orthopedium, Delft, the Netherlands; OLVG Hosp, Amsterdam, the Netherlands)

Acta Orthop 86:432-439, 2015

Background and Purpose.—Poor outcomes have been linked to errors in rotational alignment of total knee arthroplasty components. The aims of this study were to determine the correlation between rotational alignment and outcome, to review the success of revision for malrotated total knee arthroplasty, and to determine whether evidence-based guidelines for malrotated total knee arthroplasty can be proposed.

Patients and Methods.—We conducted a systematic review including all studies reporting on both rotational alignment and functional outcome. Comparable studies were used in a correlation analysis and results of revision were analyzed separately.

Results.—846 studies were identified, 25 of which met the inclusion criteria. From this selection, 11 studies could be included in the correlation analysis. A medium positive correlation ($\rho = 0.44$, 95% CI: 0.27–0.59) and a large positive correlation ($\rho = 0.68$, 95% CI: 0.64–0.73) were found between external rotation of the tibial component and the femoral component, respectively, and the Knee Society score. Revision for malrotation gave positive results in all 6 studies in this field.

Interpretation.—Medium and large positive correlations were found between tibial and femoral component rotational alignment on the one hand and better functional outcome on the other. Revision of malrotated total knee arthroplasty may be successful. However, a clear cutoff point for revision for malrotated total knee arthroplasty components could not be identified.

▶ This study is included because it highlights one of the most important technical considerations in knee replacement: proper rotational alignment of both components. The findings are straightforward in demonstrating the functional relevance as well as the correlation with reoperation for excessive rotational malalignment. Unfortunately, the review of the literature does not provide the threshold above which the rotational position becomes symptomatic or requires revision. Additionally, despite the advances in computer navigation, rotational alignment remains somewhat elusive to being amenable to improvement with these systems.

B. F. Morrey, MD

Low Albumin Levels, More Than Morbid Obesity, Are Associated With Complications After TKA

Nelson CL, Elkassabany NM, Kamath AF, et al (Univ of Pennsylvania, Philadelphia)

Clin Orthop Relat Res 473:3163-3172, 2015

Background.—Morbid obesity and malnutrition are thought to be associated with more frequent perioperative complications after TKA. However, morbid obesity and malnutrition often are co-occurring conditions. Therefore it is important to understand whether morbid obesity, malnutrition, or both are independently associated with more frequent perioperative complications. In addition, assessing the magnitude of an increase in complications and whether these complications are major or minor is important for both conditions.

Questions/Purposes.—We asked: (1) Is morbid obesity independently associated with more frequent major perioperative complications after

TKA? (2) Are major perioperative complications after TKA more prevalent among patients with a low serum albumin?

Methods.—The National Surgical Quality Improvement Program (NSQIP) database was analyzed from 2006 to 2013. Patients were grouped as morbidly obese (BMI ≥ 40 kg/m^2) or nonmorbidly obese (BMI ≥ 18.5 kg/m^2 to < 40 kg/m^2), or by low serum albumin (serum albumin level < 3.5 mg/dL) or normal serum albumin (serum albumin level < 3.5 mg/dL). The study cohort included 77,785 patients, including 35,573 patients with a serum albumin level of 3.5 g/dL or greater and 1570 patients with a serum albumin level less than 3.5 g/dL. Therefore, serum albumin levels were available for only 37,173 of the 77,785 of the patients (48%). There were 66,382 patients with a BMI between 18.5 kg/m^2 and 40 kg/m^2 and 11,403 patients with a BMI greater than 40 kg/m^2. Data were recorded on patient mortality along with 21 complications reported in the NSQIP. We also developed three composite complication variables to represent risk of any infections, cardiac or pulmonary complications, and any major complications. For each complication, multivariate logistic regression analysis was performed. Independent variables included patient age, sex, race, BMI, American Society of Anesthesiologists classification, year of surgery, and Charlson comorbidity index score.

Results.—Mortality was not increased in the morbidly obese group (0.14% vs 0.14%; $p = 0.942$). Patients who were morbidly obese were more likely to have progressive renal insufficiency (0.30% vs 0.10%; odds ratio [OR], 2.47; 95% CI, 1.27–4.29; $p < 0.001$), superficial infection (1.07% vs 0.55%; OR, 1.87; 95% CI, 1.39–2.51; $p < 0.001$), and sepsis (0.36% vs 0.23%; OR, 1.70; 95% CI, 1.04–2.53; $p = 0.034$) compared with patients who were not morbidly obese. Patients who were morbidly obese were less likely to require blood transfusion (8.68% vs 12.06%; OR, 0.70; 95% CI, 0.63–0.77; $p < 0.001$) compared with patients who were not morbidly obese. Morbid obesity was not associated with any of the other 21 perioperative complications recorded in the NSQIP database. With respect to the composite complication variables, patients who were morbidly obese had an increased risk of any infection (3.31% vs 2.41%; OR, 1.38; 95% CI, 1.16–1.64; $p < 0.001$) but not for cardiopulmonary or any major complication. The group with low serum albumin had higher mortality than the group with normal serum albumin (0.64% vs 0.15%; OR, 3.17; 95% CI, 1.58–6.35; $p = 0.001$). Patients in the low serum albumin group were more likely to have a superficial surgical site infection (1.27% vs 0.64%; OR, 1.27; 95% CI, 1.09–2.75; $p = 0.020$); deep surgical site infection (0.38% vs 0.12%; OR, 3.64; 95% CI, 1.54–8.63; $p = 0.003$); organ space surgical site infection (0.45% vs 0.15%; OR, 2.71; 95% CI, 1.23–5.97; $p = 0.013$); pneumonia (1.21 vs 0.29%; OR, 3.55; 95% CI, 2.14–5.89; $p < 0.001$); require unplanned intubation (0.51% vs 0.17%, OR, 2.24; 95% CI, 1.07–4.69; $p = 0.033$); and remain on a ventilator more than 48 hours (0.38% vs 0.07%; OR, 4.03; 95% CI, 1.64–9.90; $p = 0.002$). They are more likely to have progressive renal insufficiency (0.45% vs 0.12%; OR, 2.71;

95% CI, 1.21–6.07; $p = 0.015$); acute renal failure (0.32% vs 0.06%; OR, 5.19; 95% CI, 1.96–13.73; $p = 0.001$); cardiac arrest requiring cardiopulmonary resuscitation (0.19% vs 0.12%; OR, 3.74; 95% CI, 1.50–9.28; $p = 0.005$); and septic shock (0.38% vs 0.08%; OR, 4.4; 95% CI, 1.74–11.09; $p = 0.002$). Patients in the low serum albumin group also were more likely to require blood transfusion (17.8% vs 12.4%; OR, 1.56; 95% CI, 1.35–1.81; $p < 0.001$). In addition, among the three composite complication variables, any infection (5.0% vs 2.4%; OR, 2.0; 95% CI, 1.53–2.61; $p < 0.001$) and any major complication (2.4% vs 1.3%; OR, 1.41; 95% CI, 1.00–1.97; $p = 0.050$) were more prevalent among the patients with low serum albumin. There was no difference for cardiopulmonary complications.

Conclusions.—Morbid obesity is not independently associated with the majority of perioperative complications measured by the NSQIP and was associated only with increases in progressive renal insufficiency, superficial surgical site infection, and sepsis among the 21 perioperative variables measured. However, low serum albumin was associated with increased mortality and multiple additional major perioperative complications after TKA. Low serum albumin, more so than morbid obesity, is associated with major perioperative complications. This is an important finding, as low serum albumin may be more modifiable than morbid obesity in patients who are immobile or have advanced knee osteoarthritis.

Level of Evidence.—Level III, prognostic study (Fig 2).

▶ I'm not too sure how much value this investigation will be to the orthopaedic surgeon, but it should be useful. We can't do much about the ever-increasing number of obese and morbidly obese patient who walks through the door.

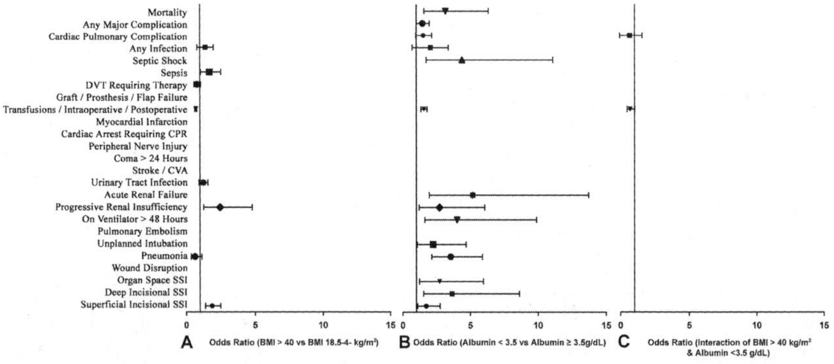

FIGURE 2.—A–C Odds ratios with 95% CIs are shown for mortality and selected perioperative complications of (A) morbid obesity versus nonmorbid obesity, (B) serum albumin level less than 3.5 g/dL versus serum albumin level of 3.5 g/dL or greater, and (C) the interaction of morbid obesity and serum albumin level less than 3.5 g/dL. DVT = deep venous thrombosis; CPR = cardiopulmonary resuscitation; CVA = cerebrovascular accident; SSI = surgical site infection. (Reprinted from Nelson CL, Elkassabany NM, Kamath AF, et al. Low albumin levels, more than morbid obesity, are associated with complications after TKA. *Clin Orthop Relat Res.* 2015;473:3163-3172, with permission from The Association of Bone and Joint Surgeons.)

But we can correct albumin deficiency. This interesting investigation of the independent impact of these 2 factors clearly indicated the low albumin condition is the dominant variable in most medical perioperative complications (Fig 2). So the special feature of this article is that it offers a new insight that may be of value, and it is actionable: we may be able to use these data to lessen postoperative medical complications.

B. F. Morrey, MD

Recurrent Hemarthroses After TKA Treated With an Intraarticular Injection of Yttrium-90

Fine S, Klestov A (Greenslopes Private Hosp, Brisbane, Australia; Royal Brisbane and Women's Hosp, Herston, Australia)
Clin Orthop Relat Res 474:850-853, 2016

Background.—Recurrent hemarthroses after a TKA are uncommon and usually respond to nonoperative treatment or intervention using angiographic embolization or synovectomy. However, in rare circumstances, the problem can be resistant to treatment.

Case Description.—We report the case of a patient who had recurrent hemarthroses after a TKA. During the first 18 months after surgery, the patient experienced 48 episodes consistent with bleeding into the knee. The bleeding episodes recurred despite use of traditional treatments, including arthroscopy, open synovectomy and embolization of a small, false aneurysm. The patient ultimately received an intraarticular injection of yttrium-90 silica/citrate, and the hemarthroses ceased soon after the injection. At last review, 25 months after the injection, the patient had experienced no additional bleeding episodes.

Literature Review.—On review of the literature, we found only one other report in which yttrium-90 was used successfully in a similar situation.

Clinical Relevance.—Yttrium-90 may be considered a treatment option in patients with recurrent hemarthroses after TKA, especially when the condition has not responded to more traditional treatments. The long-term risk of treatment with yttrium-90 for recurrent hemarthroses after a TKA remains unclear.

► We very rarely include case reports in the Year Book. The reason for this exception is that recurrent hemarthrosis can pose a very difficult problem; fortunately, it is uncommon. The evaluation can be extensive, including arteriograms. The use of ytirium-90 is a simple and attractive option that is simple to administer. This has been suggested as a chemical synovectomy at the elbow, but the proximity of the ulnar nerve and its effect on cartilage has made me reluctant to use it in this joint. I would be less concerned about these issues at the knee.

B. F. Morrey, MD

Diabetes is associated with persistent pain after hip and knee replacement

Rajamäki TJ, Jämsen E, Puolakka PA, et al (Univ of Tampere, Finland; et al)

Acta Orthop 86:586-593, 2015

Background and Purpose.—In some patients, for unknown reasons pain persists after joint replacement, especially in the knee. We determined the prevalence of persistent pain following primary hip or knee replacement and its association with disorders of glucose metabolism, metabolic syndrome (MetS), and obesity.

Patients and Methods.—The incidence of pain in the operated joint was surveyed 1–2 years after primary hip replacement (74 patients (4 bilateral)) or primary knee replacement (119 patients (19 bilateral)) in 193 osteoarthritis patients who had participated in a prospective study on perioperative hyperglycemia. Of the 155 patients who completed the survey, 21 had undergone further joint replacement surgery during the follow-up and were excluded, leaving 134 patients for analysis. Persistent pain was defined as daily pain in the operated joint that had lasted over 3 months. Factors associated with persistent pain were evaluated using binary logistic regression with adjustment for age, sex, and operated joint.

Results.—49 of the 134 patients (37%) had a painful joint and 18 of them (14%) had persistent pain. A greater proportion of knee patients than hip patients had a painful joint (46% vs. 24%; $p = 0.01$) and persistent pain (20% vs. 4%; $p = 0.007$). Previously diagnosed diabetes was strongly associated with persistent pain (5/19 vs. 13/115 in those without; adjusted OR = 8, 95% CI: 2–38) whereas MetS and obesity were not. However, severely obese patients (BMI $\geq$ 35) had a painful joint (but not persistent pain) more often than patients with BMI < 30 (14/21 vs. 18/71; adjusted OR = 5, 95% CI: 2–15).

Interpretation.—Previously diagnosed diabetes is a risk factor for persistent pain in the operated joint 1–2 years after primary hip or knee replacement.

▶ This article carries a larger message than the specific focus of the study. Despite the often-quoted statistics of 95% satisfactory results for hip and knee replacement at 5 to 10 years, this refers to survival of the implant, not freedom from pain. A growing body of literature recognizes the frequency of pain after surgery. This study documents that residual joint pain occurs in as many as 46% patients, twice as common in the knee. Also, persistent pain, that is, continuous pain for more than 3 months, occurs 5 times more frequently in the knee. The focus of the study is important, documenting that those with diabetes have statistically more persistent pain; those with a body mass index > 35 have residual but not persistent pain. For me, the take-home message is to advise patients with diabetes that they may not have the same pain relief as patients without this diagnosis. This finding is news to me.

B. F. Morrey, MD

Clinical value of SPECT/CT in the painful total knee arthroplasty (TKA): a prospective study in a consecutive series of 100 TKA

Hirschmann MT, Amsler F, Rasch H (Kantonsspital Baselland (Bruderholz, Liestal, Laufen), Switzerland; Amsler Consulting, Basel, Switzerland; Kantonsspital Baselland, Bruderholz, Switzerland)

Eur J Nucl Med Mol Imaging 42:1869-1882, 2015

Purpose.—Bone single photon emission computed tomography (SPECT)/CT is considered as beneficial in unhappy patients with pain, stiffness or swelling after total knee arthroplasty (TKA). The purpose of this study was to identify typical patterns of bone tracer uptake (BTU), distribution and intensity values in patients after TKA. The above findings were correlated with the type and fixation of TKA, the time from TKA and intraoperative findings at revision surgery.

Methods.—A total of 100 knees of 84 consecutive patients (mean age ± SD 70 ± 11 years) after TKA with persistent knee pain were prospectively included. All patients underwent clinical examination, standardized radiographs and ^{99m}Tchydroxymethane diphosphonate (HDP) SPECT/CT as part of a routine diagnostic algorithm. The diagnosis before and after SPECT/CT and final treatment were recorded. TKA component position was determined on 3-D reconstructed images. Intensity and anatomical distribution of BTU was determined. Maximum intensity values were recorded as well as ratios in relation to the proximal midshaft of the femur. Univariate analyses (chi-square test, Pearson's correlation and *t* test for independent samples) were performed ($p < 0.05$).

Results.—SPECT/CT changed the clinical diagnosis and final treatment in 85/100 (85%) knees. Intraoperative findings confirmed the preoperative SPECT/CT diagnosis in 32/33 knees (97%). TKA loosening as well as progression of patellofemoral osteoarthritis (OA) was correctly diagnosed in 100% of knees. Typical patterns of BTU for specific pathologies were identified. Loose femoral TKA components significantly correlated with increased BTU at the lateral femoral regions ($p < 0.05$). Loose tibial TKA components significantly correlated with increased BTU at all tibial regions ($p < 0.05$) and around the tibial peg ($p > 0.01$).

Conclusion.—The diagnostic benefits of SPECT/CT in patients after TKA have been proven. Typical pathology-related BTU patterns were identified, which will improve reporting quality. Due to the benefits in establishing the correct diagnosis, SPECT/CT should be part of the routine diagnostic algorithm for patients with pain after TKA.

▶ Diagnosing the cause of pain in the total knee arthroplasty patient can be difficult. In most instances, the concern is infection or loosening. When the plane films are not diagnostic, and when the blood work is not suggestive, I personally use the T99 bone scan extensively, and without question the single photon emission computed tomography scan is the most sensitive to show a response if one exists. This prospective, level I study confirms the value of the SPECT to accurately diagnose the cause of the pain. The message is clear: perform this study if there is a painful knee without obvious cause.

B. F. Morrey, MD

Intra-articular infusion: a direct approach to treatment of infected total knee arthroplasty

Whiteside LA, Roy ME, Nayfeh TA (Missouri Bone and Joint Res Foundation, St. Louis; Medstar Haarbor Orthopaedics, Baltimore, MD)

Bone Joint J 98-B:31-36, 2016

Bactericidal levels of antibiotics are difficult to achieve in infected total joint arthroplasty when intravenous antibiotics or antibiotic-loaded cement spacers are used, but intraarticular (IA) delivery of antibiotics has been effective in several studies. This paper describes a protocol for IA delivery of antibiotics in infected knee arthroplasty, and summarises the results of a pharmacokinetic study and two clinical follow-up studies of especially difficult groups: methicillin-resistant *Staphylococcus aureus* and failed two-stage revision. In the pharmacokinetic study, the mean synovial vancomycin peak level was 9242 (3956 to 32 150; SD 7608 μg/mL) among the 11 patients studied. Serum trough level ranged from 4.2 to 25.2 μg/mL (mean, 12.3 μg/mL; average of 9.6% of the joint trough value), which exceeded minimal inhibitory concentration. The success rate exceeded 95% in the two clinical groups. IA delivery of antibiotics is shown to be safe and effective, and is now the first option for treatment of infected total joint arthroplasty in our institution.

▶ This may appear to represent a new approach to the infected total knee. Some may remember "closed continuous irrigation" as treatment of septic joints before the era of joint replacement. The important issues to be considered is that this is a complex protocol but is documented to have a greater than 90% success rate, even in the face of resistant organisms. It is a costly process, but as a single-staged adjunct it is less expensive treatment than the cost of a 2-staged replacement. The complication rate, to date is low, but the sample size is relatively small. Finally, the ultimate standard today is the blended outcome of lack of recurrence and high-quality function. A single-staged replacement offers the best chance for a good functional outcome. It will be important to observe if others adopt this approach.

B. F. Morrey, MD

Functional outcomes of acutely infected knee arthroplasty: a comparison of different surgical treatment options

Dzaja I, Howard J, Somerville L, et al (Western Univ, London, Ontario, Canada; London Health Sciences Centre, Ontario, Canada)

Can J Surg 58:402-407, 2015

Background.—An infected total knee arthroplasty (TKA) can be treated with irrigation and débridement with polyethylene exchange (IDPE) or a 2-staged revision (2SR). Although research has examined infection eradication rates of both treatments, patient outcomes have not been reported. We examined patient-reported outcomes following treatment compared with matched, noninfected controls.

Methods.—We retrospectively identified patients with infected TKAs who had undergone the index procedure between May 1991 and November 2011. Patient-reported outcomes included the 12-item Short Form Health Survey, Western Ontario and McMaster Universities Arthritis Index, and Knee Society Scores as well as range of motion. Patients with noninfected primary TKAs matched by age and age-adjusted Charlson Comorbidity Index score were used as controls. Intention-to-treat groups of 2SR and IDPE were used, with the IDPE group subdivided into successful and unsuccessful groups.

Results.—We included 145 patients with infected TKAs with mean follow-up of 64.2 months and 145 controls with a mean follow-up of 35.4 months in our analysis. Outcomes of the controls and the successful IDPE groups were equivalent. The 2SR cohort had lower scores in all categories than controls. There was a 39% success rate in eradicating infection with IDPE. Patients in whom IDPE failed had lower scores in all categories than controls. There was no difference between the failed IDPE group and the 2SR group.

Conclusion.—Controversy regarding treatment options for acutely infected TKA has been focused on infection eradication. However, functional outcomes following treatment need to be taken into consideration. Patients whose infections were successfully treated with IDPE had equivalent outcomes to controls.

► This retrospective study provides additional clinical data that support the growing clinical practice to treat infected joints with a 1-stage procedure, or, as in some instances, 2 stage but with retention of the implant. The numerous outcome measures focus on posttreatment function, not just freedom form infection. This well-done study clearly documents 2 important findings. The control of infection is comparable between the single-stage debridement and poly exchange and the 2-staged revision. Importantly, the functional outcome is comparable to the uninfected knee. This study further strengthens the justification of the practice we and others have adopted for the past 10 to 15 years.

B. F. Morrey, MD

75% success rate after open debridement, exchange of tibial insert, and antibiotics in knee prosthetic joint infections: Report on 145 cases from the Swedish Knee Arthroplasty Register

Holmberg A, Thórhallsdóttir VG, Robertsson O, et al (Lund Univ, Sweden; Univ of Iceland, Reykjavík; et al)

Acta Orthop 86:457-462, 2015

Background and Purpose.—Prosthetic joint infection (PJI) is a leading cause of early revision after total knee arthroplasty (TKA). Open debridement with exchange of tibial insert allows treatment of infection with retention of fixed components. We investigated the success rate of this procedure in the treatment of knee PJIs in a nationwide material, and determined whether the results were affected by microbiology, antibiotic treatment, or timing of debridement.

Patients and Methods.—145 primary TKAs revised for the first time, due to infection, with debridement and exchange of the tibial insert were identified in the Swedish Knee Arthroplasty Register (SKAR). *Staphylococcus aureus* was the most common pathogen (37%) followed by coagulase-negative staphylococci (CNS) (23%). Failure was defined as death before the end of antibiotic treatment, revision of major components due to infection, life-long antibiotic treatment, or chronic infection.

Results.—The overall healing rate was 75%. The type of infecting pathogen did not statistically significantly affect outcome. Staphylococcal infections treated without a combination of antibiotics including rifampin had a higher failure rate than those treated with rifampin (RR = 4, 95% CI: 2–10). In the 16 cases with more than 3 weeks of symptoms before treatment, the healing rate was 62%, as compared to 77% in the other cases ($p = 0.2$). The few patients with a revision model of prosthesis at primary operation had a high failure rate (5 of 8).

Interpretation.—Good results can be achieved by open debridement with exchange of tibial insert. It is important to use an antibiotic combination including rifampin in staphylococcal infections.

► I was attracted to this article because it is aligned with our current treatment of total elbow infections. It is useful to develop treatments that pose a lower morbidity to the patient, have better functional results, and decrease costs. A 1-stage debridement, replacing only the ultra-high-molecular-weight polyethylene satisfies these goals. The only statistical factor that influenced the 75% success rate was the use of rifampin in those with staph infection. Of note, the authors considered long-term suppression as a failure, a rather strict criteria for success. Also I would consider a 62% success rate in those with symptoms at more than 3 weeks to be clinically significant compared with 77% treated within 3 weeks, even though it is not statistically significant.

B. F. Morrey, MD

Can Good Infection Control Be Obtained in One-stage Exchange of the Infected TKA to a Rotating Hinge Design? 10-year Results

Zahar A, Kendoff DO, Klatte TO, et al (Ctr for Septic Surgery, Hamburg, Germany; Univ Med Ctr Hamburg-Eppendorf, Germany)

Clin Orthop Relat Res 474:81-87, 2016

Background.—Prosthetic joint infection (PJI) occurs in 1% to 2% of total knee arthroplasties (TKAs). Although two-stage exchange is the preferred management method of patients with chronic PJI in TKA in North America, one-stage exchange is an alternative treatment method, but long-term studies of this approach have not been conducted.

Questions/Purposes.—We reviewed our minimum 9-year results of 70 patients who underwent one-stage exchange arthroplasty with a rotating hinge design to determine: (1) What was the proportion of patients free of infection? (2) What was the patient rate of survival free of any reoperation? (3) What were the clinical outcomes as measured by Hospital for Special Surgery scores? (4) What proportion of patients developed radiographic evidence of loosening?

Methods.—All one-stage revision TKAs for infection between January 1 and December 31, 2002, with a minimum 9-year followup (mean, 10 years; range, 9–11 years), in which patients had been seen within the last 1 year, were included in this retrospective review. During that period, 11 patients with infected TKAs were treated with other approaches (including two-stage approaches in eight); the general indication for one-stage revision was the diagnosis of PJI with a known causative organism. Exclusion criteria were culture-negative preoperative aspiration, known allergy to local antibiotics or bone cement, or cases in which radical débridement was impossible as a result of the involvement of important anatomical structures. Eighty-one patients with PJI were seen during this period; 70 underwent one-stage exchange using our strict protocol and were reimplanted with a rotating hinge TKA. Eleven patients (15.7%) were lost to followup. Hospital for Special Surgery scores were recorded and all radiographs were evaluated for prosthetic loosening. Failure was defined as revision surgery for infection or any other cause.

Results.—Our 10-year infection-free survival was 93% (mean, 4.1; 95% confidence interval [CI], 89%–96%; $p < 0.007$); and the patient 10-year survival rate free of revision for other causes was 91% (mean, 5.2; 95% CI, 86%–95%; $p < 0.002$). Mean Hospital for Special Surgery knee score at last followup was 69.6 (± 22.5 SD; range, 22–100) and the mean improvement in Hospital for Special Surgery knee score from preoperative to most recent followup was 35 (± 24.2 SD; range, 13–99). Evidence of radiographic loosening was seen in 11 patients at last followup, whereby in six patients, there was need for revision surgery.

Conclusions.—Our study results showed an overall infection control rate of 93% and good clinical results using our one-stage approach, which combines aggressive débridement of the collateral ligaments and posterior capsule with a rotating hinge implant. These results are comparable with two-stage techniques at a followup of 10 years; further research into one-stage exchange techniques for PJI in TKA appears warranted.

Level of Evidence.—Level IV, therapeutic study.

▶ This is one of the studies I have been waiting to see. There is clearly a growing desire not to just control infection but also preserve function in the patient with an infected knee replacement. The technique was developed and popularized by the ENDO clinic in Germany. The long-term documentation of both efficacy to treat the infection and to preserve function is documented at 90%. This rivals the efficacy of 2-staged treatment and is far superior from a functional perspective. This is the kind of study that is, or should be, a practice changer. But recognition of the details of this technique are essential before adoption.

B. F. Morrey, MD

Local Bone Quality Affects the Outcome of Prosthetic Total Knee Arthroplasty

Huang C-C, Jiang C-C, Hsieh C-H, et al (Natl Taiwan Univ Yunlin Branch; Natl Taiwan Univ Hosp, Taipei)

J Orthop Res 34:240-248, 2016

Osteoporosis and osteoarthritis commonly coexist in the elderly. In patients undergoing prosthetic total knee arthroplasty (TKA), the bone quality around the knee joint may affect the safety of prosthetic implantation and consequently satisfaction with the surgical outcome. We recruited 50 postmenopausal women undergoing TKA for primary osteoarthritis; 43 completed the study protocol. The bone quality parameters of the operated knee, including bone mineral density assessed using dual-energy X-ray absorptiometry and microarchitecture variables assessed using micro-computed tomography, were determined. Surgical outcomes were assessed according to immediate (<1 week) postoperative pain quantified using the visual analog scale and knee function quantified using the Knee Injury and Osteoarthritis Outcome Score (KOOS) at 2 and 6 months postoperatively. The influence of bone quality parameters on surgical outcomes was analyzed using simple and multiple regression analyses. Volumetric bone mineral density ($R^2 = 0.187–0.234$, $p < 0.01$), the structural model index ($R^2 = 0.103–0.181$, $p < 0.05$), and trabecular separation ($R^2 = 0.289–0.424$, $p < 0.05$) were significantly associated with postoperative pain and improvement according to the KOOS. In conclusion, local bone quality, including mineral content and microarchitecture, affects the surgical outcome of TKA.

▶ Despite the generally accepted truth that the total knee arthroplasty is one of the most successful of all procedures, we continue to be aware of patients who do not have the outcome we would want and expect. In my experience, residual pain, although not common, is often of unknown etiology.

I have always been suspicious of osteoporosis as being associated with loosening, but it never occurred to me to consider bone quality as being correlated to pain in the well-fixed implant. This is a careful and well-done study, so in my opinion, the conclusions can be believed and applied immediately. Simply advise your patient with marked osteoporosis that she or he may experience some pain after surgery due to poor quality bone. Very helpful.

B. F. Morrey, MD

Pain after total knee arthroplasty: a narrative review focusing on the stratification of patients at risk for persistent pain

Lavand'homme P, Thienpont E (Univ Hosp Saint-Luc, Brussels, Belgium)

Bone Joint J 97-B:45-48, 2015

The patient with a painful arthritic knee awaiting total knee arthroplasty (TKA) requires a multidisciplinary approach. Optimal control of acute post-operative pain and the prevention of chronic persistent pain remains a challenge. The aim of this paper is to evaluate whether stratification of patients can help identify those who are at particular risk for severe acute or chronic pain.

Intense acute post-operative pain, which is itself a risk factor for chronic pain, is more common in younger, obese female patients and those suffering from central pain sensitisation. Pre-operative pain, in the knee or elsewhere in the body, predisposes to central sensitisation. Pain due to osteoarthritis of the knee may also trigger neuropathic pain and may be associated with chronic medication like opioids, leading to a state of nociceptive sensitisation called 'opioid-induced hyperalgesia'. Finally, genetic and personality related risk factors may also put patients at a higher risk for the development of chronic pain.

Those identified as at risk for chronic pain would benefit from specific peri-operative management including reduction in opioid intake preoperatively, the peri-operative use of antihyperalgesic drugs such as ketamine and gabapentinoids, and a close post-operative follow-up in a dedicated chronic pain clinic.

▶ Without question, residual pain remains the bane of knee joint replacement surgery. Although this occurs in a relatively few patients, when there is no obvious cause that can be addressed, the situation is frustrating both for the physician and patient. This literature review highlights the relationship of preoperative pain sensation and residual pain. The intensity of pain before surgery, especially if dissociated somewhat from the objective pathology, is a clear red flag. It is also noteworthy to recognize that intense pain, beyond what is considered "typical" is correlated to chronic postoperative pain. The key is to recognize the patient at risk who exhibits preoperatively chronic pain in other anatomic regions, anxiety, and helplessness. These patients should be counseled on the probability of chronic pain after surgery, and efforts should be taken to avoid opoid medication postoperatively.

B. F. Morrey, MD

Outcomes of Varus Valgus Constrained Versus Rotating-Hinge Implants in Total Knee Arthroplasty

Malcolm TL, Bederman SS, Schwarzkopf R (Univ of California, Irvine)
Orthopedics 39:e140-e148, 2016

The stability of a total knee arthroplasty is determined by the ability of the prosthesis components in concert with supportive bone and soft tissue structures to sufficiently resist deforming forces transmitted across the knee joint. Constrained prostheses are used in unstable knees due to their ability to resist varus and valgus transformative forces across the knee. Constraint requires inherent rigidity, which can facilitate early implant failure. The purpose of this study was to describe the comparative indications for surgery and postoperative outcomes of varus valgus constrained knee (VVK) and rotating-hinge knee (RHK) total knee arthroplasty prostheses. Seven retrospective observational studies describing 544 VVK and 254 RHK patients with an average follow-up of 66 months (range, 7-197 months) were evaluated. Patients in both groups experienced similar failure rates ($P = .74$), ranges of motion ($P = .81$), and Knee Society function scores ($P = .29$). Average Knee Society knee scores were 4.2 points higher in VVK patients compared with RHK patients, indicating minimal mid-term clinical differences may exist ($P < .0001$). Absent collateral ligament support is an almost universal indication for RHK implantation vs VVK. Constrained device implantation is routinely guided by inherent stability of the knee, and, when performed, similar postoperative outcomes can be achieved with VVK and RHK prostheses (Fig 6).

► With the high percentage of successful primary knee replacements, the failure mode described in this meta-analysis is not encountered with great frequency. It therefore comes as no surprise that the 7 qualifying studies represent only about 2% to 3% of the surveyed literature. The important parameter of survival was found to be similar in the 2 stabilizing designs. However, the indication of linked rotating devices is different than that for the more simple varus valgus stabilizing designs. The takeaway is that both work reasonably well considering their intended purpose. Of note, the main distinguishing requirement of

Study or Subgroup	Varus Valgus Mean	SD	Total	Rotating Hinge Mean	SD	Total	Weight	Mean Difference IV, Fixed, 95% CI
Fuchs 2004	61.8	14.5	16	61.5	15.5	10	23.8%	0.30 [-11.65, 12.25]
Hwang 2010	85	9.04	15	81	8.96	13	76.2%	4.00 [-2.68, 10.68]
Total (95% CI)			**31**			**23**	**100.0%**	**3.12 [-2.71, 8.95]**

Heterogeneity: $Chi^2 = 0.28$, $df = 1$ ($P = 0.60$); $I^2 = 0\%$
Test for overall effect: $Z = 1.05$ ($P = 0.29$)

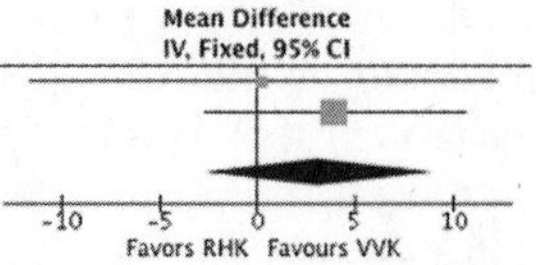

FIGURE 6.—Knee Society function score. Excluded studies were those not reporting postoperative Knee Society function scores for varus valgus knee (VVK) and rotating-hinge knee (RHK) prostheses. (Reprinted from Malcolm TL, Bederman SS, Schwarzkopf R. Outcomes of varus valgus constrained versus rotating-hinge implants in total knee arthroplasty. *Orthopedics*. 2016;39:e140-e148, with permission from SLACK Incorporated.)

the linked implant is a posteriorly unstable knee. However, in spite of this, note that the functional outcome is much better with the varus/valgus stabilizing design (Fig 6). This is to be expected because the soft tissue deficiency is not as severe in these patients.

B. F. Morrey, MD

Comparison of US and Canadian Perioperative Outcomes and Hospital Efficiency After Total Hip and Knee Arthroplasty

Hart A, Bergeron SG, Epure L, et al (Jewish General Hosp, Montréal, Québec, Canada; et al)
JAMA Surg 150:990-998, 2015

Importance.—The combination of an aging population, growing number of medical interventions, and surging economic burden of health care has renewed interest in reevaluating and exploring new health care models.

Objectives.—To compare the performance of the US and Canadian health care systems by assessing major complications following primary total hip arthroplasty (THA) and total knee arthroplasty (TKA) and to measure the efficiency of both health care models by comparing the postoperative length of stay.

Design, Setting, and Participants.—With patients grouped according to the country where they underwent surgery, we queried the National Surgical Quality Improvement Program database to identify 55 335 Canadian and US patients who underwent primary elective THA or TKA between January 1, 2011, and December 31, 2012.

Main Outcomes and Measures.—Differences in patient demographics, as well as the rate of 30-day major complications and length of stay, were compared between patients hospitalized in the United States and Canada.

Results.—Baseline characteristics were similar between the groups. Most US patients underwent general anesthesia (THA, 61.8%; TKA, 59.4%); Canadian patients received more regional anesthesia (THA, 78.7%; TKA, 81.0%). Patients in the United States received more transfusions postoperatively (THA, 9.0% more; TKA, 6.4% more; $P < .001$) and had shorter hospitalizations (THA, 1.4 days less; TKA, 1.3 days less; $P < .001$) with a greater proportion of patients discharged to rehabilitation facilities (THA, 21.6% more; TKA, 26.6% more; $P < .001$). With results reported as incidence rate ratios (95% CIs), after adjusting for all other variables, risk factors, and adverse outcomes, having surgery in Canada increased the postoperative length of stay by 57% (1.57 [1.53-1.61]) for THA and 49% (1.49 [1.46-1.52]) for TKA. With results reported as odds ratios (95% CIs), major complications were significantly more common in Canada following TKA (1.65 [1.31-2.07]) but not THA (1.09 [0.79-1.51]).

Conclusions and Relevance.—The rate of major complications was significantly higher in Canada following TKA, but there was no significant difference following THA. Patients undergoing the procedures in US hospitals also had substantially shorter lengths of hospital stay, perhaps reflecting more efficient postoperative care and discharge planning in those facilities.

▶ I was interested in this topic but did not anticipate the findings. As long as I can remember the US health system has been held to a comparison with the ideal: the Canadian health system. I know from my practice that many Canadians came to Mayo for treatment.

I was thus amazed that this analysis, which has adequate numbers and methodology, actually demonstrates better quality, in some ways, in the US treatment of the total knee arthroplasty (TKA) patient than that of the Canadian patient. The efficiency of total hip arthroplasty is similar. The key is that the length of stay after TKA is statistically less in the United States than that in Canada. The quality is similar. This suggests that in the US we are in fact doing something right.

B. F. Morrey, MD

Better survival of hybrid total knee arthroplasty compared to cemented arthroplasty: A report from the Norwegian Arthroplasty Register 1999–2012

Petursson G, Fenstad AM, Havelin LI, et al (Lovisenberg Diakonale Hosp, Oslo, Norway; Haukeland Univ Hosp, Bergen, Norway; et al)
Acta Orthop 86:714-720, 2015

Background and Purpose.—There have been few comparative studies on total knee replacement (TKR) with cemented tibia and uncemented femur (hybrid TKR). Previous studies have not shown any difference in revision rate between cemented and hybrid fixation, but these studies had few hybrid prostheses. We have evaluated the outcome of hybrid TKR based on data from the Norwegian Arthroplasty Register (NAR).

Patients and Methods.—We compared 4,585 hybrid TKRs to 20,095 cemented TKRs with risk of revision for any cause as the primary endpoint. We included primary TKRs without patella resurfacing that were reported to the NAR during the years 1999–2012. To minimize the possible confounding effect of prosthesis brands, only brands that were used both as hybrids and cemented in more than 200 cases were included. Kaplan-Meier survival analysis and Cox regression analysis were done with adjustment for age, sex, and preoperative diagnosis. To include death as a competing risk, cumulative incidence function estimates were calculated.

Results.—Estimated survival at 11 years was 94.3% (95% CI: 93.9–94.7) in the cemented TKR group and 96.3% (CI: 95.3–97.3) in the hybrid TKR group. The adjusted Cox regression analysis showed a lower risk of revision in the hybrid group (relative risk = 0.58, CI: 0.48–0.72, $p < 0.001$). The hybrid group included 3 brands of prostheses: LCS classic, LCS complete, and Profix. Profix hybrid TKR had lower risk of revision than cemented TKR, but the LCS classic and LCS complete did not. Kaplan-Meier estimated survival at 11 years was 96.8% (CI: 95.6–98.0) in the hybrid Profix group and 95.2% (CI: 94.6–95.8) in the cemented Profix group. Mean operating time was 17 min longer in the cemented group.

Interpretation.—Survivorship of the hybrid TKR at 11 years was better than that for cemented TKR, or the same, depending on the brand of prosthesis. Hybrid fixation appears to be a safe and time-efficient alternative to cemented fixation in total knee replacement surgery.

▶ This contribution is an excellent example of the ongoing and added value of registry studies. This Norwegian study provides data that are contrary to what is generally believed; uncemented knees have a higher failure rate than cemented ones. The study includes approximately 20 000 cemented and 5000 uncemented femoral component (hybrid) knee replacements. With a greater than 10-year follow-up period, the Kaplan-Meier survival calculation is slightly (2%) but statistically better in the hybrid than the cemented replacement. It is noted, however, that this difference does appear to be design specific. Although it may not change the practice, it does justify either fixation choice. The next question is which of the 2 options provides the most reliable revision, should that be necessary. But it is noted the survival of either option is about 95% at 10 years.

B. F. Morrey, MD

A Randomized, Controlled Trial of Total Knee Replacement

Skou ST, Roos EM, Laursen MB, et al (Univ of Southern Denmark, Odense; Aalborg Univ Hosp, Denmark; et al)

N Engl J Med 373:1597-1606, 2015

Background.—More than 670,000 total knee replacements are performed annually in the United States; however, high-quality evidence to support the effectiveness of the procedure, as compared with nonsurgical interventions, is lacking.

Methods.—In this randomized, controlled trial, we enrolled 100 patients with moderate-to-severe knee osteoarthritis who were eligible for unilateral total knee replacement. Patients were randomly assigned to undergo total knee replacement followed by 12 weeks of nonsurgical treatment (total-knee-replacement group) or to receive only the 12 weeks of nonsurgical treatment (nonsurgical-treatment group), which was delivered by physiotherapists and dietitians and consisted of exercise, education, dietary advice, use of insoles, and pain medication. The primary outcome was the change from baseline to 12 months in the mean score on four Knee Injury and Osteoarthritis Outcome Score subscales, covering pain, symptoms, activities of daily living, and quality of life ($KOOS_4$); scores range from 0 (worst) to 100 (best).

Results.—A total of 95 patients completed the 12-month follow-up assessment. In the nonsurgical-treatment group, 13 patients (26%) underwent total knee replacement before the 12-month follow-up; in the total-knee-replacement group, 1 patient (2%) received only nonsurgical treatment. In the intention-to-treat analysis, the total-knee-replacement group had greater improvement in the $KOOS_4$ score than did the nonsurgical-treatment group (32.5 vs. 16.0; adjusted mean difference, 15.8 [95% confidence interval, 10.0 to 21.5]). The total-knee-replacement group had a higher number of serious adverse events than did the nonsurgical-treatment group (24 vs. 6, $P = 0.005$).

Conclusions.—In patients with knee osteoarthritis who were eligible for unilateral total knee replacement, treatment with total knee replacement followed by nonsurgical treatment resulted in greater pain relief and functional improvement after 12 months than did nonsurgical treatment alone. However, total knee replacement was associated with a higher number of serious adverse events than was nonsurgical treatment, and most patients who were assigned to receive nonsurgical treatment alone did not undergo total knee replacement before the 12-month follow-up. (Funded by the Obel Family Foundation and others; MEDIC ClinicalTrials.gov number, NCT01410409.)

▶ This article is included because it would seem to prove the obvious: total knee replacement is an effective procedure. This study from health science investigators in Denmark, published in the *New England Journal of Medicine*, performed a prospective ramdomized study to test the hypothesis that most orthopedic surgeons would feel is unnecessary. Nonetheless at 1 year, the demonstration of improved function of those with total knee replacement was affirmed. They did document, not surprisingly, that those with surgery demonstrated more complications than those without surgery What's the point? Moving forward, the efficacy of orthopedic procedures will be assessed by nonsurgeons with tools with which we are unfamiliar. This will place a greater burden on our specialty to accurately document our outcomes.

B. F. Morrey, MD

9 Foot and Ankle

Introduction

This is one of the most diverse sections in this YEAR BOOK. The anatomic distribution includes the ankle, hind and mid foot and the toes. The pathology includes fracture and soft tissue injuries. The focus is on outcomes of treatment as well as patient subjective satisfaction. Management strategies include both not operative as well as description of specific operative techniques. While there is little international registry data reviewed in the foot section, a good number of the selections represent international authors. Unfortunately, unlike any other joint, replacement of the ankle, while improving, continues to be less reliable than would be desired.

Bernard F. Morrey, MD

Long-term Results After Ankle Syndesmosis Injuries

van Vlijmen N, Denk K, van Kampen A, et al (Radboud Univ Nijmegen Med Centre, The Netherlands; Flinders Univ, Bedford Park, Australia)
Orthopedics 38:e1001-e1006, 2015

Syndesmotic disruption occurs in more than 10% of ankle fractures. Operative treatment with syndesmosis screw fixation has been successfully performed for decades and is considered the gold standard of treatment. Few studies have reported the long-term outcomes of syndesmosis injuries. This study investigated long-term patient-reported, radiographic, and functional outcomes of syndesmosis injuries treated with screw fixation and subsequent timed screw removal. A retrospective cohort study was carried out at a Level I trauma center. The study group included 43 patients who were treated for ankle fractures with associated syndesmotic disruptions between December 2001 and May 2011. The study included case file reviews, self-reported questionnaires, radiologic reviews, and clinical assessments. At 5.1 (±1.76) years after injury, 60% of participants had pain, 26% had degenerative changes, 51% had loss of tibiofibular overlap, and 33% showed medial clear space widening. Retained syndesmotic positions on radiographs were linked to better self-reported outcomes. There is an inversely proportional relation between age at the

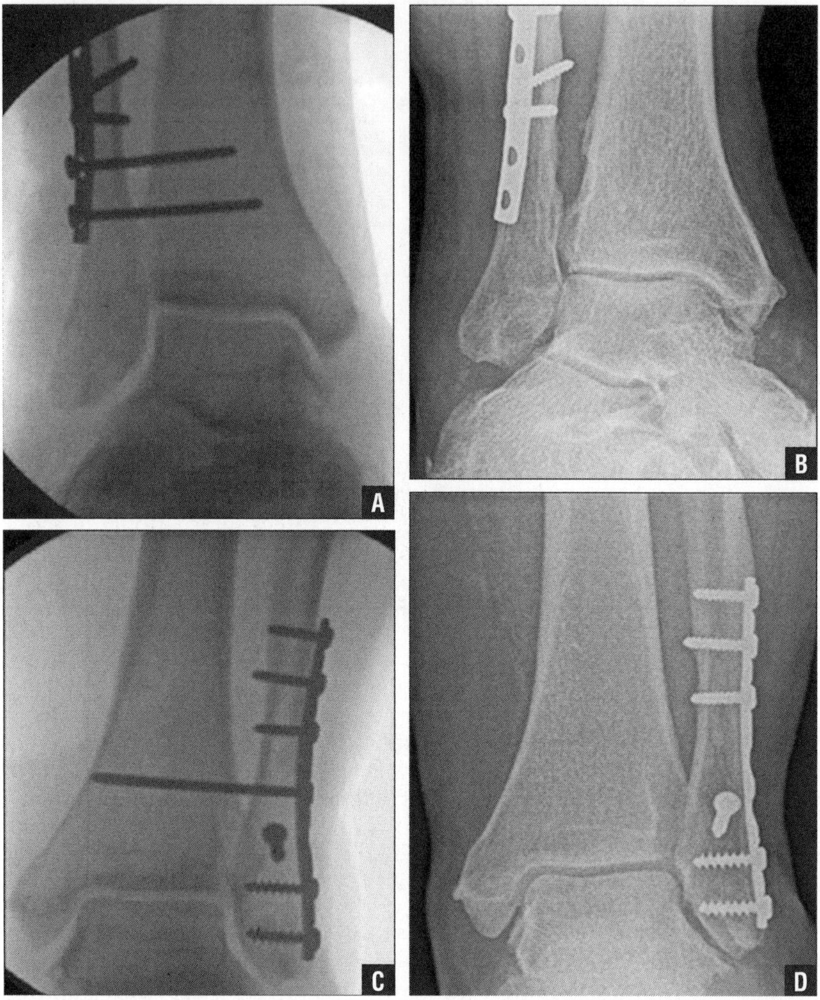

FIGURE 5.—Anteroposterior radiographs showing some widening and osteoarthritis after screw removal over time (A, B) and good outcome at final follow-up (C, D). (Reprinted from van Vlijmen N, Denk K, van Kampen A, et al. Long-term results after ankle syndesmosis injuries. *Orthopedics.* 2015;38:e1001-e1006, with permission from SLACK Incorporated.)

time of injury and satisfaction with the outcome of the ankle fracture as well as a directly proportional relation between age at the time of injury and pain compared with the preinjury state. Optimal restoration and preservation of the syndesmosis is crucial. Syndesmotic disruption is associated with poor long-term outcomes after ankle fracture. Greater age is a risk factor for chronic pain and dissatisfaction with the outcome of ankle fracture and syndesmosis injury. Therefore, patient education to facilitate realistic expectations about recovery is vital, especially in older patients (Fig 5).

▶ This study addresses an important and controversial issue regarding ankle fracture management. There are relative few data that addresses the issue of the impact of different management protocols. These issues justify the inclusion of this article in the Year Book. The methodology is retrospective, and the data are clustered retrospectively, neither of which is ideal. However, the follow-up is thorough and the duration of surveillance is adequate. The findings are of particular importance and speak for themselves. The longer period of screw maintenance of at least 3 months is correlated with less pain and better radiographic evidence of anatomic restoration (Fig 5). It is also of note that the older patient does considerably less well than the younger individual. This may influence our practice decisions with this injury.

B. F. Morrey, MD

Anatomic Reconstruction With a Semitendinosus Allograft for Chronic Lateral Ankle Instability

Dierckman BD, Ferkel RD (Southern California Orthopedic Inst, Van Nuys)

Am J Sports Med 43:1941-1950, 2015

Background.—The modified Broström procedure has been successful for most patients with chronic lateral ankle instability (CLAI); however, a subset of patients has had unsatisfactory outcomes. For those at risk of failure, anatomic reconstruction of the lateral ankle ligaments using a semitendinosus allograft to augment the modified Broström procedure is available.

Purpose.—To report the results of anatomic reconstruction of the lateral ankle with a semitendinosus allograft for the treatment of CLAI.

Study Design.—Case series; Level of evidence, 4.

Methods.—This is a retrospective review of a single surgeon's experience from 2003 to 2011 in performing anatomic lateral ankle ligament reconstruction with a semitendinosus allograft for the treatment of CLAI. Of 38 patients (40 ankles), 31 (33 ankles; 82% of patients) returned for final follow-up and constituted the study group. Preoperatively, all patients completed the American Orthopaedic Foot and Ankle Society Ankle-Hindfoot Score (AHS) and a visual analog scale (VAS) for pain and underwent plain and stress talar tilt radiographs. At the most recent follow-up, patients were evaluated by an independent surgeon and completed the postoperative AHS, Foot-Function Index (FFI), VAS for pain, Tegner activity score, and a satisfaction survey. Patients were evaluated with plain and stress talar tilt and anterior drawer radiographs.

Results.—At a mean follow-up of 38 ± 30 months (range, 24-107 months), 100% of patients were completely satisfied with the procedure. AHS values significantly improved from a mean of 60.3 ± 14.4 to

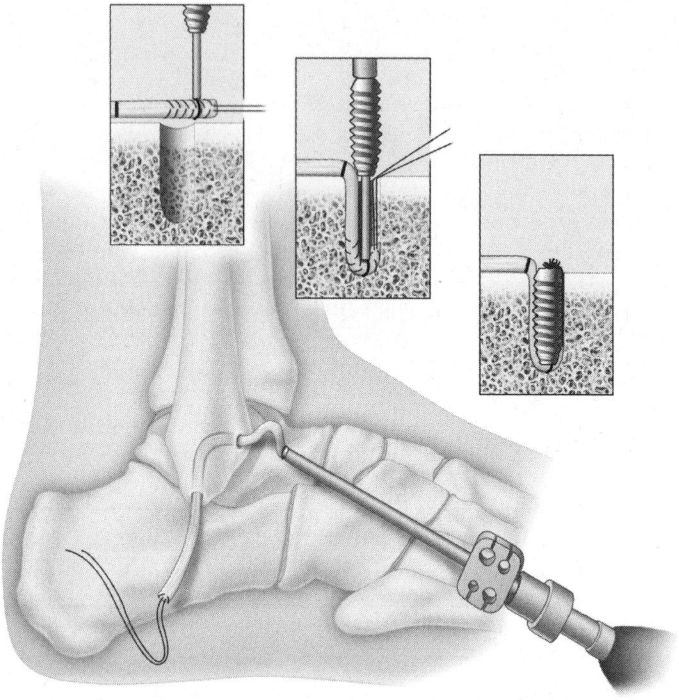

FIGURE 2.—Semitendinosus graft insertion into the talus in a right ankle. A Bio-Tenodesis screw is inserted into the talar tunnel to fixate the graft. The upper images from left to right show the sequential steps of screw fixation. (Reprinted from Dierckman BD, Ferkel RD. Anatomic reconstruction with a semitendinosus allograft for chronic lateral ankle instability. *Am J Sports Med.* 2015;43:1941-1950, with permission from The Author(s).)

87.5 ± 9.3 ($P < .0001$). VAS pain scores significantly decreased from 7.3 ± 1.3 to 1.9 ± 1.8 ($P < .0001$). Twenty-two of 31 patients (71%) either returned to or were 1 level below their previous preoperative or preinjury Tegner activity level. No patients developed arthritic changes beyond grade I on plain radiographs. On stress radiographs, the mean talar tilt decreased from 14.3° ± 5.4° to 3.1° ± 2.4°. The mean postoperative anterior tibiotalar translation was 1.8 ± 1.1 mm, with no patients having greater than 5 mm of translation.

Conclusion.—Anatomic lateral ankle ligament reconstruction with a semitendinosus allograft for the treatment of CLAI leads to high patient satisfaction, decreased pain, a stable ankle without arthritic changes, and significantly improved function (Figs 2 and 3).

► With each passing year, we review fewer and fewer technique and case studies. This article does both. But the question is important, the sample size moderate at 31 procedures, and the surveillance exceeds 3 years. The features of the technique that are of interest are that an allograft semitendinosis was used, the

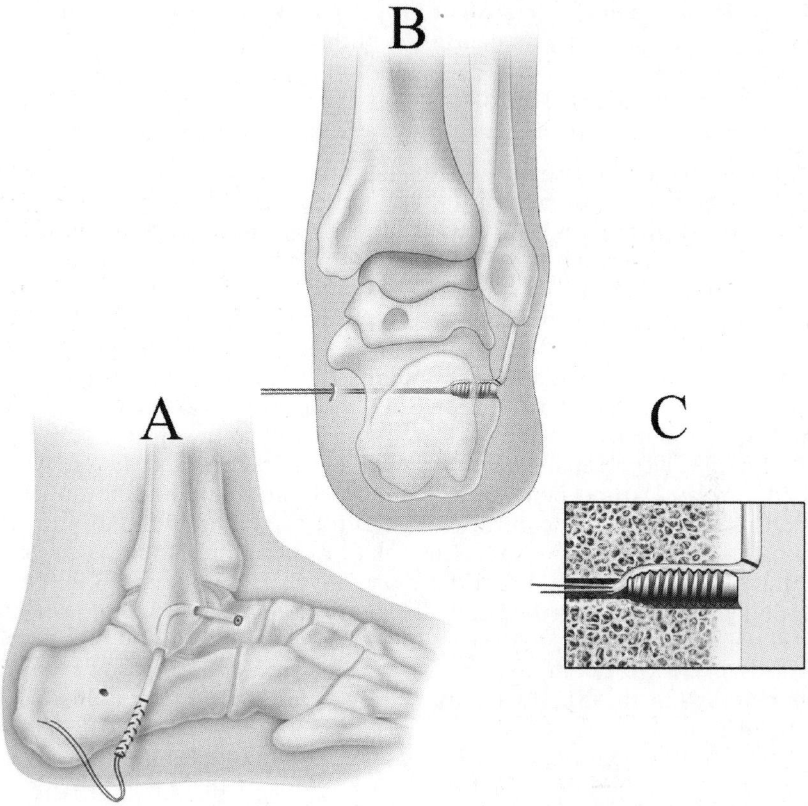

FIGURE 3.—Semitendinosus graft insertion into the calcaneus. (A) The graft is prepared for insertion into the calcaneal tunnel. (B) A posterior view of the right ankle showing the path of the suture through the calcaneus, exiting posteromedially. (C) A close-up view showing the tenodesis screw in place, fixing the graft into the calcaneal tunnel. (Reprinted from Dierckman BD, Ferkel RD. Anatomic reconstruction with a semitendinosus allograft for chronic lateral ankle instability. *Am J Sports Med.* 2015;43:1941-1950, with permission from The Author(s).)

Boström technique was followed, and the graft was secured with a tenodesis screw in the calcaneus and in the talus (Figs 2 and 3). To say the subjective outcome of 100% satisfied is impressive is an understatement. Of specific note, is the mean talar tilt of only 3 degrees. It would seem this technique, if it withstands a longer test of time, may become the standard.

B. F. Morrey, MD

A new form of surgical treatment for patients with avascular necrosis of the talus and secondary osteoarthritis of the ankle

Kodama N, Takemura Y, Ueba H, et al (Shiga Univ of Med Science, Japan)

Bone Joint J 97-B:802-808, 2015

A new method of vascularised tibial grafting has been developed for the treatment of avascular necrosis (AVN) of the talus and secondary osteoarthritis (OA) of the ankle. We used 40 cadavers to identify the vascular anatomy of the distal tibia in order to establish how to elevate a vascularised tibial graft safely. Between 2008 and 2012, eight patients (three male, five female, mean age 50 years; 26 to 68) with isolated AVN of the talus and 12 patients (four male, eight female, mean age 58 years; 23 to 76) with secondary OA underwent vascularised bone grafting from the distal tibia either to revascularise the talus or for arthrodesis. The radiological and clinical outcomes were evaluated at a mean followup of 31 months (24 to 62). The peri-malleolar arterial arch was confirmed in the cadaveric study. A vascularised bone graft could be elevated safely using the peri-malleolar pedicle. The clinical outcomes for the group with AVN of the talus assessed with the mean Mazur ankle grading scores, improved significantly from 39 points (21 to 48) pre-operatively to 81 points (73 to 90) at the final follow-up ($p = 0.01$). In all eight revascularisations, bone healing was obtained without progression to talar collapse, and union was established in 11 of 12 vascularised arthrodeses at a mean follow-up of 34 months (24 to 58). MRI showed revascularisation of the talus in all patients.

We conclude that a vascularised tibial graft can be used both for revascularisation of the talus and for the arthrodesis of the ankle in patients with OA secondary to AVN of the talus.

▶ I uncommonly review techniques in the Year Book. The effects of avascular necrosis (AVN) of the talus are so significant, and the solutions for the established process so limited, that we decided to include this article for the reader's consideration. The quality is good with cadaver studies that provide the anatomic justification. Although I think this may be a bit much for a routine fusion, in the 8 patients with established AVN, it appears to be of considerable benefit (Fig 5a, b in the original article). It does not appear to be too difficult technically. So in the young patient, it would seem this is a contribution to potentially revascularize AVN of the dome of the talus.

B. F. Morrey, MD

Factors Affecting the Outcomes of Uncomplicated Primary Open Ankle Arthrodesis

Chalayon O, Wang B, Blankenhorn B, et al (Univ of Utah, Salt Lake City; Univ of New Mexico, Albuquerque; et al)

Foot Ankle Int 36:1170-1179, 2015

Background.—The objective of this study was to identify factors influencing operative outcomes in straightforward, uncomplicated open ankle fusions.

Methods.—We reviewed all primary open ankle fusions conducted at 1 institution over an 11-year period to identify straightforward, uncomplicated open ankle fusions. Inclusion required a minimum of 6 months follow-up. Patients were excluded for neuropathic arthropathy, insensate limb, failed total ankle replacement, simultaneous arthrodesis of the subtalar joint, or fusions performed within 1 year of injury to salvage failed fixation and painful function due to (1) open fractures, (2) segmental bone loss greater than 1 cm, (3) infection, or (4) talar body fractures. The primary outcome variable was radiographic union at 6 months. Other operative complications were analyzed as secondary outcomes. Five hundred twenty-eight ankle fusion surgeries were performed on 440 patients at 1 institution during the study period. Two hundred fifteen surgeries met inclusion/exclusion eligibility criteria for uncomplicated open ankle fusions.

Results.—The overall union rate was 91%. In this cohort of uncomplicated open ankle fusions, bivariate analysis over a broad range of potential factors and further focused multivariate analysis found that nonunion was more than 3 times more likely to occur after previous subtalar fusion, and 2 times more likely to occur in patients with preoperative varus ankle alignment. The rate of reoperation was 19%, with nonunion revision as the leading reason, followed by hardware removal and incision and drainage for presumed infection. Diabetes was not a significant risk factor of either deep or superficial infection.

Conclusion.—Open ankle fusion failed in 9% of uncomplicated ankles with arthritis. Patients who had an open ankle fusion done after previous subtalar joint fusion, as well as those who had preoperative varus ankle alignment, had a significantly higher rate of nonunion.

Level of Evidence.—Level III, retrospective comparative study (Table 4).

▶ I was impressed with the large experience from a single institution with approximately 500 cases in just over a decade. The topic is a good one: adverse factors predicting nonunion. The data were surprising to me: only prior subtalar fusion or varus hindfoot deformity were statistically related to nonunion (Table 4). The rate of 9% nonunion is a little higher than one might expect from an institution with so much experience. It was also of interest

TABLE 4.—Risk Ratio for Each Predictor Variable Tested for an Association With Nonunion of Fusion Using Univariable Poisson Regression Model (n = 215 surgeries, n = 209 patients)

Risk Factor	No. of Surgeries	No. With Nonunion (%)	Risk Ratio	95% CI	*P* Value
Patient factors					
Age, per I y increase	215		1.00	0.97-1.03	.96
Female sex	100	8 (8)	0.75	0.29-1.91	.54
Diabetes	26	2 (8)	0.79	0.17-3.63	.76
Cardiovascular disease and hypertension	103	9 (9)	0.89	0.37-2.15	.79
Smoker	47	5 (11)	1.21	0.42-3.53	.72
Alcohol use	78	6 (8)	0.75	0.29-1.96	.56
Illicit drug use	6	2 (33)	5.31	0.91-31.00	.06
Etiology					
Nontrauma	55	8 (15)	[Referent]		
Posttraumatic	160	12 (8)	0.52	0.21-1.26	.15
Limiting to subgroup of patients with posttraumatic arthritis					
Late fusion (occurs > I y after trauma)	154	11 (7)	[Referent]		
Early fusion (occurs within I y after trauma)	6	1 (17)	2.33	0.30-18.08	.42
Weight, per kg increase			1.00	0.98-1.02	.94
BMI					
Underweight (BMI < 18.5)	1	1 (100)	11.75	1.31-105.14	.03
Normal (BMI 18.5-25)	47	4 (9)	[Referent]		
Overweight (BMI 25.0-29.9)	56	4 (7)	0.84	0.21-3.36	.80
Obese (BMI 30-34.9)	58	5 (9)	1.01	0.27-3.77	.98
Morbidly obese (BMI ≥ 35)	48	5 (10)	1.22	0.33-4.56	.76
ASA class, per score increase			1.08	0.46-2.51	.87
Preop. bone loss	53	6 (11)	1.31	0.50-3.41	.58
Preop. osteoporosis	64	9 (14)	1.93	0.80-4.66	.14
Preop. infection	8	1 (13)	1.36	0.18-10.17	.76
Previous subtalar fusion	15	4 (27)	4.18	1.19-14.65	.03
Preop. alignment (clinical)					
Neutral	79	3 (4)	[Referent]		
Varus[a]	70	10 (14)	4.22	1.11-16.02	.03
Valgus[a]	55	6 (11)	3.10	0.74-12.98	.12
Unknown	11	1 (9)			
Moment arm (min/max), mm					
Varus (−86.3/−10)	37	2 (5)	0.50	0.10-2.56	.40
Neutral (−10/10)	46	5 (11)	[Referent]		
Valgus (10/47)	31	5 (16)	1.48	0.43-5.13	.53
Tibial-calcaneus axis angle (min/max), degrees					
Varus (−54/−10)	54	5 (9)	1.18	0.09-15.30	.90
Neutral	47	4 (9)	[Referent]		
Valgus (10/31)	13	3 (23)	11.29	0.32-396.03	.18
Talar tilting angle (min/max), degrees					
Varus (−77/−10)	40	7 (18)	2.31	0.88-6.07	.09
Neutral (−10/10)	132	10 (8)	[Referent]		
Valgus (10/37)	30	2 (7)	0.88	0.19-4.02	.87
Absolute value of talar tilting					
Angle, degrees					
< 10	132	10 (8)	[Referent]		
10-19.9	34	5 (15)	1.94	0.66-5.68	.23
> 20	36	4 (11)	1.47	0.46-4.68	.52
Operative factors					
Distal syndesmosis fusion included	153	12 (8)	0.61	0.25-1.49	.28
Approach					

(Continued)

TABLE 4. *(continued)*

Risk Factor	No. of Surgeries	No. With Nonunion (%)	Risk Ratio	95% CI	*P* Value
Open lateral malleolus fused as onlay	141	11 (8)	[Referent]		
Open lateral malleolus removed	10	2 (20)	2.56	0.57-11.56	.22
Anterior approach	47	4 (9)	1.09	0.35-3.43	.88
Posterior approach	10	1 (10)	1.28	0.17-9.93	.81
Mini open	7	2 (29)	3.66	0.81-16.52	.09
Implant					
Screws without plate	147	14 (10)	[Referent]		
Lateral plate	7	0 (0)	[b]		
Anterior plate	47	3 (6)	0.62	0.18-2.11	.44
Posterior plate	10	1 (10)	1.06	0.14-8.00	.95
External fixator	8	2 (25)	2.82	0.65-12.22	.17
Bone graft/substitute					
None	8	1 (13)	1.41	0.16-12.11	.75
Any bone graft	207	19 (9)	[Referent]		

Abbreviations: ASA class, American Society of Anesthesiologists Physical Status classification; BMI, body mass index; CI, confidence interval; Preop., preoperative.

[a]Risk ratio calculated after elimination of patients with "unknown" alignment.

[b]All patients receiving these treatments had successful union, so risk ratio could not be estimated.

Reprinted from Chalayon O, Wang B, Blankenhorn B, et al. Factors affecting the outcomes of uncomplicated primary open ankle arthrodesis. *Foot Ankle Int.* 2015;36:1170-1179, with permission from The Author(s).

that smoking and obesity were not found to be risk factors for nonunion. This is difficult to understand.

B. F. Morrey, MD

Long-Term Outcome of Open Plantar Fascia Release

MacInnes A, Roberts SC, Kimpton J, et al (Ninewells Hosp, Dundee, Scotland; Woodend Hosp, Aberdeen, Scotland; Univ Hosps South Manchester, England)
Foot Ankle Int 37:17-23, 2016

Background.—Plantar fasciitis is thought to be a self-limiting condition best treated by conservative measures, but despite this many patients have a prolonged duration of symptoms and surgery may be indicated. Partial plantar fascial release is reported to have a short-term success rate of up to 80%, but anecdotally this was not thought to represent our local experience.

Methods.—An audit of long-term patient-reported outcomes following open partial plantar fascia release was performed. A total of 30 patients (33 feet) were identified over a 10-year period and case notes were reviewed. Patients were contacted by letter and invited to complete 2 validated patient-reported outcome score questionnaires (Visual Analog Scale—Foot and Ankle [VAS-FA] and Manchester Oxford Foot Questionnaire [MOXFQ]). Responses were received from 24 patients

(26 feet). The average ages were 42.4 (range 24-61) for male and 46.2 (range 33-60) for female patients, with a female/male ratio of 2.7:1. The average duration of treatment prior to operative intervention was 3.1 years (range 1-5). Preoperatively, our cohort underwent a range of conservative measures. All patients were reviewed postoperatively, and average time from surgery to completion of questionnaires was 80 months (range 14-130).

Results.—The outcomes were worse in patients who had received preoperative steroid injections and this was found to be statistically significant. The mean MOXFQ score was 33.6 ± 3.9 (0-64). Mean VAS-FA score was 57.8 ± 4.9 (24-100).

Conclusion.—This study found a negative correlation between duration of follow-up and outcome, in both MOXFQ and VAS-FA, showing that patients continued to improve many years postoperatively. The authors also found worse outcomes with preoperative steroid injections, better outcomes in older patients, and a weak gender bias, suggesting results in men were better than those in women. A prolonged recovery period and generally poor outcomes leads the authors to suggest that open plantar fascia release is of questionable clinical value and that patients may improve in the natural course of the disease, in spite of surgery.

Level of Evidence.—Level III, comparative study (Fig 4).

▶ Having spent 7 years in the Mayo Clinic foot clinic, I came to hate plantar fasciitis. I felt I had little to offer these poor patients except cortisone. One

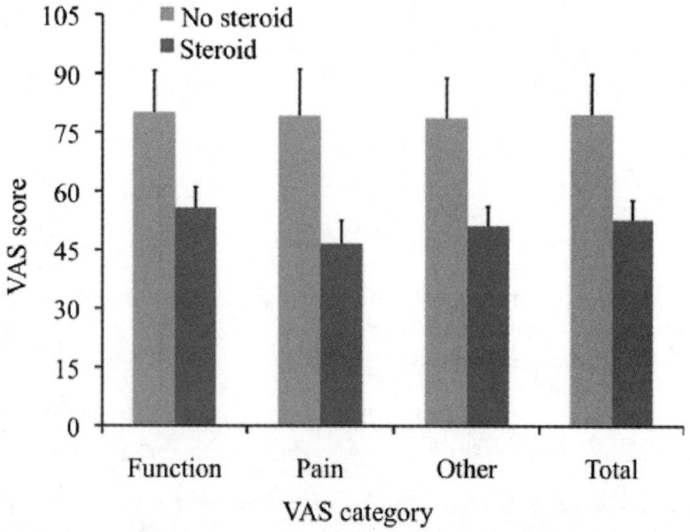

FIGURE 4.—Graph comparing Visual Analog Scale–Foot and Ankle scores of patients who underwent preoperative steriod injection against patients who did not. (Reprinted from MacInnes A, Roberts SC, Kimpton J, et al. Long-term outcome of open plantar fascia release. *Foot Ankle Int.* 2016;37:17-23, with permission from The Author(s).)

problem was that I was reluctant to offer surgery because of the lack of a predictable outcome and prolonged morbidity—at least in my experience. This article is worthwhile in that the effects of open release are carefully studied, and the authors conclude that surgery should be avoided if possible. The data support this conclusion. Of special note is only 30 procedures were done over a 10-year period. Hence the conclusions are predicated on a careful selection process. Finally, of particular note is the adverse effect of cortisone injections on all postoperative parameters studied (Fig 4). So, the bottom line is that steroid and surgery are to be avoided. What to do? I feel the percutaneous ultrasonic fasciotomy may be a solution. Time will tell.

B. F. Morrey, MD

A Biomechanical Comparison of an Open Repair and 3 Minimally Invasive Percutaneous Achilles Tendon Repair Techniques During a Simulated, Progressive Rehabilitation Protocol

Clanton TO, Haytmanek CT, Williams BT, et al (Steadman Philippon Res Inst, Vail, CO; et al)

Am J Sports Med 43:1957-1964, 2015

Background.—While the nonoperative management of Achilles tendon ruptures is a viable option, surgical repair is preferred in healthy and active populations. Recently, minimally invasive percutaneous repair methods with assistive devices have been developed.

Hypothesis/Purpose.—The purpose of this study was to biomechanically analyze 3 commercially available, minimally invasive percutaneous techniques compared with an open Achilles repair during a simulated, progressive rehabilitation program. It was hypothesized that no significant biomechanical differences would exist between repair techniques.

Study Design.—Controlled laboratory study.

Methods.—A simulated, midsubstance Achilles rupture was created 6 cm proximal to the calcaneal insertion in 33 fresh-frozen cadaveric ankles. Specimens were then randomly allocated to 1 of 4 different Achilles repair techniques: (1) open repair, (2) the Achillon Achilles Tendon Suture System, (3) the PARS Achilles Jig System, or (4) an Achilles Midsubstance SpeedBridge Repair variation. Repairs were subjected to a cyclic loading protocol representative of progressive postoperative rehabilitation: 250 cycles at 1 Hz for each loading range: 20-100 N, 20-200 N, 20-300 N, and 20-400 N.

Results.—The open repair technique demonstrated significantly less elongation (5.2 ± 1.1 mm) when compared with all minimally invasive percutaneous repair methods after 250 cycles ($P < .05$). No significant differences were observed after 250 cycles between the Achillon, PARS, or SpeedBridge repairs, with mean displacements of 9.9 ± 2.2 mm, 12.2 ± 4.4 mm, and 10.0 ± 3.9 mm, respectively. When examined over smaller cyclic intervals, the majority of elongation, regardless of repair,

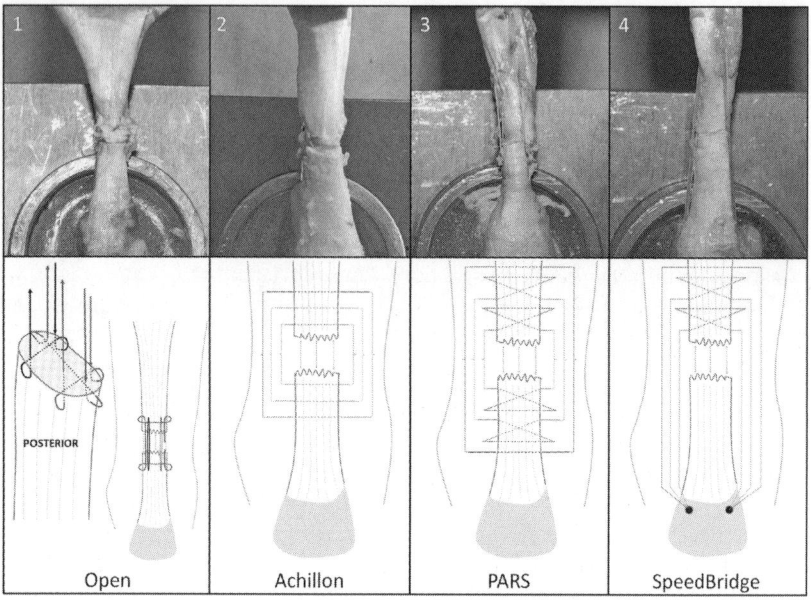

FIGURE 1.—Photographs and simplified schematic diagrams illustrating the 4 different repair constructs and suture configurations: (1) open repair, (2) the Achillon Achilles Tendon Suture System (Integra LifeSciences Corp), (3) the PARS Achilles Jig System (Arthrex Inc), and (4) an Achilles Midsubstance SpeedBridge Repair variation (Arthrex Inc). Crossed sutures for the PARS and SpeedBridge repairs indicate those that were performed in a locking fashion. (Reprinted from Clanton TO, Haytmanek CT, Williams BT, et al. A biomechanical comparison of an open repair and 3 minimally invasive percutaneous achilles tendon repair techniques during a simulated, progressive rehabilitation protocol. *Am J Sports Med.* 2015;43:1957-1964, with permission from The Author(s).)

occurred within the first 10 cycles. Within the first 10 cycles, open repairs achieved 71.2% of the total elongation observed after 250 cycles. Corresponding values for the Achillon, PARS, and SpeedBridge repairs were 81.8%, 77.9%, and 69.0%, respectively. No significant differences were observed in the total number of cycles to failure between minimally invasive percutaneous repairs and open repairs. Minor differences in the mechanism of failure were noted; however, the majority of all repairs failed at the suture-tendon interface.

Conclusion.—Minimally invasive percutaneous repair techniques demonstrated a susceptibility to significant early repair elongation when compared with open repairs. However, the ultimate strengths of repairs (cycles to failure) were comparable across all techniques.

Clinical Relevance.—The reduced early elongation of open repairs suggests that patients treated with this technique may be able to progress through an earlier and/or more aggressive postoperative rehabilitation protocol with a lower risk of early irrevocable repair elongation or gapping about the repair site. However, in cases where cosmesis or wound-healing complications are of significant concern, minimally invasive percutaneous techniques provide a biomechanically reasonable alternative based on their repair strengths (cycles to failure). These repairs may need to be protected longer postoperatively to allow for biological healing and avoid early repair elongation and potential gapping between the healing tendon ends (Fig 1).

▶ The optimal management of Achilles rupture remains unabated. Although nonoperative treatment is viable, most recommend repair in the active or athletic patient. The authors studied the initial stability of a classic open procedure and 3 less invasive repair techniques (Fig 1). The findings are worthwhile. The open procedure does provide statistically significant initial resistance to elongation, but after the full cyclic run out, there is no difference among any of the repairs. Of note also is that all 3 of the less invasive repairs show comparable strength. The authors correctly observe that the value of the findings is to consider an open procedure only if an aggressive rehabilitation program is anticipated.

B. F. Morrey, MD

Effectiveness of customised foot orthoses for Achilles tendinopathy: a randomised controlled trial

Munteanu SE, Scott LA, Bonanno DR, et al (La Trobe Univ, Melbourne, Victoria, Australia; et al)

Br J Sports Med 49:989-994, 2015

Aim.—To evaluate the effectiveness of customised foot orthoses in chronic mid-portion Achilles tendinopathy.

Methods.—This was a participant-blinded, parallel-group randomised controlled trial at a single centre (La Trobe University, Melbourne, Australia). One hundred and forty participants aged 18–55 years with mid-portion Achilles tendinopathy were randomised to receive eccentric calf muscle exercises with either customised foot orthoses (intervention group) or sham foot orthoses (control group). Allocation to intervention was concealed. The Victorian Institute of Sports Assessment-Achilles (VISA-A) questionnaire was completed at baseline, then at 1, 3, 6 and 12 months, with 3 months being the primary end point. Differences between groups were analysed using intention to treat with analysis of covariance.

Results.—After randomisation into the customised foot orthoses group (n = 67) or sham foot orthoses group (n = 73), there was 70.7% follow-up of participants at 3 months. There were no significant differences between groups at any time point. At 3 months, the mean (SD) VISA-A score was 82.1 (16.3) and 79.2 (20.0) points for the customised and sham foot orthosis groups, respectively (adjusted mean difference (95% CI)=2.6 (−2.9 to 8.0), $p = 0.353$). There were no clinically meaningful differences between groups in any of the secondary outcome measures.

Conclusions.—Customised foot orthoses, prescribed according to the protocol in this study, are no more effective than sham foot orthoses for reducing symptoms and improving function in people with mid-portion Achilles tendinopathy undergoing an eccentric calf muscle exercise programme.

Trial Registration Number.—Australian New Zealand Clinical Trials Registry: number ACTRN12609000829213.

▶ This well conceived and executed randomized controlled trial (RCT) caught my attention because of the findings and conclusion. Although I cannot distinguish between my bias or my informed opinion, I have long felt the customized orthoses, so often prescribed for a multitude of aliments, were, for the most part, ineffective. I do not doubt footwear modification is effective in helping to manage many conditions, but the added value of the custom device is the question. This study clearly shows that for a midsubstance Achilles problem, no value is realized.

B. F. Morrey, MD

"Angle to Be Corrected" in Preoperative Evaluation for Hallux Valgus Surgery: Analysis of a New Angular Measurement

Ortiz C, Wagner P, Vela O, et al (Clínica Alemana-Universidad del Desarrollo, Santiago, Chile)

Foot Ankle Int 37:172-177, 2016

Background.—The most common methods for assessing severity of hallux valgus deformity and the effects of an operative procedure are the angular measurements in weightbearing radiographs, specifically the hallux valgus angle and intermetatarsal angle (IMA). Our objective was to analyze the interobserver variability in hallux valgus patients of a new angle called the "angle to be corrected" (ATC), and to compare its capacity to differentiate between different deformities against IMA.

Methods.—We included 28 symptomatic hallux valgus patients with 48 weightbearing foot x-rays. Three trained observers measured the 1 to 2 IMA and the ATC. We then identified retrospectively 45 hallux valgus patients, which were divided into 3 operative technique groups having used the ATC as reference, and analyzed the capacity of the IMA to differentiate between them.

Results.—The IMA average value was 13.6 degrees, and there was a significant difference between observer 3 and observer 1 ($P = .001$). The average value for the ATC was 8.9 degrees, and there was no difference between observers. Both angles showed a high intraclass correlation. Regarding the capacity to differentiate between operative technique groups, the ATC was different between the 3 operative technique groups analyzed, but the IMA showed differences only between 2.

Conclusions.—The ATC was at least as reliable as the intermetatarsal angle for hallux valgus angular measurements, showing a high intraclass correlation with no interobserver difference. It can be suggested that the ATC was better than the IMA to stratify hallux valgus patients when deciding between different operative treatments.

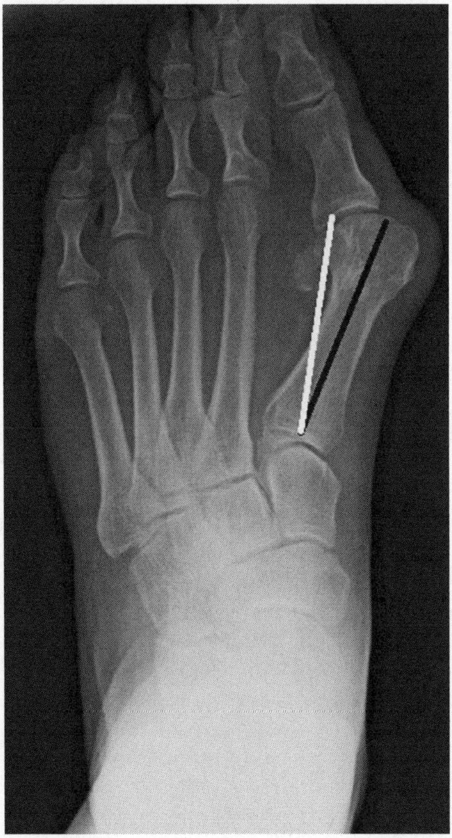

FIGURE 1.—Anteroposterior x-ray of a hallux valgus patient. Lines drawn represent the angle to be corrected (ATC). The black line represents the first metatarsal bone axis, passing through the midline of the base and of the head of the metatarsal. The white line starts at the same starting point as the metatarsal axis, but its distal end goes through the midpoint of the sesamoid complex, that is, the mid-distance between the medial and lateral sesamoid. (Reprinted from Ortiz C, Wagner P, Vela O, et al. "Angle to be corrected" in preoperative evaluation for hallux valgus surgery: analysis of a new angular measurement. *Foot Ankle Int.* 2016;37:172-177, with permission from The Author(s).)

Level of Evidence.—Level III, comparative study (Fig 1).

▶ I was attracted to this article because I thought it offered a new and apparently useful clinical parameter on which to formulate a surgical plan for hallux valgus deformity. The so-called angle to be corrected is reliably identified by multiple observers and is defined by a line down the midportion of the first metatarsal shaft and a line from the proximal point of this line proceeding distally to bisect the space between the 2 sesamoids (Fig 1). The authors demonstrate both a high degree of interobserver reliability and also the ability to differentiate the degree of correction after various procedures. Very interesting concept.

B. F. Morrey, MD

Outcome of Distal First Metatarsal Osteotomy Shortening in Hallux Rigidus Grades II and III

Ceccarini P, Ceccarini A, Rinonapoli G, et al (Univ of Perugia, Italy)
Foot Ankle Int 36:1469-1474, 2015

Background.—Existing techniques for operative treatment of hallux rigidus commonly combine skeletal and soft tissue interventions to obtain long-lasting relief of pain. To date, operative treatments include implant arthroplasty, cheilectomy, various osteotomies, nonimplant arthroplasty, and arthrodesis. We assessed a technique that respects the anatomy and joint function and used a shortening osteotomy of the head of the first metatarsal.

Methods.—We evaluated a series of 40 consecutive patients affected by grade II and III hallux rigidus, aged 32 to 79 years, who had undergone surgery from January 2010 to January 2014. All patients were evaluated clinically and radiographically, preoperatively and postoperatively, and underwent a final follow-up at a mean of 35.4 (range = 12-51) months. For the clinical evaluation, the American Orthopaedic Foot & Ankle Society (AOFAS) clinical rating scale for the hallux metatarsophalangeal-interphalangeal joints was used.

Results.—A patient survey revealed excellent and good overall satisfaction in 90% of the sample. Postoperative results included a significant increase ($P < .001$) in the median global AOFAS score, from 39 (range = 25-60) to 84 (range = 78-94).

Conclusions.—The technique of a shortening osteotomy of the first metatarsal head appeared to be useful for the correction of stiffness, pain relief, and an improvement in range of motion. Other advantages were that it preserved the integrity of the metatarsophalangeal joint and led to a rapid functional recovery.

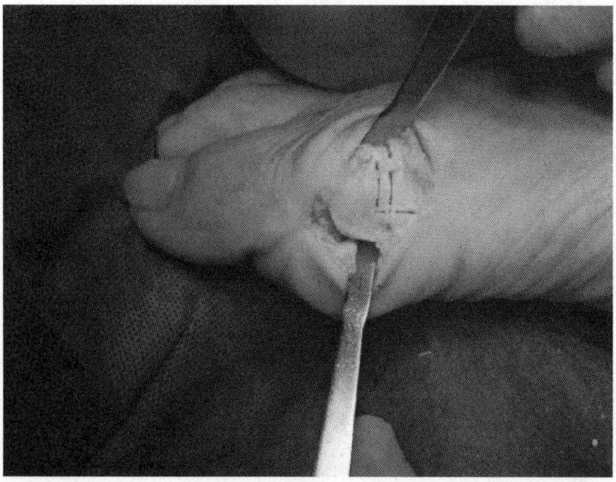

FIGURE 1.—Osteotomy shortening. (Reprinted from Ceccarini P, Ceccarini A, Rinonapoli G, et al. Outcome of distal first metatarsal osteotomy shortening in hallux rigidus grades II and III. *Foot Ankle Int.* 2015;36:1469-1474, with permission from The Author(s).)

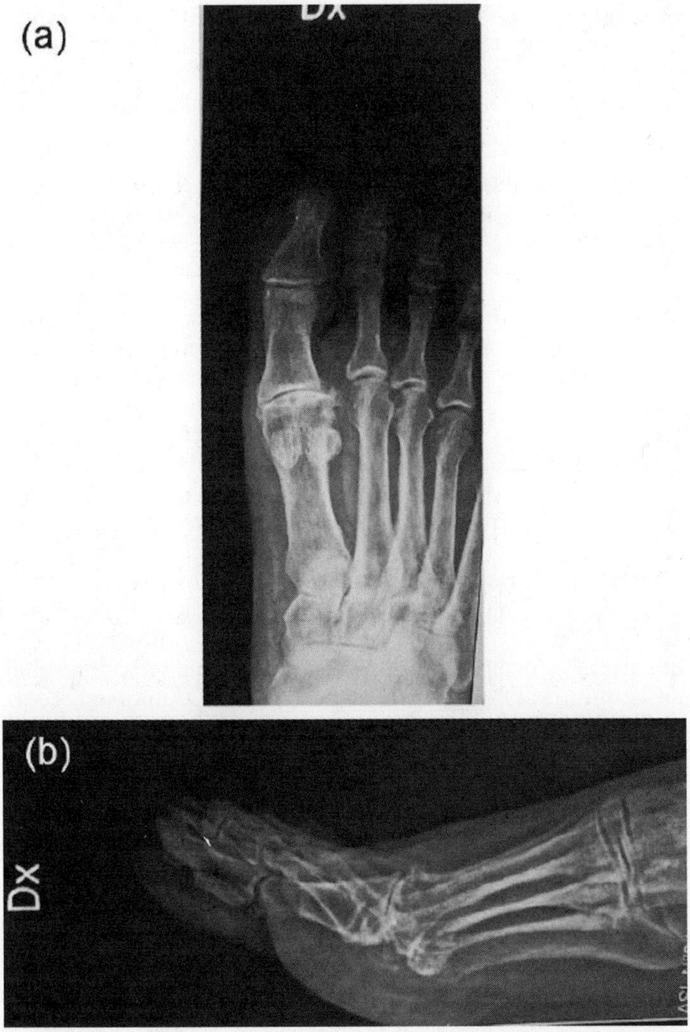

FIGURE 2.—Preoperative grade III hallux rigidus in anteroposterior and lateral views. (Reprinted from Ceccarini P, Ceccarini A, Rinonapoli G, et al. Outcome of distal first metatarsal osteotomy shortening in hallux rigidus grades II and III. *Foot Ankle Int.* 2015;36:1469-1474, with permission from The Author(s).)

Level of Evidence.—Level IV, retrospective case series (Figs 1 and 2).

▶ As may have been well noted, few case series are reviewed in the YEAR BOOK these days. I included this because this osteotomy seems to be simple and effective with a very good 90% positive response at 3 years average. It would have been helpful if the author provided a drawing instead of Fig 1. The example provided is of interest because it shows the recommended shortening very clearly of about 3 mm, but what I found interesting is that the joint space was reconstituted to a great extent Fig 2. The authors indicate this is to be reserved for Grade 2 and 3 disease and that lateral translation of the shaft can be performed if needed.

B. F. Morrey, MD

Effect of Obesity on Outcome of Hallux Valgus Surgery

Chen JY, Lee MJH, Rikhraj K, et al (Singapore General Hosp)

Foot Ankle Int 36:1078-1083, 2015

Background.—Obesity is a global epidemic, but its effect on foot and ankle surgeries is not well defined. This study aimed to investigate the influence of obesity on functional outcome scores, incidence of postoperative surgical site infection (SSI), and repeat surgery after hallux valgus (HV) corrective surgery.

Methods.—Between January 2007 and December 2011, 452 patients who underwent HV corrective surgery at a tertiary hospital were evaluated. They were categorized into 2 groups based on their body mass index (BMI): (1) BMI less than 30 kg/m^2 (control); (2) BMI 30 kg/m^2 or more (obese). The patients were prospectively followed for 2 years.

Results.—Patients in the obese group were significantly older by 4 years (95% CI, 1-7 years) ($P = .043$). The preoperative American Orthopaedic Foot & Ankle Society Hallux Metatarsophalangeal-Interphalangeal (AOFAS Hallux MTP-IP) Scale and Physical Component Score were 6 points (95% CI, 1-11 points) and 3 points (95% CI, 1-6 points) poorer, respectively, in the obese group ($P = .014$ and $P = .032$, respectively). However, the Visual Analog Scale, AOFAS Hallux MTP-IP Scale, Physical Component Score, and Mental Component Score were comparable between the 2 groups at 6 months and 2 years of follow-up (all $P > .05$). Eleven patients (3%) in the control group and 1 patient in the obese group (2%) developed postoperative SSI ($P = .777$). Nine patients (2%) in the control group and 7 patients in the obese group (14%) required repeat surgery for complications ($P < .001$).

Conclusion.—The authors conclude that while it is important to warn obese patients of the significantly higher risk of repeat surgery, these patients should not be excluded from undergoing HV surgery.

Level of Evidence.—Level III, retrospective comparative series.

▶ I was surprised to learn of the adverse effect of obesity on the outcome of total elbow replacement. Hence, I could hardly be surprised at these findings. It should be noted that the threshold of a body mass index (BMI) of 30 is, by today's standards a rather mild form of obesity. In hip and knee surgery the effect of obesity is hardly detectible at a BMI of 30 and becomes manifest only at 40 or 45! Similar to virtually all other studies, this work documents that those with obesity do benefit from the procedure but pay a higher price in complications and reoperations.

B. F. Morrey, MD

Comparison of two classification systems in predicting the outcome of diabetic foot ulcers: the Wagner grade and the Saint Elian Wound score systems

Huang Y, Xie T, Cao Y, et al (Shanghai Jiao Tong Univ School of Medicine, China; Shanghai TCM-integrated Hosp, China; et al)

Wound Repair Regen 23:379-385, 2015

The aim of the study was to compare two systems of classification in a consecutive population with diabetic foot ulcers: the Wagner grade and the Saint Elian Wound Score System (SEWSS). Sociodemographic information, patient-related and ulcer-related data at first presentation was recorded, and the patients were followed up until wound healing or accepting major amputation or for 24 weeks. One hundred eighty-six patients were included in the study, of which 172 patients were completely followed up. Among the remaining 172 patients, 53.5% ($n = 92$) were healed without minor amputation, 32% ($n = 55$) were healed with minor amputation, 9.3% ($n = 16$) were not healed at study termination,

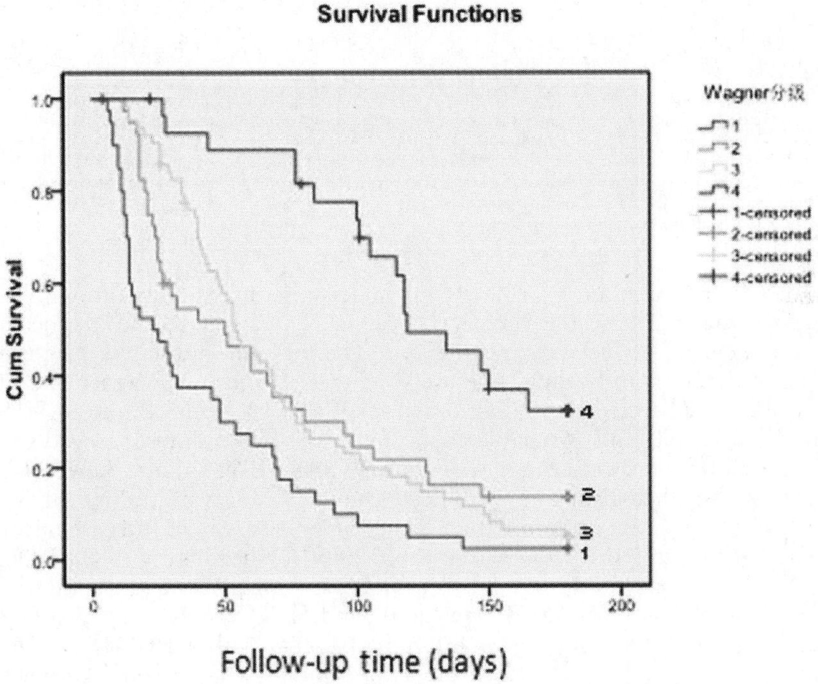

FIGURE 2.—Kaplan–Meier survival probability analyses for wound healing success by days and Wagner grade from 1 to 4 for a maximum follow-up period of 24 weeks. [Color figure can be viewed in the online issue, which is available at wileyonlinelibrary.com.] (Reprinted from Huang Y, Xie T, Cao Y, et al. Comparison of two classification systems in predicting the outcome of diabetic foot ulcers: The Wagner grade and the Saint Elian Wound score systems. *Wound Repair Regen.* 2015;23:379-385, with permission from the Wound Healing Society.)

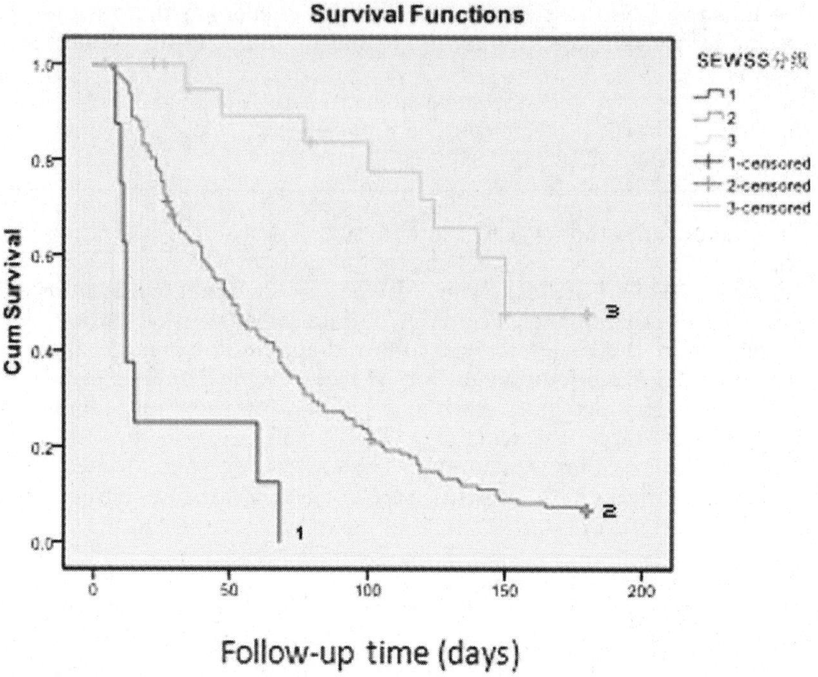

FIGURE 3.—Kaplan–Meier survival probability analyses for wound healing success by days and SWESS grade from I to III for a maximum follow-up period of 24 weeks. [Color figure can be viewed in the online issue, which is available at wileyonlinelibrary.com.] (Reprinted from Huang Y, Xie T, Cao Y, et al. Comparison of two classification systems in predicting the outcome of diabetic foot ulcers: The Wagner grade and the Saint Elian Wound score systems. *Wound Repair Regen.* 2015;23:379-385, with permission from the Wound Healing Society.)

3.5% ($n = 6$) died and 1.7% ($n = 3$) underwent major amputation. The median healing time for Wagner 1, Wagner 2, Wagner 3, and Wagner 4 were 23, 50, 54, 119 days, respectively. The log-rank test showed significant differences in healing time for Wagner 1, Wagner 2, Wagner 3, and Wagner 4; The median healing time for SEWSS I, SEWSS II and SEWSS III were 12, 51, and 150 days, respectively. The log-rank test showed significant differences in healing time for SEWSS I, SEWSS II and SEWSS III. Cox regression analysis showed a decreasing probability of healing with or without minor amputation with a higher SEWSS value, an increase in the SEWSS by one score reduced the probability for healing by 24%. ROC analysis showed Wagner 3 and a cut-point 17 of SEWSS had the highest Youden's index. Both the Wagner grade and SEWSS system were associated with the ulcer healing time for the patients with active DFUs. The SEWSS score makes it a better prediction tool of DFU outcome synthetically (Figs 2 and 3).

▶ I have been interested in this topic since I was in the foot clinic at Mayo in my early career. I have become reintroduced to the topic because I am involved in an instrument that treats diabetic foot ulcers. This condition costs society millions of dollars to treat and exacts a comparable toll on the part of the patient. To introduce a new treatment, it is critically important to understand the extent of the pathology being treated—hence, this study. As mentioned, the Meggitt Wagner classification from the university of Texas is the gold standard and classifies into 4 groups based on depth, infection, and gangrene. The newer Saint Elian Wound Score System (SEWSS) system considers perfusion, size, depth, infection, and sensation, and thus is more complex. The analysis clearly shows that the latter system is more accurate to predict successful treatment of healing the ulcer (Figs 2 and 3). The concern is whether the SEWSS system is too complex for the clinician to adopt. But this is an important issue. Plus, the nature of the treatment should be factored in, and this may be changing in the near future.

B. F. Morrey, MD

A systematic review and meta-analysis of débridement methods for chronic diabetic foot ulcers

Elraiyah T, Domecq JP, Prutsky G, et al (Mayo Clinic, Rochester, MN; et al)

J Vasc Surg 63:37S-45S.e1-2, 2016

Background.—Several methods of débridement of diabetic foot ulcers are currently used. The relative efficacy of these methods is not well established.

Methods.—This systematic review and meta-analysis was conducted to find the best available evidence for the effect of débridement on diabetic foot wound outcomes. We searched MEDLINE, Embase, Cochrane Central Register of Controlled Trials, Web of Science, and Scopus through October 2011 for randomized controlled studies (RCTs) and observational comparative studies.

Results.—We identified 11 RCTs and three nonrandomized studies reporting on 800 patients. The risk of bias was moderate overall. Meta-analysis of three RCTs showed that autolytic débridement significantly increased the healing rate (relative risk [RR], 1.89; 95% confidence interval [CI] 1.35-2.64). Meta-analysis of four studies (one RCT) showed that larval débridement reduced amputation (RR, 0.43; 95% CI, 0.21-0.88) but did not increase complete healing (RR, 1.27; 95% CI, 0.84-1.91). Surgical débridement was associated with shorter healing time compared with conventional wound care (one RCT). Insufficient evidence was found for comparisons between autolytic and larval débridement (one RCT), between ultrasound-guided and surgical débridement, and between hydrosurgical and surgical débridement.

Conclusions.—The available literature supports the efficacy of several débridement methods, including surgical, autolytic, and larval débridement. Comparative effectiveness evidence between these methods and supportive evidence for other methods is of low quality due to methodologic limitations and imprecision. Hence, the choice of débridement method at the present time should be based on the available expertise, patient preferences, the clinical context and cost.

▶ With the problem of diabetes reaching epidemic proportions around the world, this topic regarding a major complication of the disease is of particular relevance. This meta-analysis reveals a 2% analysis rate from a screen of 700 articles. The analysis itself is more focused on statistical methodology and accuracy than clinical characteristics of those undergoing treatment. For example, the criteria for success is primarily a decrease in size of the wound, not complete healing. Of note also is that no mention is made of recurrence, which is really the ultimate discriminator. All this said, the one "truth" is that traditional sharp debridement, ultrasonic, or larval methods are all effective with insufficient granularity to indicate whether one is better than another. They are all better than nonoperative management, given that all studies did have specific inclusion criteria for the surgery, but this was highly variable among the studies.

B. F. Morrey, MD

A systematic review and meta-analysis of off-loading methods for diabetic foot ulcers

Elraiyah T, Prutsky G, Domecq JP, et al (Mayo Clinic, Rochester, MN; et al)

J Vasc Surg 63:59S-68S.e1-2, 2016

Background.—Increased plantar foot pressure is one of several key factors that lead to diabetic foot ulcers. Multiple methods have been proposed to relieve this pressure and thus enhance wound healing and potentially prevent relapse. We aimed in this systematic review to find the best available evidence for off-loading methods.

Methods.—We searched MEDLINE, Embase, Cochrane CENTRAL, Web of Science, and Scopus through October 2011. Pairs of independent reviewers selected studies and extracted data. Predefined outcomes of interest included complete wound healing, time to complete wound healing, amputation, infection, and relapse rates.

Results.—We identified 19 interventional studies, of which 13 were randomized controlled trials, including data from 1605 patients with diabetic foot ulcers using an off-loading method. The risk of bias in the included studies was moderate. This analysis demonstrated improved wound healing with total contact casting over removable cast walker, therapeutic shoes, and conventional therapy. There was no advantage of irremovable cast walkers over total contact casting. There was improved healing with half-shoe compared with conventional wound care. Therapeutic shoes and insoles reduced relapse rate in comparison with regular footwear. Data were sparse regarding other off-loading methods.

Conclusions.—Although based on low-quality evidence (ie, evidence warranting lower certainty), benefits are demonstrated for use of total

Study name	Statistics for each study				
		Lower	upper	Z-Value	p-Value
Faglia, 2010	-4.400	-6.550	-2.250	-4.011	0.000
Armstrong, 2001	-16.900	-21.044	-12.756	-7.993	0.000
Van De Weg, 2008	-31.000	-48.946	-13.054	-3.386	0.001
Piaggesi, 2007	-1.500	-18.559	15.559	-0.172	0.863
Time to complete healing, I² = 91%	**-12.359**	**-22.626**	**-2.092**	**-2.359**	**0.018**

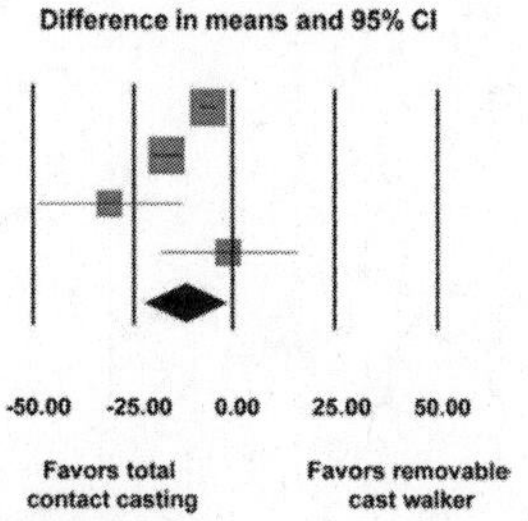

FIGURE 3.—Total contact casting (TCC) vs removable cast walker (RCW), time to heal in days. *CI*, Confidence interval. (Reprinted from Elraiyah T, Prutsky G, Domecq JP, et al. A systematic review and meta-analysis of off-loading methods for diabetic foot ulcers. *J Vasc Surg.* 2016;63:59S-68S.e1-2, with permission from the Society for Vascular Surgery.)

contact casting and irremovable cast walkers in the treatment of diabetic foot ulcers. Reduced relapse rate is demonstrated with various therapeutic shoes and insoles in comparison with regular footwear (Fig 3).

▶ As noted elsewhere in this section, any insight into the optimal management of the diabetic foot ulcer is of great clinical value because of the considerable burden of the disease and this particular complication from all perspectives. The meta-analysis does provide some useful insights. The gold standard of treatment is offloading, but not all modalities are of equal benefit. The best effect is seen with total contact casts and nonremovable cast walkers. However, removable cast walkers do statistically worse than the total contact cast (Fig 3). Although special shoes are less effective to heal the ulcer, they are effective in avoiding a recurrence. This article provides good practical and clinically useful information.

B. F. Morrey, MD

Effect of Obesity on Clinical and Radiographic Outcomes Following Reconstruction of Stage II Adult Acquired Flatfoot Deformity

Soukup DS, MacMahon A, Burket JC, et al (Hosp for Special Surgery, NY)
Foot Ankle Int 37:245-254, 2016

Background.—Obesity is a known risk factor for the development of adult acquired flatfoot deformity (AAFD), but obesity's effects on outcomes following AAFD reconstruction are unknown. We hypothesized that obesity would negatively impact outcomes following joint-preserving stage II AAFD reconstruction.

Methods.—This retrospective study compared the outcomes of normal-weight (18.5 kg/m^2 $\leq$ BMI < 25 kg/m^2), overweight (25 kg/m^2 $\leq$ BMI < 30 kg/m^2), and obese (BMI $\geq$ 30 kg/m^2) patients after AAFD reconstruction. Clinical outcome measures included the Foot and Ankle Outcome Score (FAOS), Short-Form 12 (SF-12), and Numeric Rating Scale

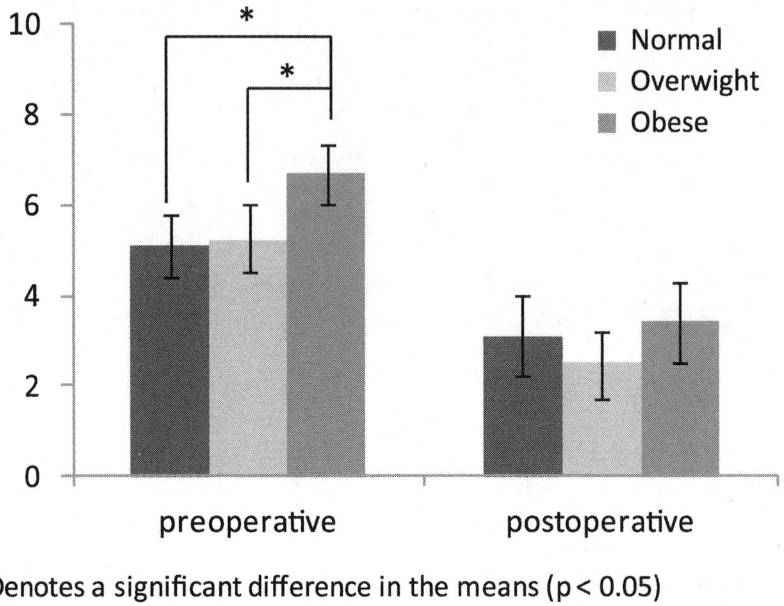

FIGURE 4.—Mean preoperative and postoperative NRS Pain scores. Error bars represent 95% confidence intervals. (See Supplemental Table 2 for complete NRS Pain data.) *Editor's Note*: Please refer to original journal article for full references. (Soukup DS, MacMahon A, Burket JC, et al. Effect of obesity on clinical and radiographic outcomes following reconstruction of stage II adult acquired flatfoot deformity. *Foot Ankle Int.* 2016;37:245-254, with permission from The Author(s).)

of Pain (NRS Pain) administered preoperatively and at least 1 year postoperatively. Anteroposterior and lateral radiographs were taken preoperatively and at least 6 months postoperatively. Pre- to postoperative changes in outcome measures were assessed within BMI classes. Preoperative, postoperative, and pre- to postoperative changes in outcomes were compared among BMI classes. There were 41 normal-weight patients, 39 overweight patients, and 44 obese patients with a mean age of 56 years, FAOS follow-up of 2.9 years, and radiographic follow-up of 2.1 years. Demographics and reconstructive procedures were comparable among the 3 BMI classes.

Results.—All outcomes significantly increased pre- to postoperatively in the 3 groups with the exception of the FAOS Symptoms subscale for normal-weight patients ($P = .340$) and SF-12 Mental Component score for all 3 BMI classes ($P > .999$). Preoperatively, obese patients had more symptoms than normal-weight patients, scoring 12 points lower on the FAOS Symptoms subscore ($P = .008$). Obese patients also scored 11 points lower preoperatively on the SF-12 Overall score ($P = .028$) and had 31% greater pain than normal-weight patients ($P = .003$). There were no differences among the 3 BMI classes in any postoperative outcomes assessed.

Conclusion.—Although obese patients had significantly worse symptoms, overall health, and NRS pain scores preoperatively, the short-term clinical and radiographic outcomes of stage II AAFD reconstruction were similar for normal-weight, overweight, and obese patients. We suggest that joint-preserving reconstruction remains a viable alternative to fusion of the triple joint complex for the treatment of overweight and obese stage II AAFD patients.

Level of Evidence.—Level III, retrospective cohort study (Fig 4).

▶ The study considers an interesting aspect of the effectiveness of surgery on the obese patient. Recognizing that obese patients are a at greater risk for flat foot, do they do less well with surgery? The cohort was stratified into 3 groups each with about 45 patients: nonoverweight; overweight body mass index 25 to 30; obese > 35. Using clinical assessment tools both general and anatomic specific as well as pre- and postprocedure radiographs the findings were consistent. The obese patient had more problems and pain before surgery and consistently improved with surgery. Of interest the pattern of improvement was similar for all 3 groups, including those with a BMI > 35 (Fig 4). This refuted the authors' hypothesis. The shortcoming of the study is the usual one: short overall follow-up of less that 3 years. Nonetheless, useful information for the short term.

B. F. Morrey, MD

An Ankle-Foot Orthosis With a Lateral Extension Reduces Forefoot Abduction in Subjects With Stage II Posterior Tibial Tendon Dysfunction

Neville C, Bucklin M, Ordway N, et al (SUNY Upstate Med Univ, Syracuse, NY; et al)

J Orthop Sports Phys Ther 46:26-33, 2016

Study Design.—Controlled laboratory, repeated measures.

Background.—Posterior tibial tendon dysfunction is a common musculoskeletal problem that includes tendon degeneration and collapse of the medial arch of the foot (flatfoot deformity). Ankle-foot orthoses (AFOs) typically are used to correct flatfoot deformity. Correction of flatfoot deformity involves increasing forefoot adduction, forefoot plantar flexion, and hindfoot inversion.

Objectives.—To test whether a foot orthosis with a lateral extension reduces forefoot abduction in patients with stage II posterior tibial tendon dysfunction while walking.

Methods.—The gait of 15 participants with stage II posterior tibial tendon dysfunction was evaluated under 3 conditions: a standard AFO, an AFO with a lateral extension, and a shoe-only control condition. Kinematic variables of interest were evaluated at designated time points in the gait cycle and included hindfoot inversion/eversion, forefoot plantar flexion/dorsiflexion, and forefoot abduction/adduction. A 3-by-4, repeated-measures analysis of variance (brace condition by gait phase) was used to compare variables across conditions.

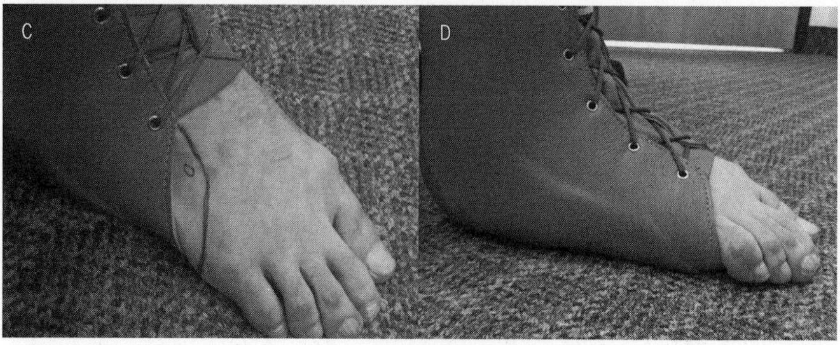

FIGURE 1.—The standard-length AFO (C). The AFO with lateral extension (D). Abbreviation: AFO, ankle-foot orthosis. (Reprinted from Neville C, Bucklin M, Ordway N, et al. An ankle-foot orthosis with a lateral extension reduces forefoot abduction in subjects with stage II posterior Tibial tendon dysfunction. *J Orthop Sports Phys Ther* 2016;46:26-33, with permission from Journal of Orthopaedic & Sports Physical Therapy.)

Results.—The AFO with a lateral extension resulted in a significantly greater change in forefoot adduction compared to the standard AFO (2.6°, $P = .02$) and shoe-only conditions (4.1°, $P < .01$) across all phases of stance. Forefoot plantar flexion was significantly increased when comparing the standard AFO and AFO with a lateral extension to the shoe-only condition. The AFO with the lateral extension also demonstrated significantly increased hindfoot inversion during the loading response and terminal stance phases.

Conclusion.—Off-the-shelf and standard AFOs have been shown to improve forefoot plantar flexion and hindfoot eversion, but not forefoot adduction. A lateral extension added to a standard AFO along the forefoot significantly improved forefoot adduction in participants with posterior tibial tendon dysfunction while walking (Fig 1).

▶ The authors note the 3% prevalence and the considerable problem with progressive flatfoot deformity associated with dysfunction or rupture of the posterior tibial tendon. In an effort to avoid the end-stage condition requiring surgery, shoe modifications and orthoses are the standard treatment. This study demonstrates a simple modification of a standard orthotic brace currently used for this condition can result in even greater effectiveness.

(Fig 1C, D). Although the study cohort of 15 patients is rather small, the fact that measurable improvement was noted would seem to validate the adaption of this modification. My only question is the long-term tolerance of this device.

B. F. Morrey, MD

Fifth metatarsal fractures – Is routine follow-up necessary?

Ferguson KB, McGlynn J, Jenkins P, et al (Glasgow Royal Infirmary, Glasgow, Scotland, United Kingdom)

Injury 46:1664-1668, 2015

Background.—Fifth metatarsal fractures are common, and the outcome with conservative treatment is generally very satisfactory. Operative treatment is only used for selected injuries, particularly stress fractures. Traditionally these patients are routinely reviewed at a fracture clinic, mainly due to the perceived risk of non-union with a Jones' fracture. In 2011 we introduced a standardised protocol to promote weight bearing as pain allowed with an elasticated support or a removable boot. Patients were discharged with structured advice and a help-line number to access care if required, but no further face-to-face review was arranged. More complex cases were reviewed at a "virtual clinic." Our hypothesis was that the introduction of this standardised protocol would be safe, patient-centred and significantly reduce unnecessary outpatient clinic review.

Patients and Methods.—We audited fracture clinic attendance and outcomes 1 year before and 1 year after the protocol was introduced in 2011. All radiographs taken at the Emergency Department (ED) presentation were reviewed and classified independently for validation.

Results.—From 2009 to 2010, 279 patients who presented to the ED with fifth metatarsal fractures were referred to a fracture clinic. Of these 279 patients, 267 (96%) attended the fracture clinic, resulting in an overall total of 491 outpatient attendances. Three (1%) were treated operatively for delayed/non-union.

From 2011 to 2012, 339 patients presented to the ED with fifth metatarsal fractures – only 67 (20%) were referred to a fracture clinic. 62 (18%) attended clinic appointments with 102 appointments in total. Five (1%) required operative intervention.

Conclusion.—Our study showed no added clinical value for routine outpatient follow-up of fifth metatarsal fractures. Patients can be safely discharged and allowed to bear weight at the time of initial ED presentation if they are provided with appropriate information and ready access to experienced fracture clinic staff (Fig 2).

▶ This study caught my eye because it goes in the direction of our future treatment trends. By carefully assessing the outcome of closely and loosely supervised treatment of the fifth metatarsal fracture, the authors are able to definitively answer the question they asked: is routine clinical surveillance of this fracture warranted? No. The 1% rate of each group proves this point. The dramatic reduction in medical resources achieved with the management protocol followed in this study is truly impressive (Fig 2). I would hope this

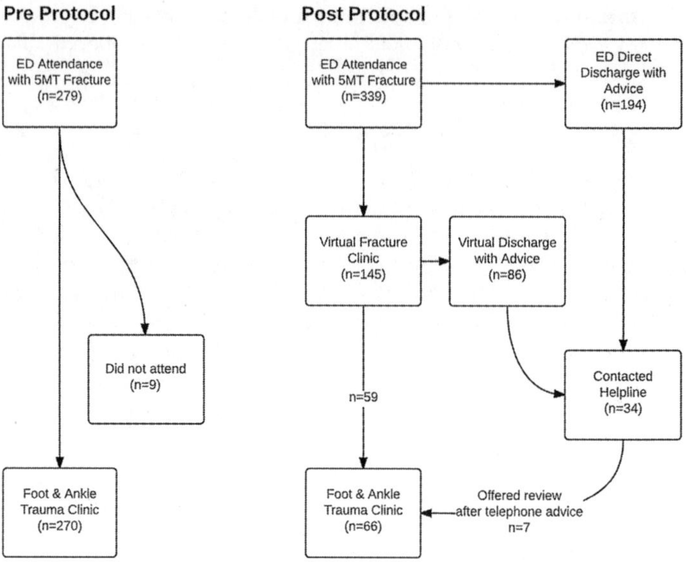

FIGURE 2.—Discharge outcome from emergency department. (Reprinted from Ferguson KB, McGlynn J, Jenkins P, et al. Fifth metatarsal fractures – is routine follow-up necessary? *Injury.* 2015;46:1664-1668, with permission from Elsevier.)

insight, gained in the United Kingdom, could travel to the North American practice.

B. F. Morrey, MD

Outcome After Salvage Arthrodesis for Failed Total Ankle Replacement

Kamrad I, Henricson A, Magnusson H, et al (Lund Univ and Skåne Univ Hosp, Malmö, Sweden; Falu Central Hosp, Sweden)
Foot Ankle Int 37:255-261, 2016

Background.—In cases with total ankle replacement (TAR) failure, a decision between revision TAR and salvage arthrodesis (SA) must be made. In a previous study, we analyzed revision TAR and found low functional outcome and satisfaction. The aims of the current study were to analyze SA concerning failure rate and patient-related outcome measures (PROMs).

Methods.—Until September 2014, a total of 1110 primary TARs were recorded in the Swedish Ankle Registry. Of the 188 failures, 118 were revised with SA (and 70 with revision TAR). Patient- and implant-specific data for SA cases were analyzed as well as arthrodesis techniques. Failure of SA was defined as repeat arthrodesis or amputation. Generic and region-specific PROMs of 68 patients alive with a solid unilateral SA performed more than 1 year before were analyzed.

Results.—The first-attempt solid arthrodesis rate of SA was 90%. Overall, 25 of 53 (47%) patients were very satisfied or satisfied. Mean Self-reported Foot and Ankle Score (SEFAS) was 22 (95% confidence interval 20-24), Euro Qol—5 Dimensions 0.57 (0.49-0.65), Euro Qol—Visual Analogue Scale 59 (53-64), Short Form-36 physical 34 (31-37) and mental 50 (46-54). The scores and satisfaction were similar to those after revision TAR but the reoperation rate was significantly lower in SA ($P < .05$).

Conclusion.—Salvage arthrodesis after failed TAR had a solid arthrodesis rate of 90% at first attempt, but similar to revision TAR, less than 50% of the patients were satisfied and the functional scores were low. Until studies show true benefit of revision TAR over SA, we favor SA for failed TAR.

Level of Evidence.—Level IV, retrospective case series.

▶ This is an interesting registry study comparing ankle arthrodesis to revision arthroplasty for failed total ankle arthroplasty. I was first struck by the extremely high revision rate of 15%. The sobering reality is that despite a 90% fusion rate with the initial attempt, only 50% patients were satisfied with the salvage procedure. This is identical to the rate satisfied with revision as a salvage for failure of the primary replacement. The authors correctly recommend arthrodesis as the salvage of choice at this time, noting the lower ($P < .05$) reoperation rate in the arthrodesis cohort. In addition, the likelihood of additional reoperations going forward is higher in the revision group. Message: fusion is the treatment of choice as a salvage for failed total ankle replacement, but it is far from an ideal salvage.

B. F. Morrey, MD

10 Sports Medicine

Introduction

Just as we are careful not to allow the rotator cuff topic to dominate the shoulder section, even more so do we guard against this being an anterior cruciate exclusive review. Topics relating to variations of technique have, for the most part, been avoided in favor of outcomes-oriented contributions. The ongoing concern regarding concussion is again reflected in this year's reviews, as are topics of more general interest. Some upper extremity sports issues are included here instead of in the shoulder section. Also, topics regarding the foot and ankle are reviewed in this section. It is hoped this will provide a useful balance of information that will be of value in one's care of the serious or not so serious athlete. The quality of the studies in the sports literature appears to be increasing over the years.

Bernard F. Morrey, MD

Levels of Evidence in the Clinical Sports Medicine Literature: Are We Getting Better Over Time?

Grant HM, Tjoumakaris FP, Maltenfort MG, et al (Jefferson Med College, Philadelphia, PA; Thomas Jefferson Univ, Philadelphia, PA; et al)

Am J Sports Med 42:1738-1742, 2014

Background.—There has been an increased emphasis on improving the level of evidence used as the basis for clinical treatment decisions. Several journals now require a statement of the level of evidence as a basic gauge of the study's strength.

Purpose.—To review the levels of evidence in published articles in the clinical sports medicine literature and to determine if there has been an improvement in the levels of evidence published over the past 15 years.

Study Design.—Systematic review.

Methods.—All articles from the years 1995, 2000, 2005, and 2010 in *The American Journal of Sports Medicine (AJSM)*, *Arthroscopy*, and sports medicine–related articles from *The Journal of Bone and Joint Surgery–American (JBJS-A)* were analyzed. Articles were categorized by type and ranked for level of evidence according to guidelines from the Centre for Evidence-Based Medicine. Excluded were animal, cadaveric, and basic science articles; editorials; surveys; special topics; letters to the editor; and correspondence. Statistical analysis was performed with chi-square.

Results.—A total of 1580 articles over the 4 periods met the inclusion criteria. The percentage of level 1 and 2 studies increased from 6.8% to 12.6%, 22.9%, and 23.5%, respectively ($P < .0001$), while level 4 and 5 studies decreased from 78.9% to 72.4%, 63.9%, and 53.0% ($P < .0001$). *JBJS-A* had a significant increase in level 1 and 2 studies (4.1%, 5.1%, 28.2%, 27.8%; $P < .0001$), as did *AJSM* (9.4%, 17.1%, 36.1%, 30.1%; $P < .0001$). *Arthroscopy* showed no significant change over time. Diagnostic, therapeutic, and prognostic studies all showed significant increases in level 1 and 2 studies over time ($P < .05$).

Conclusion.—There has been a statistically significant increase in the percentage of level 1 and 2 studies published in the sports medicine literature over the past 15 years, particularly in *JBJS-A* and *AJSM*. The largest increase was seen in diagnostic studies, while therapeutic and prognostic studies demonstrated modest improvement. The emphasis on increasing levels of evidence to guide treatment decisions for sports medicine patients may be taking effect.

▶ This represents a trend type study with a critically and relevant question: is the level of evidence improving in the orthopedic literature? The answer is yes. The improvements were most dramatic 15 and 10 years ago, and although the rate of change is slowing, the trends continue. Of interest that is this trend is very similar in the 2 major sources of orthopedic information: the *Journal of Bone and Joint Surgery* and the *American Journal of Sports Medicine*. It is important to understand the need for higher quality studies to allow confidence in the recommendations that may improve patient care. However, the actual correlation with clinically relevant practice improvement is still lacking at this time.

B. F. Morrey, MD

Gaze Stabilization Test Asymmetry Score as an Indicator of Previous Concussion in a Cohort of Collegiate Football Players

Honaker JA, Criter RE, Patterson JN, et al (Univ of Nebraska-Lincoln)
Clin J Sport Med 25:361-366, 2015

Objective.—Vestibular dysfunction may lead to decreased visual acuity with head movements, which may impede athletic performance and result in injury. The purpose of this study was to test the hypothesis that athletes with history of concussion would have differences in gaze stabilization test (GST) as compared with those without a history of concussion.

Design.—Cross-sectional, descriptive.

Setting.—University Athletic Medicine Facility.

Participants.—Fifteen collegiate football players with a history of concussion, 25 collegiate football players without a history of concussion.

Intervention.—Participants completed the dizziness handicap inventory (DHI), static visual acuity, perception time test, active yaw plane GST, stability evaluation test (SET), and a bedside oculomotor examination.

Main Outcome Measures.—Independent samples t test was used to compare GST, SET, and DHI scores per group, with Bonferroni-adjusted alpha at $P < 0.01$. Receiver operating characteristic curve analysis and area under the curve (AUC) were used to assess the clinical performance of the GST and SET.

Results.—Athletes with previous concussion had a larger GST asymmetry score [mean (M) = 12.40, SD = 9.09] than those without concussion (M = 4.92, SD = 4.67; t (18.70) = −2.955, $P = 0.008$, 95% CI, −12.79 to −2.18, $d = -1.37$). Clinical performance of the GST (AUC = 0.77) was better than the SET (AUC = 0.61).

Conclusions.—Results suggest peripheral vestibular or vestibular–visual interaction deficits in collegiate athletes with a history of concussion. The results support further research on the use of GST for sport-related concussion evaluation and monitoring.

Clinical Relevance.—Inclusion of objective vestibular tests in the concussion protocol may reveal the presence of peripheral vestibular or visual—vestibular deficits. Therefore, the GST may add an important perspective on the effects of concussion.

▶ We have made an effort over the past several years to highlight the increasing awareness of the presence of and long-term significance of concussion in the athlete. Because I care for high school athletes, I feel an increased responsibility to protect these young people while not depriving them of an activity that is so important to their physical, emotional, and intellectual development. Hence, this study caught my attention. Although the protocol to allow an athlete to return to competition is much improved over the past few years, we constantly seek the discriminating factor that helps define the player at risk. The observation of the effectiveness of gaze stabilization and its correlation to residual vestibular deficiency may be that test. Further study will be enlightening.

B. F. Morrey, MD

Management of Sport-Related Concussion in the Pediatric and Adolescent Population

Provance AJ, Engelman GH, Terhune EB, et al (Children's Hosp Colorado, Aurora; Rocky Vista Univ, Parker, CO; Georgetown Univ School of Medicine, Washington, DC; et al)

Orthopedics 39:24-30, 2016

Concussions make up nearly 10% of all high school athletic injuries. Recent changes in concussion management guidelines and legislation aim to make concussion care more standardized and safe but simultaneously pose a challenge for the primary care and sports medicine physician.

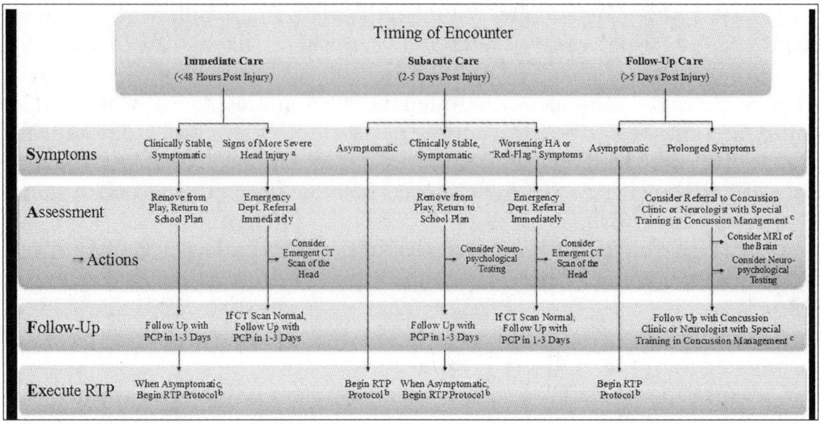

FIGURE 1.—SAFE (Symptoms, Assessment, Follow-up, Execute return-to-play) protocol for concussion management. [a]Loss of consciousness greater than 5 seconds, signs of altered mental status, palpable skull fracture, scalp hematoma, severe mechanism of injury, signs of basilar skull fracture, history of vomiting or severe headache. [b]Only begin return-to-play protocol once patient is completely asymptomatic for 24 hours. [c]May also be indicated in patients who have sustained multiple concussions within a short time frame, have identified comorbidities, or have more concerning symptoms of a moderate traumatic brain injury. Abbreviations: CT, computed tomography; HA, headache; MRI, magnetic resonance imaging; PCP, primary care physician; RTP, return to play. (Reprinted from Provance AJ, Engelman GH, Terhune EB, et al. Management of sport-related concussion in the pediatric and adolescent population. *Orthopedics*. 2016;39:24-30, with permission from SLACK Incorporated.)

Pediatric and adolescent concussions may cause anxiety for the treating physician due to concerns over return-to-play decisions, academic issues, and the potential for second impact syndrome. Determining when to refer a patient to an emergency department acutely, to an outpatient concussion clinic, or to other subspecialists may be a difficult decision for the primary care physician. The aim of this article is to review current evidence regarding concussion treatment and return-to-school and return-to-play recommendations to provide the primary care and sports medicine physician with practical guidelines for managing concussions (Fig 1).

▶ Review articles such as this are difficult to effectively summarize. The topic is ever increasing in the medical community and in the public's awareness. Fortunately guidelines have now been developed that help with the 2 main issues facing the local team doctor: when can the player safely return to sport? and when should I refer the patient for specialized assessment? The so-called SAFE (Symptoms, Assessment, Follow-up, Execute) guidelines are helpful in determining when a patient should return to sport. Today there are standardized protocols that must be followed to fulfill these requirements (Fig 1). The issue of when to refer is less clear, but the guidelines demonstrated in the figure are helpful. Note the temporal thresholds of 48 hours, 5 days, and 10 days. The implication is the patient requires close monitoring over this time period.

B. F. Morrey, MD

Family Physicians with a Certificate of Added Qualifications (CAQs) in Sports Medicine Spend the Majority of Their Time Practicing Sports Medicine

Rankin WM, Cochrane A, Puffer JC (Univ of Kentucky, Lexington; American Board of Family Medicine, Lexington)

J Am Board Fam Med 28:695-696, 2015

While family physicians holding certificates of added qualifications in sports medicine practice in multiple settings, little is currently known about the proportion of their time devoted exclusively to the practice of sports medicine. We found that most spend a majority of their time doing so, and this number has been increasing over the past decade.

▶ This is a simple, brief, and informative article. Many orthopedic surgeons may not know that since 1993, a certificate of added qualifications in sports medicine exists for the family practitioner. There are 1875 such trained physicians, and importantly, more than 50% have an exclusive sports medicine practice. The numbers have been increasing over the past decade. I recently had occasion to personally interact with many of these physicians and am impressed with their knowledge base and care, especially with the massive volume of minor injuries and chronic overuse tendinopathy.

B. F. Morrey, MD

Cheerleading Injuries in United States High Schools

Currie DW, Fields SK, Patterson MJ, et al (Colorado School of Public Health, Aurora; Univ of Colorado—Denver; Lemak Sports Medicine, Birmingham, AL; et al)

Pediatrics 137:1-9, 2016

Background and Objectives.—Approximately 400 000 students participate in US high school cheerleading annually, including 123 386 involved in competitive spirit squads. The degree of athleticism and the difficulty of cheerleading skills have increased in recent decades, renewing safety concerns. This study describes the epidemiology of high school cheerleading injuries and compares cheerleading injury rates and patterns relative to other sports.

Methods.—Data collected by the longitudinal, National High School Sports-Related Injury Surveillance Study from 2009/2010 through 2013/2014 were analyzed.

Results.—Injury rates in cheerleading ranked 18th of 22 sports, with an overall injury rate of 0.71 per 1000 athlete-exposures (AEs). Competition (0.85) and practice (0.76) injury rates were similar, whereas performance rates were lower (0.49). Although 96.8% of injured cheerleaders were girls, the overall injury rate was higher in boys (1.33 vs 0.69, rate ratio [RR]: 1.93, 95% confidence interval [CI]: 1.30–2.88). Although concussions were the most common cheerleading injury (31.1% of injuries), concussion rates were significantly lower in cheerleading (2.21 per 10 000 athlete-exposures) than all other sports combined (3.78; RR: 0.58, 95% CI: 0.51–0.66) and all other girls' sports (2.70; RR: 0.82, 95% CI: 0.72–0.93). Over half of all injuries occurred during stunts (53.2%).

Conclusions.—Although safety remains a concern among cheerleaders, overall injury rates are lower than most other high school sports. Although overall injury rates are relatively low, cheerleading injuries may be more severe when they do occur. A detailed knowledge of cheerleading injury patterns relative to other sports is needed to drive targeted, evidence-based prevention efforts.

▶ I must confess that this study was of interest because my daughter was a high school cheerleader and did engage in competitive events. It is actually comforting to see the rate of injury ranks as 18 of 22 sports and to know the rate has not significantly increased in the past 5 years. This is helpful because we all know of instances of a devastating injury having occurred to cheerleaders. The most worrisome is that of paralysis, frequently related to the "pyramid" or a variation of it. Concussion is also relatively uncommon, but 5% of injuries prevent return to sport that season, and 2.5% are career-ending. Of interest and possibly not surprisingly, the frequency of injury is greater in males than females.

B. F. Morrey, MD

A Qualitative Investigation of Return to Sport After Arthroscopic Bankart Repair: Beyond Stability

Tjong VK, Devitt BM, Murnaghan ML, et al (Univ of Toronto, Ontario, Canada; et al)
Am J Sports Med 43:2005-2011, 2015

Background.—Arthroscopic shoulder stabilization is known to have excellent functional results, but many patients do not return to their preinjury level of sport, with return to play rates reported between 48% and 100% despite good outcome scores.

Purpose.—To understand specific subjective psychosocial factors influencing a patient's decision to return to sport after arthroscopic shoulder stabilization.

Study Design.—Case series; Level of evidence, 4.

Methods.—Semistructured qualitative interviews were conducted with patients aged 18 to 40 years who had undergone primary arthroscopic shoulder stabilization and had a minimum 2-year follow-up. All patients participated in sport before surgery without any further revision operations or shoulder injuries. Qualitative data analysis was performed in accordance with the Strauss and Corbin theory to derive codes, categories, and themes. Preinjury and current sport participation was defined by type, level of competition, and the Brophy/Marx shoulder activity score. Patient-reported pain and shoulder function were also obtained.

Results.—A total of 25 patients were interviewed, revealing that fear of reinjury, shifts in priority, mood, social support, and self-motivation were found to greatly influence the decision to return to sport both in patients who had and had not returned to their preinjury level of play. Patients also described fear of sporting incompetence, self-awareness issues, recommendations from physical therapists, and degree of confidence as less common considerations affecting their return to sport.

Conclusion.—In spite of excellent functional outcomes, extrinsic and intrinsic factors such as competing interests, kinesiophobia, age, and internal stressors and motivators can have a major effect on a patient's decision to return to sport after arthroscopic shoulder stabilization. The qualitative methods used in this study provide a unique patient-derived perspective into postoperative recovery and highlight the necessity to recognize and address subjective and psychosocial factors rather than objective functional outcome scores alone as contributing to a patient's decision to return to play.

▶ This contribution address a common problem with a different question and methodology. The gold standard of all sports articles is "return to sport," ideally at the same level. We all know there are many variables that influence this as an end point or as a measure of success of the procedure. For the shoulder, the authors demonstrate the true complexity of the issue and note motivation and perceived status as being major factors that determine the return to full activity. Although the sample size is small, the methodology appears to provide valid conclusions. Going forward, these more subjective variables should be given additional consideration when determining whether to operate and what is the true impact of the procedure.

B. F. Morrey, MD

Distal Biceps Tendon Ruptures: An Epidemiological Analysis Using a Large Population Database

Kelly MP, Perkinson SG, Ablove RH, et al (Univ of Wisconsin, Madison; Mayo Clinic Health System, Owatonna, MN; State Univ of New York at Buffalo, NY)
Am J Sports Med 43:2012-2017, 2015

Background.—The incidence of distal biceps tendon ruptures was studied more than 10 years ago in a small patient cohort. Recent diagnostic advancements have improved the ability to detect this rare injury.

Hypothesis.—The incidence of distal biceps tendon ruptures will be significantly greater than previously reported.

Study Design.—Descriptive epidemiologic study.

TABLE 2.—Demographic Data[a]

	Current Study	Safran and Graham[12]	*P* Value[b]
Male sex	88/92 (95.7)	13/14 (92.8)	.52
Obesity[c]	46/69 (66.7)	5/14 (35.7)	.04
Labor-intensive job	43/87 (49.4)	4/14 (28.6)	.16
Dominant limb	38/73 (52.1)	12/14 (85.7)	.04

Editor's Note: Please refer to original journal article for full references.
[a]Data are reported as No./total (%).
[b]Fisher exact test.
[c]University of Wisconsin data: body mass index >30. Safran and Graham data: labeled by primary care physician.
Reprinted from Kelly MP, Perkinson SG, Ablove RH, et al. Distal biceps tendon ruptures: an epidemiological analysis using a large population database. *Am J Sports Med.* 2015;43:2012-2017, with permission from The Author(s).

Methods.—A query of the PearlDiver Technologies national database containing public and private insurance patients was used to estimate the national incidence of distal biceps tendon ruptures in the United States. A retrospective chart review of our local population identified demographic groups and risk factors that increased likelihood of injury.

Results.—The estimated national incidence of distal biceps tendon rupture was 2.55 per 100,000 patient-years. The local incidence was 5.35 per 100,000 patient-years. The mean and median ages of patients in our regional cohort were 46.3 and 46 years, respectively. Males composed the majority of the injured population (national 95%, regional 96%). Smoking and elevated body mass index were found to be associated with increased likelihood of injury, while diabetes mellitus showed no association.

Conclusion.—The incidence of distal biceps tendon ruptures in this study was higher than previously reported (Table 2).

▶ Distal biceps tendon rupture, once thought of to be rare, is well recognized to be more common than previously documented. This study reveals that the frequency may be twice as common, 5.35 versus 2.55 in 100 000, than heretofore documented. Some of the difference is an ever increasing recognition due to a higher index of suspicion and better imaging diagnostic techniques. I found the demographics in Table 2 of interest because they document the statistical relevance of the common associated factors: gender, activity, and extremity dominance. The corollary to this study is the recognition that we have reliable techniques to treat the condition safely and effectively.

B. F. Morrey, MD

Microfracture and Osteochondral Autograft Transplantation Are Cost-effective Treatments for Articular Cartilage Lesions of the Distal Femur

Miller DJ, Smith MV, Matava MJ, et al (Northwest Orthopaedic and Sports Medicine, Richland, WA; Washington Univ, St Louis, MO)

Am J Sports Med 43:2175-2181, 2015

Background.—Multiple techniques have been suggested for the treatment of isolated knee articular cartilage injuries. For smaller lesions (<2-5 cm^2), microfracture and osteochondral autograft transplantation (OAT) are commonly used options. With an increasing focus on health care efficiency, analyzing the cost-effectiveness of treatment modalities has become increasingly important.

Purpose/Hypothesis.—The purpose of this study was to analyze the costs and outcomes of microfracture and OAT to compare their cost-effectiveness. The hypothesis was that microfracture would be more cost-effective.

Study Design.—Economic and decision analysis; Level of evidence, 2.

Methods.—A literature search was performed to identify studies comparing microfracture and OAT for the treatment of articular cartilage lesions of the distal femur in an adult population. Data from these studies including surgical time, failure rates, revision surgeries, outcome scores, and return to athletics were then incorporated into a constructed cost model using standard accounting methodology. The model was based on actual 2013 cost figures (in US dollars) for all procedure, operating room, and instrumentation costs.

Results.—Three studies, with a mean follow-up of 8.7 years, met the inclusion criteria of having evidence level 1 or 2 comparing microfracture and OAT. There was a cumulative 28.6% reoperation rate among patients undergoing microfracture compared with 12.5% among patients undergoing OAT. While both groups demonstrated significant improvements compared with preoperative levels, the only significant differences in any outcome score reported between the 2 procedures were the International Cartilage Repair Society (ICRS) score and patient-reported return to their previous sports activity level. While microfracture had a lower initial cost ($3100), these savings lessened over 1 year ($1843) and 10 years ($996). Microfracture was more cost-effective when comparing Lysholm and Hospital for Special Surgery scores, whereas OAT was more cost-effective when comparing Tegner and ICRS scores. There was a significantly lower cost for return to play in athletes after OAT versus microfracture at 1 year ($11,428 vs $16,953, respectively), 3 years ($12,856 vs $38,000, respectively), and 10 years ($32,141 vs $60,799, respectively).

Conclusion.—Published level 1 and 2 clinical studies with a 10-year follow-up demonstrated that the net cost and cost-effectiveness of microfracture and OAT are comparable for the treatment of isolated articular cartilage lesions of the distal femur.

TABLE 3.—Cost Comparison[a]

	Initial	Total Net Cost 1 y	10 y
Microfracture	$7220	$8769	$10,483
OAT	$10,320	$10,612	$11,479
Difference	−$3100	−$1843	−$996

OAT, osteochondral autograft transplantation.
[a]Costs are based on 2013 US dollars.
Reprinted from Miller DJ, Smith MV, Matava MJ, et al. Microfracture and osteochondral autograft transplantation are cost-effective treatments for articular cartilage lesions of the distal femur. *Am J Sports Med.* 2015;43:2175-2181, with permission from The Author(s).

TABLE 4.—Cost of Return to Play[a]

	Return to Play, y 1	3	10
Microfracture	$16,953	$38,000	$60,799
OAT	$11,427.84	$12,856.42	$32,141.05

OAT, osteochondral autograft transplantation.
[a]Costs are based on 2013 US dollars.
Reprinted from Miller DJ, Smith MV, Matava MJ, et al. Microfracture and osteochondral autograft transplantation are cost-effective treatments for articular cartilage lesions of the distal femur. *Am J Sports Med.* 2015;43:2175-2181, with permission from The Author(s).

Clinical Relevance.—Given similar clinical outcomes, microfracture and OAT are both viable, cost-effective first-line treatment options for these injuries (Tables 3 and 4).

▶ In my opinion, this is an excellent article because it addresses an important question, employs current state-of-the-art methodology, and focuses on cost-effectiveness of disparate treatment options for femoral chondral lesions. Note that the literature is actually quiet on the subject of cost-effectiveness of the 2 most common treatment options: microfracture and osteochondral autograft transplantation (OAT). In sum, the cost-effectiveness depends on what is being measured. In broad terms, the OAT procedure is about $1000 more costly at 1 and 10 years (Table 3). However, if one is dealing with an individual that requires a high performance level, the OAT is half as costly, and in this instance, the difference is about $30,000 (Table 4). Hence, which is the most cost-effective procedure is stratified according to the level of activity required by the patient.

B. F. Morrey, MD

Is Sport Activity Possible After Arthroscopic Meniscal Allograft Transplantation? Midterm Results in Active Patients

Zaffagnini S, Grassi A, Marcheggiani Muccioli GM, et al (Istituto Ortopedico Rizzoli, Bologna, Italy)

Am J Sports Med 44:625-632, 2016

Background.—Meniscal allograft transplantation (MAT) has produced good to excellent results in the general population; however, few investigations have examined MAT in athletes and sport-related outcomes.

Purpose.—To report midterm clinical outcomes of MAT and the rate of return to sport in a physically active population.

Study Design.—Case series; Level of evidence, 4.

Methods.—The study included all physically active patients who underwent arthroscopic MAT without bone plugs and had a minimum of 2 years of follow-up at a single institution. Clinical evaluation was performed with the Knee injury and Osteoarthritis Outcome Score (KOOS), the Tegner activity scale, and a 0- to 100-point subjective scale for knee function and satisfaction. Outcomes evaluated included ability to return to sport, time to return to sport, level of sport activity upon return compared with preinjury level, and level of decrease in sport participation or reasons for not returning to sport participation. Comparisons were made between patients who did or did not return to sport and between patients who returned to the same level or a decreased level. Regression analysis was performed to determine the variables affecting the outcomes.

Results.—Eighty-nine patients, whose mean ± SD age at surgery was 38.5 ± 11.2 years, were evaluated to a mean follow-up of 4.2 ± 1.9 years. Total KOOS improved from a mean ± SD of 39.5 ± 18.5 preoperatively to 84.7 ± 14.8 at the latest follow-up ($P < .001$). The Tegner score improved significantly from a median of 2 (interquartile range [IQR], 1-4) preoperatively to a median of 4 (IQR, 3-6) at the latest follow-up ($P < .001$), although it did not reach the preinjury level of 6 (IQR, 5-7) ($P < .001$). Older age at surgery was correlated with the worst clinical results. Sixty-six patients (74%) were able to return to sport after 8.6 ± 4.1 months. Forty-four (49%) returned to the same level as preinjury. Patients who did not return to sport activity and those who reduced their activity level at follow-up had inferior subjective outcomes compared with those who returned to sport and those who returned to their preinjury levels, respectively. Only 11 patients (12%) underwent a surgical procedure during the follow-up period.

Conclusion.—Arthroscopic MAT without bone plugs improved knee function and reduced pain, allowing sport resumption in 74% of patients and return to the preinjury activity level in 49% of patients at midterm follow-up. Of all the demographic and surgical variables, only age at surgery seemed to affect outcomes.

▶ This is one of the few studies I have seen that addresses this topic, and I was frankly, interested in their findings. There is value in all the procedures being done at a single institution, and the follow-up instruments are validated allowing one to have confidence in the findings. The simple message is that, given the inclusion criteria, 75% returned to sport in less than a year, and 50% returned to the same level as preinjury. This is pretty good. The surveillance of almost 100 patients followed for at least 2 years (mean 4 years) also provides strength to their conclusion.

B. F. Morrey, MD

Meniscus Suture Repair: Minimum 10-Year Outcomes in Patients Younger Than 40 Years Compared with Patients 40 and Older

Steadman JR, Matheny LM, Singleton SB, et al (Steadman Philippon Res Inst, Vail, CO)
Am J Sports Med 43:2222-2227, 2015

Background.—Few studies have compared outcomes after meniscus suture repair in patients younger than 40 years versus patients 40 years and older.

Purpose.—To document failure rates and long-term outcomes after meniscus suture repair by a single surgeon, using the inside-out technique, at a minimum 10-year follow-up in patients younger than 40 years versus those 40 years and older.

Study Design.—Cohort study; Level of evidence, 3.

Methods.—This study included all patients 18 years or older who underwent meniscus suture repair with the inside-out technique by a single surgeon between January 1992 and December 2003. Patients were divided into 2 cohorts according to age: <40 years (cohort 1) and ≥40 years (cohort 2). If patients underwent subsequent knee surgery, all subsequent reports, whether performed by the original treating surgeon or by a different surgeon elsewhere, were reviewed by 2 independent reviewers not involved in the primary care of the patients. Reviewers classified surgeries as failures if the subsequent surgery treated the same area of the meniscus as repaired in the index surgery. Patients completed a subjective questionnaire at minimum of 10 years after arthroscopy. Outcomes measures included Lysholm, Tegner, and patient satisfaction with outcome. All data were collected prospectively.

Results.—The surgeon performed 339 meniscus repairs between 1992 and 2003. The study included 181 knees in 178 patients, who had a mean age of 33 years (range, 18-70 years). Cohort 1 contained 136 knees; 16 patients (12%) were lost to follow-up and 47 (35%) underwent a subsequent knee arthroscopy. Cohort 2 contained 45 knees; 2 patients (4.4%) were lost to follow-up, 3 patients had a total knee arthroplasty, and 12 patients (28%) underwent a subsequent knee arthroscopy. In cohort 1, the meniscus repair failure rate was 5.5% (6/110), and in cohort 2 it was 5.3% (2/38) (P =.927). There was no significant difference in failure rate based on which meniscus was repaired (P =.257), concomitant anterior cruciate ligament (ACL) reconstruction (P =.092), or microfracture (P =.674). Average follow-up time for cohort 1 was 16.1 years (range, 10.0-21.9 years), with 82% follow-up (n = 73/89); average follow-up time for cohort 2 was 16.2 years (range, 10.1-21.0 years), with 93% follow-up (n = 28/30). There were no significant differences in outcomes scores after meniscus suture repair based on age cohort or meniscus side, presence of an ACL tear, or concomitant microfracture procedure.

Conclusion.—Meniscus repair failure rate was not different in patients who were younger than 40 years versus those who were 40 years or older at time of meniscus index surgery. Patients who underwent meniscus suture repair had high function and high patient satisfaction at an average of 16 years after meniscus suture repair, and no differences were seen based on age (Fig 1).

▶ This is a really important contribution because it provides the clinician important information that is different from my perception and what has been generally accepted as true: meniscus repair is equally effective in those under and over 40 years of age. Note the marked differences in the cohort sizes—3 times as many patients younger compared with older than 40 years—suggesting the careful selection criteria employed. The strengths of the study are that

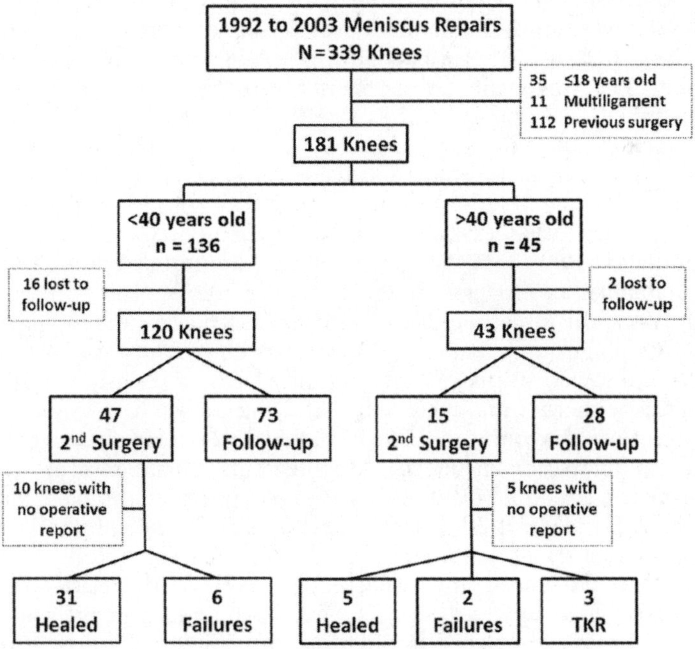

FIGURE 1.—Flow chart describing patient cohorts and patient selection. TKR, total knee replacement. (Reprinted from Steadman JR, Matheny LM, Singleton SB, et al. Meniscus suture repair: minimum 10-year outcomes in patients younger than 40 years compared with patients 40 and older. *Am J Sports Med.* 2015;43:2222-2227, with permission from The Author(s).)

the procedures were all done by 1 surgeon over a 12-year period with considerable follow-up periods averaging more than 15 years. The overall success rate of 95% is impressive (Fig 1). Finally, it is surprising the outcome was not influenced by the presence of an anterior cruciate ligament injury or concurrent microfracture. This is a landmark experience in my opinion.

B. F. Morrey, MD

Age-Related Risk Factors for Revision Anterior Cruciate Ligament Reconstruction: A Cohort Study of 21,304 Patients From the Kaiser Permanente Anterior Cruciate Ligament Registry

Maletis GB, Chen J, Inacio MCS, et al (Kaiser Permanente Baldwin Park, CA; Kaiser Permanente, San Diego, CA; et al)

Am J Sports Med 44:331-336, 2016

Background.—It is not clear whether risk factors for revision anterior cruciate ligament reconstruction (ACLR) are the same throughout patients' lives.

Purpose.—To assess (1) the risk of revision ACLR by age and (2) age-specific risk factors for revision ACLR.

Study Design.—Cohort study; Level of evidence, 2.

Methods.—A cohort study using patients having undergone primary ACLR who were registered in the Kaiser Permanente ACLR Registry (February 2005 to June 2013) was conducted. Aseptic revision was the main endpoint. Age was evaluated as a risk factor for revision. The cohort was stratified into 4 age groups: <21, 21-30, 31-40, and >40 years. Graft type, sex, body mass index (BMI), and race were assessed as revision risk factors within each group. Survival analyses were conducted.

Results.—Of the 21,304 patients evaluated, 7026 (33%) patients were aged <21 years, 5762 (27%) were 21-30 years, 4656 (22%) were 31-40 years, and 3860 (18%) were >40 years. Allografts were used in 8671 (41%) patients, hamstring autografts in 6823 (32%), and bone–patellar tendon–bone (BPTB) autografts in 5260 (25%). The 5-year revision probability was highest in patients <21 years old (9.0%; 95% CI, 8.0%-10.1%) and lowest in those >40 years old (1.9%; 95% CI, 1.3%-2.7%). Compared with patients aged >40 years, the adjusted revision risk for patients aged <21 years was 7.76 (95% CI, 5.52-10.90). In patients aged <21 years, a lower revision risk was seen in female patients (hazard ratio [HR], 0.76; 95% CI, 0.61-0.93) compared with male patients, patients with a BMI of 30-35 kg/m^2 (HR, 0.75; 95% CI, 0.59-0.95) and BMI >35 kg/m^2 (HR, 0.49; 95% CI, 0.34-0.70) compared with those with a BMI <30 kg/m^2, and black patients (HR, 0.55, 95% CI, 0.36-0.85) compared with white patients. Sex, BMI, and race were not associated with the risk of revision in older patients. In patients ≤40 years old, those with allografts had a higher risk of revision than those with BPTB autografts (HR, 2.69, 2.35, and 3.04 for patients aged <21, 21-30, and 31-40 years, respectively). Patients <21 years old with hamstring

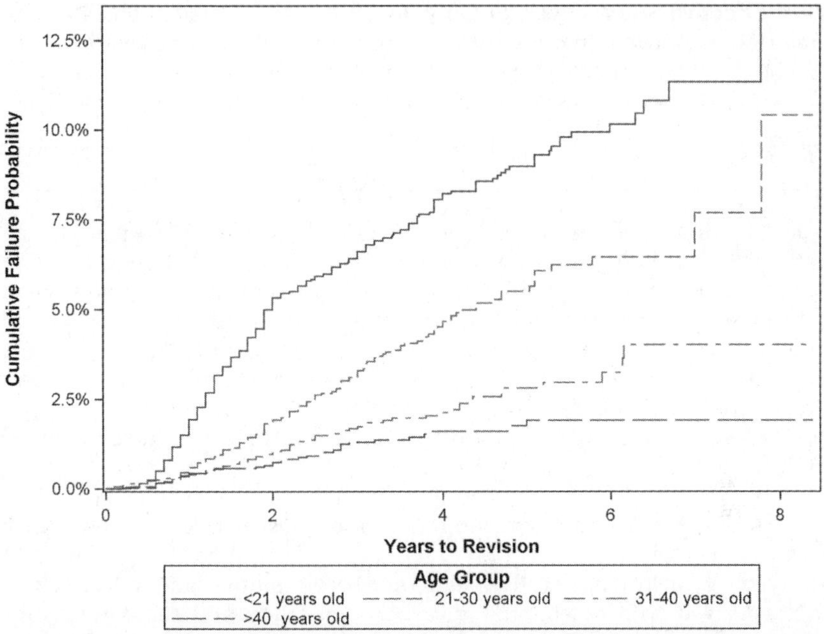

FIGURE 1.—Kaplan-Meier curve for cumulative failure probability estimates of patients with primary anterior cruciate ligament reconstruction by patient age group. (Reprinted from Maletis GB, Chen J, Inacio MCS, et al. Age-related risk factors for revision anterior cruciate ligament reconstruction: a cohort study of 21,304 patients from the Kaiser Permanente anterior cruciate ligament registry. *Am J Sports Med.* 2016;44:331-336, with permission from The Author(s).)

autografts had a 1.61 times (95% CI, 1.20-2.17) higher risk of revision than did patients with BPTB autografts; these differences were not identified in older patients.

Conclusion.—Age at the time of ACLR surgery is a strong risk factor for revision ACLR. Other risk factors for revision ACLR, such as graft type, sex, race, and BMI, may vary in strength and significance over a patient's life. Understanding the age-related risk factors associated with revision ACLR may help with appropriate patient counseling and optimal graft choice when performing ACLR (Fig 1).

▶ This is a well conceived and executed study. While the main question is quite simple - age related risk of a revision anterior cruciate ligament (ACL) procedure, the complexity increases considerably as one considers the compounding variables, such as gender, race body mass index (BMI) and especially graft type.

The answer to the central question is clearly answered and demonstrated in Fig 1. Note the highest risk is of course in those under 21 years, but the decrease in risk by decades is not linear with the other three decade cohorts. BMI plays a role that was greater than gender. But, of interest, the bone patella bone graft outperformed other autogtaft options as well as all the allograft categories. I mention this as the BPB was the graft of choice in my practice.

B. F. Morrey, MD

Cost-Effectiveness Analysis of Early Reconstruction Versus Rehabilitation and Delayed Reconstruction for Anterior Cruciate Ligament Tears

Mather RC III, Hettrich CM, Dunn WR, et al (Duke Univ School of Medicine, Durham, NC; Univ of Iowa School of Medicine; Univ of Wisconsin Med Ctr, Madison; et al)

Am J Sports Med 42:1583-1591, 2014

Background.—An initial anterior cruciate ligament (ACL) tear can be treated with surgical reconstruction or focused rehabilitation. The KANON (Knee Anterior cruciate ligament, NON-surgical versus surgical treatment) randomized controlled trial compared rehabilitation plus early ACL reconstruction (ACLR) to rehabilitation plus optional delayed ACLR and found no difference at 2 years by an intention-to-treat analysis of total Knee injury and Osteoarthritis Outcome Score (KOOS) results.

Purpose.—To compare the cost-effectiveness of early versus delayed ACLR.

Study Design.—Economic and decision analysis; Level of evidence, 2.

Methods.—A Markov decision model was constructed for a cost-utility analysis of early reconstruction (ER) versus rehabilitation plus optional delayed reconstruction (DR). Outcome probabilities and effectiveness were derived from 2 sources: the KANON study and the Multicenter Orthopaedic Outcomes Network (MOON) database. Collectively, these 2 sources provided data from 928 ACL-injured patients. Utilities were measured by the Short Form–6 dimensions (SF-6D). Costs were estimated from a societal perspective in 2012 US dollars. Costs and utilities were discounted in accordance with the United States Panel on Cost-Effectiveness in Health and Medicine. Effectiveness was expressed in quality-adjusted life-years (QALYs) gained. Principal outcome measures were average incremental costs, incremental effectiveness (as measured by QALYs), and net health benefits. Willingness to pay was set at $50,000, which is the currently accepted standard in the United States.

Results.—In the base case, the ER group resulted in an incremental gain of 0.28 QALYs over the DR group, with a corresponding lower overall cost to society of $1572. Effectiveness gains were driven by the low utility of an unstable knee and the lower utility for the DR group. The cost of rehabilitation and the rate of additional surgery drove the increased cost of the DR group. The most sensitive variable was the rate of knee instability after initial rehabilitation. When the rate of instability falls to 51.5%, DR is less costly, and when the rate of instability falls below 18.0%, DR becomes the preferred cost-effective strategy.

Conclusion.—An economic analysis of the timing of ACLR using data exclusively from the KANON trial, MOON cohort, and national average reimbursement revealed that early ACLR was more effective (improved QALYs) at a lower cost than rehabilitation plus optional delayed ACLR.

Therefore, early ACLR should be the preferred treatment strategy from a societal health system perspective.

▶ Interesting question, interesting methodology. In the simplest of terms, is an early anterior cruciate ligament reconstruction cost-effective? The answer, I think, is pretty well defined in this study. Yes, "if . . ." The "if" is dependent on whether the reconstructive procedure is effective. If, overall, the reconstruction is at least 55% effective in attaining the goals of the procedure, it is better to reconstruct than to wait. Assuming that most have a better than 55% success rate, the answer is, reconstruct early.

B. F. Morrey, MD

Eligibility and Disqualification Recommendations for Competitive Athletes With Cardiovascular Abnormalities: Preamble, Principles, and General Considerations: A Scientific Statement From the American Heart Association and American College of Cardiology

Maron BJ, on behalf of the American Heart Association Electrocardiography and Arrhythmias Committee of the Council on Clinical Cardiology, Council on Cardiovascular Disease in the Young, Council on Cardiovascular and Stroke Nursing, Council on Functional Genomics and Translational Biology, and the American College of Cardiology ()
Circulation 132:e256-e261, 2015

Background.—The tragedy of sudden death among young athletes participating in sports has prompted a closer look at the eligibility and disqualification guidelines that are currently in place for organized competitive sports. The goal is to ensure the health and safety of young athletes and avoid sudden death while not unfairly or unnecessarily removing people from a healthy, athletic lifestyle. Three Bethesda Conferences have produced statements of criteria for eligibility and disqualification for competitive athletes with cardiovascular conditions since 1985. The American Heart Association and American College of Cardiology (AHA/ACC) offer a document based on the experience and expertise of the panelists and available scientific evidence that estimates athletes' medical risk.

Causes of Sudden Death.—Young athletes of both sexes, of minority status, and in a wide range of individual and team sports can suffer sudden death. Genetic heart diseases are the major cause of death, including hypertrophic cardiomyopathy, congenital coronary anomalies, myocarditis, aortic valve stenosis, aortic dissection/rupture, atherosclerotic coronary artery disease, ion channelopathies, and arrhythmogenic right ventricular cardiomyopathy. In addition, commotion cordis causes sudden death in more young athletes than any of the structural cardiovascular diseases. Older athletes (those over age 35 years) tend to die of atherosclerotic coronary artery disease, which is seen less often in younger sports participants.

Assessment of Risk.—Young persons who participate in competitive sports while they have cardiovascular abnormalities have limited control when exposed to extreme and unpredictable environmental conditions, such as altered blood volume, hydration, or electrolyte levels. Sport makes extreme demands on athletes and can suddenly enhance the risk for potentially lethal arrhythmias and sudden death. Removal from the lifestyle of athletic training and competition reduces the risk, but prophylactic treatment may also be undertaken for some young patients. For these reasons, risk stratification on a case-by-case basis is needed to guide medical decisions. The goal is to avoid the increased sudden death risk and make it a controllable variable by taking a conservative approach.

In practice, rather than removal from sports participation, athletes may be encouraged to change their competitive sport involvement to one that is of lower intensity. It can, however, be difficult to ask an athlete to change the position played to remain in a sport. In addition, training activities, which are often more stringent than actual play, must also be controlled and monitored sufficiently.

Role of Guidelines.—The specific recommendations offered by AHA/ACC are similar to or identical to those in the report of the 36th Bethesda Conference. Specific recommendations may be less restrictive based on data and observations that have become available since 2005. Gray areas remain, which contribute to differences of opinion between practitioners about the role of clinical judgment in specific cases. The AHA/ACC document is not intended to absolutely mandate action or to represent the general medical and legal standard of care in all cases. The recommendations do not replace individual clinical judgment and informed medical reasoning.

Some practitioners may choose to prudently deviate from the recommendations in certain situations. Athletes who are fully informed and have specific conditions may continue to engage in competitive sports in accordance with their physician's and athletic organization's recommendations. Some flexibility is desirable, as is the recognition of individual responsibility and choice. Specific medical clearance or disqualification recommendations are ultimately the responsibility of the managing physician with medically relevant knowledge of the individual patient/athlete.

Clinicians must acknowledge the complexity of the decisions in these cases and avoid being unduly influenced by the free-will desires of athletes who are willing to take on sports participation even though they face medically unreasonable risks to do so. Third-party interests, such as high schools, colleges, and professional clubs, contribute to the complexity of the process, but the paramount concern is for the athlete's health and safety when medical eligibility recommendations are made.

▶ With the current focus of the nonmusculoskeletal injury being on concussion, it is important to be aware of this initiative regarding cardiovascular risks. The important insights to me were that this effort comprised 15 separate task forces and dates back to 1985. The recommendations have been updated every decade since then. As with the head injured athlete, there are specific recommendations that qualify an athlete with a cardiovascular issue fit for play. However, as expected, the documents recognizes many gray areas requiring individual physician judgment. What I found most interesting, and frankly a little disturbing, is a formal table in the document listing all the potential conflicts of interest of the contributors. Where will this end?

B. F. Morrey, MD

Are Muscle Strength and Function of the Uninjured Lower Limb Weakened After Anterior Cruciate Ligament Injury? Two-Year Follow-up After Reconstruction

Chung KS, Ha JK, Yeom CH, et al (KEPCO Med Ctr, Seoul, Korea; Inje Univ, Seoul, Korea; et al)

Am J Sports Med 43:3013-3021, 2015

Background.—After an anterior cruciate ligament (ACL) injury, the uninjured contralateral lower limb may become weakened because of neuromuscular changes, proprioceptive deficits, and disuse of the limb; this weakness predisposes the limb to ACL injury. However, no results have been reported regarding weakness in the contralateral limb after ACL injury.

Hypothesis.—Muscle strength and functional status of the contralateral lower limb are reduced after unilateral ACL injury.

Study Design.—Cohort study; Level of evidence, 3.

Methods.—The ACL group consisted of 75 patients who underwent primary unilateral ACL reconstruction and were followed at 3, 6, 12, and 24 months postoperatively. A group of 75 healthy individuals (controls) were matched one-to-one with the ACL group for age, sex, body mass index, and initial Tegner activity level. The side that was evaluated in each control subject corresponded to the injured limb in the matched ACL subject. Isokinetic muscle strength, including extension peak torque per body weight (EPT) and flexion peak torque per body weight (FPT), was evaluated at angular velocities of 60 and 180 deg/s. Patients were also evaluated by single-legged hop test.

Results.—Compared with the EPT at 60 deg/s in the control group (290.9 ± 40.1 N·m/kg), the value in the ACL group 24-month follow-up (276.6 ± 42.8 N·m/kg) as well as other follow-up times was significantly lower ($P < .05$), whereas the EPT at 180 deg/s and the FPT at 60 and 180 deg/s in the ACL group were significantly lower than the control group at 3-month follow-up but were restored to normal levels at final follow-up. Results from the single-legged hop test demonstrated that the ACL group performed at a significantly lower level than the control group at 24-month follow-up (158.4 ± 25.3 vs 176.3 ± 24.7 cm;

$P < .05$) as well as other follow-up times. However, both measurements improved significantly as the follow-up time progressed.

Conclusion.—After ACL injury, isokinetic extensor muscle strength and functional status of the contralateral limb were reduced, even at 24 months after ACL reconstruction. However, both measurements improved significantly as the follow-up time progressed. In contrast, flexion muscle strength was restored to normal levels. Therefore, care should be taken to restore muscle strength and functional status in not only the ACL-reconstructed knee but also the uninjured limb.

▶ This study would seem to provide some useful clinical information. A modest sample was studied to determine the effect of strength on the noninjured extremity after anterior cruciate ligament (ACL) reconstruction. That the contralateral extremity did suffer functional loss of strength is well documented with the use of a valid control group. The study underscores the value of the current widespread practice of rehabilitating both extremities after ACL reconstruction. Of specific note is the selective weakening of the extensors, justifying the further emphasis of this muscle group in the rehabilitation process.

B. F. Morrey, MD

Anterior Cruciate Ligament Injury, Return to Play, and Reinjury in the Elite Collegiate Athlete: Analysis of an NCAA Division I Cohort

Kamath GV, Murphy T, Creighton RA, et al (Univ of North Carolina at Chapel Hill)

Am J Sports Med 42:1638-1643, 2014

Background.—Graft survivorship, reinjury rates, and career length are poorly understood after anterior cruciate ligament (ACL) reconstruction in the elite collegiate athlete. The purpose of this study was to examine the outcomes of ACL reconstruction in a National Collegiate Athletic Association (NCAA) Division I athlete cohort.

Study Design.—Case series; Level of evidence, 4.

Methods.—A retrospective chart review was performed of all Division I athletes at a single public university from 2000 to 2009 until completion of eligibility. Athletes were separated into 2 cohorts: those who underwent precollegiate ACL reconstruction (PC group) and those who underwent intracollegiate reconstruction (IC group). Graft survivorship, reoperation rates, and career length information were collected.

Results.—Thirty-five athletes were identified with precollegiate reconstruction and 54 with intracollegiate reconstruction. The PC group had a 17.1% injury rate with the original graft, with a 20.0% rate of a contralateral ACL injury. For the IC group, the reinjury rates were 1.9% with an ACL graft, with an 11.1% rate of a contralateral ACL injury after intracollegiate ACL reconstruction. The athletes in the PC group used 78% of their total eligibility (average, 3.11 years). The athletes in

TABLE 5.—Effect of Meniscal or Chondral Injury at Index ACL Reconstruction on Eligibility Used (Intracollegiate Group)[a]

	Completion of Eligibility		
	Complete	Incomplete	Total
No meniscal/chondral injury, n	15	4	19
Meniscal/chondral injury, n	14	10	24

[a]There was no statistically significant correlation between the presence of a meniscal/chondral injury and completion of eligibility after the initial ACL reconstruction ($P = .152$, χ^2 test). ACL, anterior cruciate ligament.

Reprinted from Kamath GV, Murphy T, Creighton RA, et al. Anterior cruciate ligament injury, return to play, and reinjury in the elite collegiate athlete: analysis of an NCAA division I cohort. *Am J Sports Med.* 2014;42:1638-1643, with permission from The Author(s).

the IC group used an average of 77% of their remaining NCAA eligibility; 88.3% of those in the IC group played an additional non-redshirt year after their injury. The reoperation rate for the PC group was 51.4% and was 20.4% for the IC group.

Conclusion.—Reoperation and reinjury rates are high after ACL reconstruction in the Division I athlete. Precollegiate ACL reconstruction is associated with a very high (37.1%) rate of repeat ACL reinjuries to the graft or opposite knee. The majority of athletes are able to return to play after successful reconstruction (Table 5).

▶ This report was selected because of the topic. In fact, although the study period covers almost a decade, the actual sample size is rather small. Nonetheless the central finding is of value. Those returning to sport after an anterior cruciate ligament (ACL) reconstruction are at marked risk for reinjury. This risk is greater if the ACL injury and reconstruction occurred before entering college. Regardless, the incidence of reinjury is 25% to 35%, which is considerable. What I found of particular interest is that the frequency of reinjury as a function of associated meniscus injury was 79% if there was an initial meniscus/chondral injury, compared to 58% likelihood if there had been no such injury. This 20% difference is significant clinically, but not statistically, $P = 0.152$ (Table 5). There is a message here—specifically, there is a real difference between clinical and statistical significance.

B. F. Morrey, MD

Combined Biplanar High Tibial Osteotomy, Anterior Cruciate Ligament Reconstruction, and Abrasion/Microfracture in Severe Medial Osteoarthritis of Unstable Varus Knees

Schuster P, Schulz M, Richter J (Centre for Arthroscopy and Sports Medicine, Markgröningen, Germany)

Arthroscopy 32:283-292, 2016

Purpose.—To determine survivorship and functional results of medial open-wedge high tibial osteotomy (HTO) combined with anterior cruciate ligament reconstruction (ACLR) and a chondral resurfacing (CR) procedure (abrasion/microfracture) in patients with Kellgren-Lawrence grade 3 and 4 osteoarthritis with full-thickness cartilage defects, anterior cruciate ligament (ACL) insufficiency, and varus malalignment.

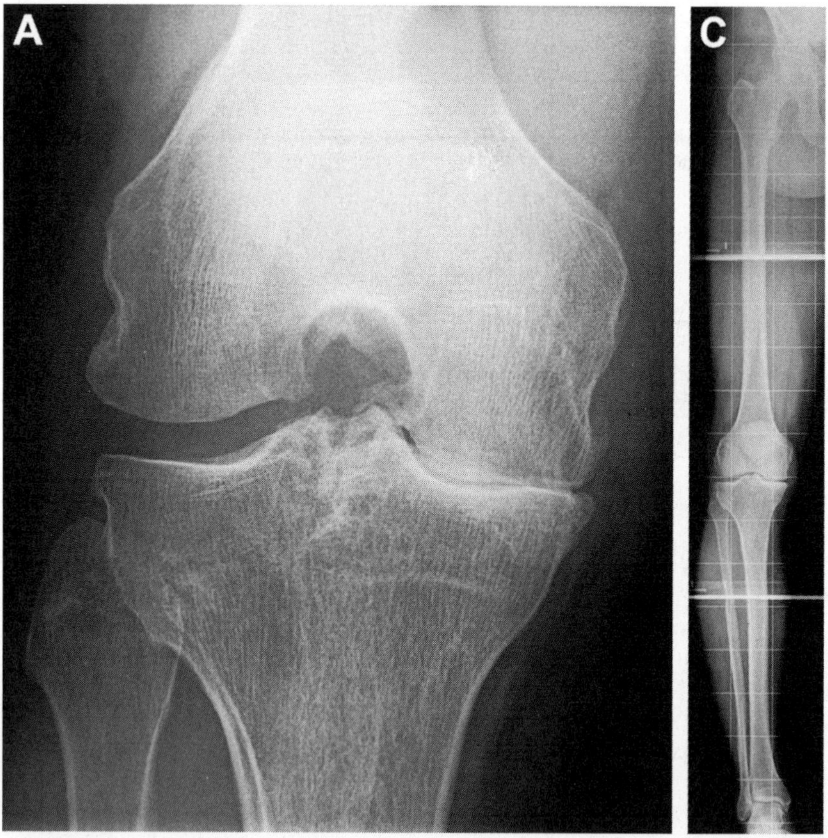

FIGURE 1.—Preoperative (A) Rosenberg, and (C) axis views of a right knee. (Reprinted from Schuster P, Schulz M, Richter J. Combined biplanar high tibial osteotomy, anterior cruciate ligament reconstruction, and abrasion/microfracture in severe medial osteoarthritis of unstable varus knees. *Arthroscopy.* 2016;32:283-292, with permission from Arthroscopy Association of North America.)

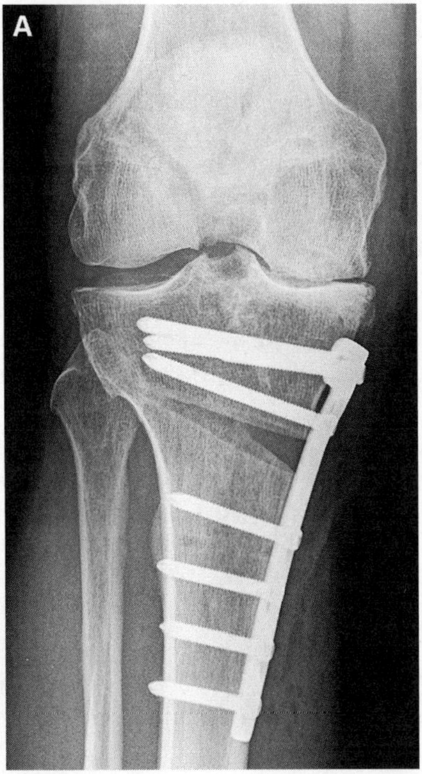

FIGURE 3.—Postoperative (A) anteroposterior views of a right knee with an angular stable plate (TomoFix) for fixation and reconstructed anterior cruciate ligament (same patient as Fig 1). The plate does not interfere with the tibial tunnel. (Reprinted from Schuster P, Schulz M, Richter J. Combined biplanar high tibial osteotomy, anterior cruciate ligament reconstruction, and abrasion/microfracture in severe medial osteoarthritis of unstable varus knees. *Arthroscopy.* 2016;32:283-292, with permission from Arthroscopy Association of North America.)

Methods.—From October 2005 to March 2009, all combined HTO (fixation with angular stable internal fixator), ACLR, and CR procedures in knees with symptomatic medial osteoarthritis (Kellgren-Lawrence grade 3 and 4), ACL insufficiency, varus malalignment (>4°), and full-thickness large-area cartilage defects were prospectively surveyed with a minimum follow-up period of 5 years regarding survival (not requiring arthroplasty), functional outcome (subjective International Knee Documentation Committee [IKDC] score), and subjective satisfaction. Clinical evaluation (objective IKDC parameters and KT-1000 [MEDmetric, San Diego, CA] measurement), radiologic evaluation, and revision arthroscopy were performed between 1 and 2 years postoperatively.

Results.—Twenty-three knees (mean age, 47.0 ± 5.8 years) were included. The rate of follow-up was 100% at 6.0 ± 0.8 years (range, 5.2 to 7.5 years), with no arthroplasty until then. The mean subjective IKDC score improved from 47.7 ± 11.1 to 72.8 ± 15.0 at 1 year,

70.9 ± 16.0 at 3 years, and 73.1 ± 16.4 at 5 years ($P < .001$). Clinical examination and revision arthroscopy were performed in 22 cases (95.5%) at 1.3 ± 0.5 years (range, 1.0 to 2.0 years). Four ACL grafts (18.1%) were insufficient, and 2 grafts (9.1%) were stable but showed signs of degeneration. Good cartilage regeneration was seen in most cases, but no correlation with subjective IKDC score was apparent ($P = .528$).

Conclusions.—HTO in combination with ACLR and a CR procedure is effective in the treatment of severe medial osteoarthritis with concomitant ACL insufficiency and varus malalignment. The effect of the CR, as well as the reason for the considerable rate of graft insufficiency, remains unclear.

Level of Evidence.—Level IV, therapeutic case series (Figs 1A, C and 3A).

▶ I have been waiting for this study to appear. I, and all of us who were trained by Mark Coventry, did hundreds of proximal tibial osteotomies. Today the proximal tibial osteotomy is all but abandoned, except in the young patient exactly as depicted in this article (Fig 1). I am pleased to see all patients survived free of TKA for at least 6 years. It is gratifying that the objective functional scores reflect a high degree of function. When we performed this procedure, we did not address the degenerative joint surface because our data suggested this is not necessary. These authors also could not demonstrate its value. My only concern is I do not feel the massive plate is necessary because it interferes with subsequent replacement (Fig 3). We had similar outcomes with a closing wedge stabilized by 1 or 2 step staples. Regardless, this is an important article dealing with a complex patient.

B. F. Morrey, MD

***CORR* Insights®: Does Combined Intra- and Extraarticular ACL Reconstruction Improve Function and Stability? A Meta-analysis**

Baumfeld J (Lahey Clinic, Peabody, MA)
Clin Orthop Relat Res 473:2619-2620, 2015

Background.—Anterior cruciate ligament (ACL) reconstruction techniques have been associated with a high success rate, but a closer look indicates results are not as good in young patients and high-level high school and collegiate athletes as in other patients. Often young, active patients are unable to return to their high level of participation and may suffer an increased rate of ACL graft rupture or contralateral ACL rupture during the first 1 to 2 years after surgery. To improve these results, orthopedic surgeons are exploring other approaches, especially more anatomic reconstructions of the ACL and double-bundle techniques or single-bundle anatomic techniques. Some studies question whether the anterolateral ligament of the knee should be addressed during surgery. This ligament is crucial in controlling internal rotation, especially in a flexed knee.

Proposed Approaches.—The risk of graft rupture and instability, as well as limitations regarding a return to athletics, may be addressed by dealing with other potential sources of instability in the knee. Adding an extra-articular procedure with an ACL intraarticular reconstruction has been proposed. A review of studies evaluating this approach has been hampered by the small number of comparative trials included, by interobserver differences, and by variability in how the ACL was reconstructed. Factors that were not well controlled include surgical approach, graft type, and graft position. In addition, fewer extra-articular reconstruction procedures are now done.

Conclusions.—Orthopedic specialists need to more effectively identify and define the causes of failure with knee reconstruction. It remains to be decided whether combining procedures with ACL reconstruction creates enough value to outweigh the risks of additional surgical time and complications. A subset of patients may be the only ones to benefit from reconstruction or repair of the anterolateral ligament of the knee or other procedures, and these individuals must be identified. Further studies are needed, including prospective randomized trials comparing current anatomic ACL reconstruction techniques with and without added anterolateral ligament reconstruction to assess whether the combined approach is worthwhile.

▶ Whether we like it or not, the sports section is synonamous with or at least dominated by articles relating to the anterior cruciate ligament. We try to avoid suggestions for a better technique in favor of evidence-based outcomes or insights as to indications and prognostic variables. The interesting feature of this insight review is the hypothesis. An extraarticular component is added because of the failures seen in a significant number of individuals, especially young active males. The author, a former Mayo resident, does a nice job of placing the review in perspective. The bottom line is, before this modification is introduced into practice, we need much more data, ideally from an adequately powered randomized controlled trial.

B. F. Morrey, MD

Functional Outcome and Graft Retention in Patients With Septic Arthritis After Anterior Cruciate Ligament Reconstruction: A Systematic Review

Makhni EC, Steinhaus ME, Mehran N, et al (Columbia Univ Med Ctr, NY; Wayne State Univ, Detroit, MI; et al)

Arthroscopy 31:1392-1401, 2015

Purpose.—To provide a comprehensive review of clinical and functional outcomes after treatment for septic arthritis after anterior cruciate ligament reconstruction.

Methods.—A systematic review of the literature was performed. Two reviewers assessed and confirmed the methodologic quality of each study. Studies that met the inclusion criteria were assessed for pertinent data, and when available, similar outcomes were combined to generate frequency-weighted means.

Results.—Nineteen studies met the inclusion and exclusion criteria for this review, reporting on a total of 203 infected knees. The mean age was 27.5 years and the mean length of follow-up was 44.2 months, with male patients comprising 88% of the population. Hamstring and bone–patellar tendon–bone autografts were used in 63% and 33% of patients, respectively, with 78% of patients retaining their grafts. The studies reported mean flexion and extension deficits of 5.8° and 1.0°, respectively, and laxity testing showed a mean difference of 1.9 mm. The studies reported mean Lysholm, International Knee Documentation Committee, and Tegner scores of 82.1, 68.2, and 5.6, respectively. Of the patients, 83% reported an ability to return to activities of daily living whereas 67% reported a return to their preinjury level of athletics. Evidence of new degenerative changes was seen in 22% of patients.

Conclusions.—Septic arthritis after anterior cruciate ligament reconstruction remains a very infrequent event, affecting 0.5% of patients. On average, outcomes in these patients are comparable with those in patients in whom infection does not develop, including postoperative range of motion, residual instability, Lysholm scores, and return to preinjury level of activity. These patients do exhibit decreased International Knee Documentation Committee scores compared with patients without septic arthritis, however. The impact of this differential is not clear, but this scoring difference suggests that septic arthritis may be associated with more severe symptoms and reduced functional outcomes. In addition, there is limited evidence suggesting that septic arthritis leads to early degenerative changes found on imaging.

Level of Evidence.—Level IV, systematic review of Level III and IV studies.

▶ Once again, a systematic review of the literature addresses an important question. With an infection rate of .5%, this type of information cannot be derived from a single practice. The useful practical information is that an infected anterior cruciate ligament can be effectively managed with debridement and graft retention. Although this group did demonstrate about 2 mm of additional laxity, little functional deficit was observed, and most returned to full activity. It should be noted that the follow-up period was brief, less than 5 years. This is too early to determine whether infection predisposes to early arthrosis, and it will be hard to evaluate because the instability component must be factored into the analysis.

B. F. Morrey, MD

Autograft Versus Allograft Anterior Cruciate Ligament Reconstruction: A Prospective, Randomized Clinical Study With a Minimum 10-Year Follow-up

Bottoni CR, Smith EL, Shaha J, et al (Tripler Army Med Ctr, Honolulu, HI; Tufts Med Ctr, Boston, MA; et al)

Am J Sports Med 43:2501-2509, 2015

Background.—The use of allografts for anterior cruciate ligament (ACL) reconstruction in young athletes is controversial. No long-term results have been published comparing tibialis posterior allografts to hamstring autografts.

Purpose.—To evaluate the long-term results of primary ACL reconstruction using either an allograft or autograft.

Study Design.—Randomized controlled trial; Level of evidence, 1.

Methods.—From June 2002 to August 2003, patients with a symptomatic ACL-deficient knee were randomized to receive either a hamstring autograft or tibialis posterior allograft. All allografts were from a single tissue bank, aseptically processed, and fresh-frozen without terminal irradiation. Graft fixation was identical in all knees. All patients followed the same postoperative rehabilitation protocol, which was blinded to the therapists. Preoperative and postoperative assessments were performed via examination and/or telephone and Internet-based questionnaire to ascertain the functional and subjective status using established knee metrics. The primary outcome measures were graft integrity, subjective knee stability, and functional status.

Results.—There were 99 patients (100 knees); 86 were men, and 95% were active-duty military. Both groups were similar in demographics and preoperative activity level. The mean and median ages of both groups were identical at 29 and 26 years, respectively. Concomitant meniscal and chondral pathologic abnormalities, microfracture, and meniscal repair performed at the time of reconstruction were similar in both groups. At a minimum of 10 years (range, 120-132 months) from surgery, 96 patients (97 knees) were contacted (2 patients were deceased, and 1 was unable to be located). There were 4 (8.3%) autograft and 13 (26.5%) allograft failures that required revision reconstruction. In the remaining patients whose graft was intact, there was no difference in the mean Single Assessment Numeric Evaluation, Tegner, or International Knee Documentation Committee scores.

Conclusion.—At a minimum of 10 years after ACL reconstruction in a young athletic population, over 80% of all grafts were intact and had maintained stability. However, those patients who had an allograft failed at a rate over 3 times higher than those with an autograft.

▶ Frankly, this report is a bit confusing and really just confirms the current status: allograft and autograft reconstruction for anterior cruciate ligament result in similar clinical outcome. The careful assessment does reveal that at 10 years autograft integrity is significantly superior to that of allograft. This has been noted in the past. However, as before, the clinical outcome is similar. So this is not definitive, but the longer term must favor the autograft. This study, although suggestive, does not validate this observation.

B. F. Morrey, MD

Increased Failure Rates After Anterior Cruciate Ligament Reconstruction With Soft-Tissue Autograft-Allograft Hybrid Grafts

Burrus MT, Werner BC, Crow AJ, et al (Univ of Virginia Health System, Charlottesville)

Arthroscopy 31:2342-2351, 2015

Purpose.—To compare the rate of failure between a group of patients who underwent anterior cruciate ligament (ACL) reconstruction with an autograft-allograft hybrid soft-tissue graft and a matched group of patients who underwent ACL reconstruction with hamstring autograft.

Methods.—From 2007 to 2012, 29 patients underwent hybrid ACL reconstruction performed by 4 fellowship-trained sports medicine surgeons at a single institution. Patients who underwent ACL reconstruction with hamstring autograft comprised the control group and were matched to patients in the hybrid group by sex, age, date of surgery, reconstruction technique, and method of femoral fixation. Graft failure was defined as revision ACL reconstruction or complete graft rupture on magnetic resonance imaging. Graft compromise was defined as magnetic resonance imaging evidence of partial graft rupture or arthroscopically identified partial graft rupture. Lysholm Knee Scoring Scale and International Knee Documentation Committee scores were obtained.

Results.—Both groups included 10 men and 19 women, with a mean postoperative follow-up period of 44.4 ± 16.9 months in the hybrid group and 48.0 ± 15.2 months in the control group. Follow-up was obtained in 25 of 29 patients (86.2%) in the hybrid group, and each was matched to 1 patient who received hamstring autograft. The failure rate was 13.8% (4 of 29 patients) in the hybrid group compared with 3.4% (1 of 29) in the control group ($P = .160$). An additional 27.6% of hybrid group patients (7 of 29) had compromised grafts as defined earlier, as compared with 1 (3.4%) of the control patients ($P = .022$). Thus the overall hybrid graft failure/compromise rate was 37.9% (11 of 29) compared with 6.9% (2 of 29) for the hamstring autograft group ($P = .005$). In the hybrid group, the Lysholm score (80.2 ± 12.1) was significantly lower than that in the control autograft ACL group (89.9 ± 11.8) ($P = .030$). The International Knee Documentation Committee score for the hybrid ACL group (71.26 ± 19.5) was significantly worse than that for the autograft ACL group (85.7 ± 13.0) ($P = .012$).

Conclusions.—Allograft-autograft hybrid hamstring ACL grafts fail or become structurally compromised at a higher rate than matched autograft hamstring controls.

Level of Evidence.—Level III, retrospective comparative study.

▶ A continuing point of discussion with soft tissue reconstruction is that of the performance difference between allo- and autograft tissue. This case-controlled study attempts to answer the question of difference between host versus an allograft/autograft hybrid anterior cruciate ligament reconstruction. The most definite end point is graft failure. The relatively small sample, $N = 25$, was followed a reasonable period of 44 months. The failure rate of the hybrid is 14% compared with 3% failure of the autograft. To me the important point is that to the surgeon, a 14% failure rate is clinically significantly different from 3%. However, the small sample size results in no statistical difference. $P = .16$. This study does not really address the question definitively, but it is strongly suggestive.

B. F. Morrey, MD

Days to Return to Participation After a Hamstrings Strain Among American Collegiate Soccer Players

Cross KM, Saliba SA, Conaway M, et al (Univ of Virginia, Charlottesville; et al)
J Athl Train 50:733-741, 2015

Context.—Among US collegiate soccer players, the incidence rate and the event characteristics of hamstrings strains differ between sexes, but comparisons in the return-to-participation (RTP) time have not been reported.

Objective.—To compare the RTP time between male and female collegiate soccer players and analyze the influence of event characteristics on the RTP time for each sex.

Design.—Descriptive epidemiology study.

Setting.—Data were collected from collegiate teams that voluntarily participated in the National Collegiate Athletic Association Injury Surveillance System.

Patients or Other Participants.—Collegiate soccer athletes who sustained 507 hamstrings strains (306 men, 201 women) during the 2004 through 2009 fall seasons.

Main Outcome Measure(s).—Nonparametric statistics were used to evaluate RTP time differences between sexes and among categories of each event characteristic (ie, time of season, practice or competition, player position). Negative binomial regression was used to model the RTP time for each sex. All analyses were performed separately for first-time and recurrent strains.

Results.—We found no differences in the RTP time between sexes for first-time (median: men = 7.0 days, women = 6.0 days; $P = .07$) or recurrent (median: men = 11 days, women = 5.5 days; $P = .06$) hamstrings strains. For male players with first-time strains, RTP time was increased when the strain occurred during competition or the in-season/postseason and varied depending on the division of play. Among female players with first-time strains, we found no differences in RTP time within characteristics. For male players with recurrent hamstrings strains, the RTP time was longer when the injury occurred during the in-season/postseason. Among female players with recurrent strains, RTP time was longer for forwards than for midfielders or defenders.

Conclusions.—Although we found no differences in the RTP time after hamstrings strains in male and female collegiate soccer players, each sex had unique event characteristics that influenced RTP time.

▶ To anyone caring for athletes at any level, the question of return to sport is central. This study inquires whether there is a difference in gender and return to play; the answer? No. The issue of the time of the season—pre, during, or post—is important, as might be expected. What we have found in our experience and in the literature is that the patient actually knows when he or she can return. Despite all the efforts to provide objective criteria, the simple question is whether you can return to a competitive level is probably the most important consideration in these patients.

B. F. Morrey, MD

11 Trauma and Amputation

Introduction

The articles in the Trauma and Amputation chapter were chosen to highlight a few areas of controversy in the orthopedic trauma literature, as well as to update the reader on commonly encountered orthopaedic trauma conditions. I have included several articles related to clavicle fracture fixation. This topic has become quite popular recently and literature is being produced on a regular basis regarding this topic. Significant controversy about operative versus nonoperative management, method of surgical treatment, and cost implications of treatment choices regarding clavicle fractures persist.

I have also attempted to provide the reader with articles on commonly encountered conditions, including ankle and hip fractures. These injuries represent a significant percentage of trauma cases that the average orthopedic surgeon will encounter, and these articles add to the knowledge base of these conditions.

I encourage the reader to review the paper related to misclassification of Pelvic ring injuries in the national drama data bank. This paper highlights a concern related to the use of "big data" to evaluate outcomes and to guide decision making, and the information and discussion are applicable to conditions far beyond pelvic ring injuries.

Stephen A. Sems, MD

Concomitant Ankle Injuries Associated With Tibial Shaft Fractures

Jung KJ, Chung CY, Park MS, et al (Soonchunhyang Univ Cheonan Hosp, Korea; Seoul Natl Univ Bundang Hosp, Kyungki, Korea; et al)

Foot Ankle Int 36:1209-1214, 2015

Background.—Ankle injuries associated with tibial shaft fractures can cause postoperative ankle pain and stiffness even when satisfactory bony union has been achieved. Although several previous studies have described these injuries, they have not been clearly defined or classified in terms of ankle injury type or need for surgical fixation.

Methods.—Seventy-one consecutive patients (mean ± SD age, 48.3 ± 16.7 years; 37 men and 34 women) with tibial shaft fractures who underwent computed tomography examination were included. Data were collected including age, sex, body mass index, fracture location of the tibia and fibula (in percentile of length), tibial fracture shape (spiral, oblique, transverse), presence and pattern of concomitant ankle injuries (on the distal tibial articular surface), and necessity for surgical fixation of ankle injuries. Factors associated with concomitant ankle injuries associated with tibial shaft fractures were analyzed by logistic regression analysis.

Results.—A total of 47 (64.7%) of the 71 tibial shaft fractures involved concomitant ankle injuries, including 8 cases of combined lateral malleolar fracture, posterior malleolar fracture, and anterior inferior tibiofibular ligament (AITFL) avulsion fracture; 9 cases of combined posterior malleolar fracture and AITFL avulsion fracture; 6 cases of combined lateral malleolar fracture and posterior malleolar fracture; 1 case of combined lateral malleolar fracture and AITFL avulsion fracture; 10 cases of posterior malleolar fracture; 7 cases of lateral malleolar fracture; 5 cases of AITFL avulsion fracture; and 1 unclassified fracture. Of these, 34 of the ankle injuries required surgical fixation. Spiral-type tibial shaft fracture was significantly associated with concomitant ankle injury ($P = .001$).

Conclusions.—Orthopaedic surgeons should be aware that tibial shaft fractures, especially spiral-type fractures, are frequently associated with ankle injuries, such as lateral malleolar fractures, posterior malleolar fractures, and AITFL avulsion fractures. A considerable portion of these cases may necessitate surgical fixation. We recommend all spiral-type tibial shaft fractures routinely undergo computed tomography examination.

Level of Evidence.—Level III, comparative series.

▶ Ankle injuries associated with tibial shaft fractures may be missed because patients do not complain of ankle pain when they have an unstable tibial shaft fracture. However, it is well recognized that these 2 injuries occur in association with each other.

This article reviews 71 tibial shaft fractures that underwent CT scans in the emergency department. During the time period of the study, all tibial shaft fractures seen in the emergency department at this institution routinely underwent CT examination. Overall, almost 65% of patients with tibial shaft fractures also had ankle injuries. This number increased to 89% for patients with spiral tibia fractures. Ankle injuries were much less common in patients with oblique or transverse tibia fractures.

When a patient presents with a distal one-third tibial shaft fracture or a spiral tibial shaft fracture, the surgeon should closely evaluate the imaging and consider obtaining a CT scan to look at concomitant ankle injuries if the plain x-rays do not reveal an obvious ankle injury.

The authors of this article performed internal fixation of ankle injuries if the fragment was greater than 25% of the articular surface and displaced more than 2 mm. Alternatively, stress examination of the ankle joint could be used after fixation of tibial shaft fractures to determine ankle instability and the need for surgical fixation of concomitant ankle injuries associated with tibial shaft fractures. In patients with ankle fractures associated with tibial shaft fractures, it is reasonable to perform fixation of the tibial shaft fracture initially and then perform stress evaluations under anesthesia to determine ankle stability and need for fixation of any ankle injuries.

S. A. Sems, MD

The Fate of the Fixed Syndesmosis Over Time

Gennis E, Koenig S, Rodericks D, et al (Boston Med Ctr, MA; ProHEALTH Care Associates, Lake Success, NY; Boston Univ Med School, MA)
Foot Ankle Int 36:1202-1208, 2015

Background.—A prior study demonstrated statistical widening of the syndesmosis within weeks of elective screw removal. However, no information is available as to the radiographic outcomes of screw retention. The aim of this study was to evaluate radiographic syndesmotic widening and talar shift over time in patients treated with syndesmotic screws and to compare screw removal with retention along with other potential risk factors that may have led to tibia-fibula diastasis after weightbearing.

Methods.—One hundred sixty-six skeletally mature patients with ankle fractures and concomitant syndesmotic injuries were treated with syndesmotic reduction and screw fixation. The syndesmosis was evaluated intraoperatively either by a stress test or direct visualization. If the syndesmosis was incompetent, it was reduced and stabilized with syndesmotic screws to maintain reduction. Anteroposterior, mortise, and lateral radiographs at presentation, postoperatively, and at follow-up after weightbearing were evaluated. We measured the medial clear space (MCS), tibia-fibula overlap (OL), and tibia-fibula clear space (CS). Screws that were retained were graded as loose/broken or intact.

Results.—The fibula shifted an insignificant amount on postoperative mortise radiographs after elective syndesmotic screw removal at 3 months or more after initial fixation, indicated by a slightly greater CS and lower OL. The MCS did not change from preoperative to postoperative screw removal. There was no change in the radiographic markers from the postoperative to final follow-up images in those whose screws became loose or broken. Likewise, there was no radiographic difference if screws remained intact versus those that were loose or broken.

Conclusion.—In contradistinction to prior work, we found that only very mild widening (0.5 mm) of the tibia-fibula space occurred after weightbearing following syndesmotic fixation. The removal of syndesmotic screws at 3 months resulted in a slightly lower OL (<1 mm) and greater CS (0.5 mm) on mortise radiographs than screw retention even if the retained screws loosened or broke. This was not associated with any talar subluxation, and these differences were not statistically significant. The mortise remained intact whether the syndesmotic screws were removed, were loosened or broken, or remained solid.

Level of Evidence.—Level IV, retrospective case series.

▶ A plethora of literature has been published over the past decade discussing syndesmotic injuries of the ankle. Evaluating all of the potential methods, protocols, and techniques of syndesmotic injury management is daunting. Variables associated with syndesmotic fixation include the number, location, and size of screws, method of exposure, methods of radiographic evaluation of reduction, and methods of evaluation of syndesmotic stability.

This article provides a radiographic evaluation of the displacement associated with removing syndesmotic screws versus retaining them. The authors found no difference in the overall radiographic parameters between screws that were broken or loose versus intact. They did find slight changes in the tibia-fibula overlap and tibia-fibula clear space when screws were removed versus retained. These changes did not appear to have any significant impact on the overall alignment of the tibiotalar joint.

The authors present a clear explanation of their thought process when managing syndesmotic injuries. Stability is determined intraoperatively via direct examination or radiography, and fixation is placed usually in a tricortical manner.

The authors describe a technique of shared decision making regarding the removal of syndesmotic screw fixation. This technique represents the ideal method for physician patient interaction. The information from this article allows the surgeon to discuss the options of syndesmotic screw fixation and removal with patients and determined on a case-by-case basis whether screws should be removed or retained. Screws that are retained have a very high (80%–90%) rate of loosening or breakage. Patients who decided to retain their syndesmotic screws should be counseled that they will most likely loosen or break with time. This will set appropriate expectations for the patient and will likely result in patients who are more satisfied with the care provided.

S. A. Sems, MD

Does Ankle Aspiration for Acute Ankle Fractures Result in Pain Relief? A Prospective Randomized Double-Blinded Placebo Controlled Trial

Ewald TJ, Holte P, Cass JR, et al (United States Air Force, Rochester, MN; Mayo Clinic, Rochester, MN)

J Orthop Trauma 29:399-403, 2015

Objectives.—Does ankle aspiration help with pain control in patients with ankle fractures?

Design.—Prospective, double-blind, randomized, placebo-controlled trial.

Setting.—Level 1 Academic Medical Center.

Patients/Participants.—Consecutive skeletally mature patients with ankle fractures.

Intervention.—Randomized between ankle aspiration and sham procedure.

Main Outcome Measurements.—Pain scores for 72 hours after injury and pain medicine usage.

Results.—Comparison between study subjects receiving ankle aspiration and sham procedure showed no significant differences in pain scores acutely in the emergency department or within 3 days after injury. There were also no statistically significant differences in pain medicine usage within 3 days after injury. Secondary outcomes, including lower leg volume, 6-month functional outcome scores, and complication rate, also showed no significant differences between subjects receiving aspiration and the sham procedure.

Conclusions.—Aspiration of acute ankle fractures does not result in decreased pain scores or opioid usage after aspiration. Aspiration of acute ankle fractures does not provide measurable clinical benefit.

Level of Evidence.—Therapeutic Level I. See Instructions for Authors for a complete description of levels of evidence.

▶ When fractures occur in an intraarticular location, a hemarthrosis is produced. Hemarthroses may distend the capsule, causing pain and limiting range of motion of the involved joint. Aspiration of the elbow after radial head fractures has been shown to result in less pain and improved motion. This technique has also been described in the hip after femoral neck fractures. Aspiration in this setting has been recommended to decrease the intracapsular pressure to promote perfusion of the femoral head.

This technique has not previously been described for use in ankle fractures. Ankle fractures are common injuries that result in significant swelling and subsequent stiffness. The contribution that hemarthrosis and capsular distension contributed to pain, swelling, and decreased function associated with ankle fracture was previously not understood. This study definitively determined that relationship.

This study is a prospective, randomized, double-blind, placebo-controlled trial. It is unique in several ways. The first is that it employed a sham procedure in the control arm. In reviewing the entirety of literature from 2015 related to orthopedic trauma, this was the only human trial encountered by this editor that employed a sham procedure in the control group. Additionally this trial was well powered; larger than the majority of single-institution randomized controlled trials; and both patient and treating surgeon were blinded to the treatment group.

This study found no difference in pain scores, narcotic use, swelling, or longer term functional outcomes between the groups. They concluded that routine aspiration of ankle fractures was not warranted as a method for pain control, swelling control, or to improve long-term functional outcomes. The reason no differences were seen is believed to be related to the fact that ankle fractures are not purely intracapsular fractures. Ankle fractures by rule involve the joint, but the fracture extends beyond the capsule. Therefore, hemarthrosis is not contained in a closed space, as are radial head fractures and femoral neck fractures.

This study did not use injection of local anesthetics into the joint after aspiration. Injection of local anesthetic would likely reduce pain associated with ankle fractures, and it is reasonable to consider performing this procedure in the acute setting. This study was able to decisively conclude that aspiration of the ankle hemarthrosis in the setting of an acute ankle fracture provides no appreciable benefit, and there is no role for the routine aspiration of acute ankle fracture–associated hemarthrosis.

S. A. Sems, MD

Life-and limb-threatening infections following the use of an external fixator

Jauregui JJ, Bor N, Thakral R (Sinai Hosp of Baltimore, MD; et al)
Bone Joint J 97-B:1296-1300, 2015

External fixation is widely used in orthopaedic and trauma surgery. Infections around pin or wire sites, which are usually localised, non-invasive, and are easily managed, are common. Occasionally, more serious invasive complications such as necrotising fasciitis (NF) and toxic shock syndrome (TSS) may occur.

We retrospectively reviewed all patients who underwent external fixation between 1997 and 2012 in our limb lengthening and reconstruction programme. A total of eight patients (seven female and one male) with a mean age of 20 years (5 to 45) in which pin/wire track infections became limb- or life-threatening were identified. Of these, four were due to TSS and four to NF. Their management is described. A satisfactory outcome was obtained with early diagnosis and aggressive medical and surgical treatment.

Clinicians caring for patients who have external fixation and in whom infection has developed should be aware of the possibility of these more serious complications. Early diagnosis and aggressive treatment are required in order to obtain a satisfactory outcome.

▶ External fixation is commonly used in the treatment of traumatized patients with skeletal injuries. Additionally, this technology is useful in the treatment of deformity correction and limb lengthening after orthopedic trauma or other acquired or congenital conditions. This article reviews 8 cases of severe infections after external fixator applications.

Six of the 8 patients in this series develop infections within 90 days of their surgical procedure. Two other patients develop infections several months after their procedure. The authors managed the infections with debridement of the pin sites or surgical wound, while leaving the external fixation in place unless the bone had already consolidated and the fixator could be removed without creating skeletal instability.

The authors propose a modification to the Dahl classification for wire and pin site infections. This modification adds a grade 6 classification, which includes systemic signs and necrotizing fasciitis. The authors recommend intravenous antibiotic treatment and surgical debridement but suggest that the external fixator does not necessarily need to be removed entirely.

This series describes the most severe types of infections associated with external fixation. The number of patients that were treated with external fixation during this time period by these authors was not mentioned in the article, so determining the incidence of this type of infection is not possible. Fortunately, this is a rare occurrence. In the setting of severe soft tissue infection or systemic involvement of an infection associated with an extra fix it, urgent debridement should be performed, but the external fixator may be retained throughout the course of treatment.

S. A. Sems, MD

Hexapod external fixator closed distraction in the management of stiff hypertrophic tibial nonunions

Ferreira N, Marais LC, Aldous C (Univ of KwaZulu-Natal, Pietermaritzburg, South Africa)

Bone Joint J 97-B:1417-1422, 2015

Tibial nonunion represents a spectrum of conditions which are challenging to treat, and optimal management remains unclear despite its high rate of incidence. We present 44 consecutive patients with 46 stiff tibial nonunions, treated with hexapod external fixators and distraction to achieve union and gradual deformity correction. There were 31 men and 13 women with a mean age of 35 years (18 to 68) and a mean follow-up of 12 months (6 to 40). No tibial osteotomies or bone graft procedures were performed. Bony union was achieved after the initial surgery in 41 (89.1%) tibias. Four persistent nonunions united after repeat treatment with closed hexapod distraction, resulting in bony union in 45 (97.8%) patients. The mean time to union was 23 weeks (11 to 49). Leg-length was restored to within 1 cm of the contralateral side in all tibias. Mechanical alignment was restored to within 5° of normal in 42 (91.3%) tibias. Closed distraction of stiff tibial nonunions can predictably lead to union without further surgery or bone graft. In addition to generating the required distraction to achieve union, hexapod circular external fixators can accurately correct concurrent deformities and limb-length discrepancies.

▶ Tibia fractures have a relatively high rate of nonunion because of the high-energy nature of these fractures in conjunction with their poor soft tissue envelope. Treatment of nonunion of the tibia is complicated by these same factors, as well as the difficulty in accurately classifying the nonunion type. Nonunions are typically classified based on their mobility, bone formation, bone loss, and presence of infection. Techniques that work well for one type of nonunion may not be appropriate for a different type. This study reports on 46 stiff hypertrophic nonunions treated with a hexapod external fixator.

The authors provide a nice description of their technique including the "rings first" method of frame application. The authors distracted the nonunion to obtain limb length equality. If there was no bone loss, the fracture site was distracted by 3 mm to promote the healing.

The patients wore the fixators for a mean of 23 weeks. Union was achieved in almost 90% of the cases with initial treatment. Five patients failed their initial treatment and were retreated with the same technique and obtained union. The authors indicate that they believe the failures were due to early external fixator removal. The described technique for frame removal included dynamization of the frame and examination of the nonunion site for pain with stress, followed by 2 weeks of full weight bearing in the dynamized frame.

Circular external fixators are powerful tools that allow correction of deformities, full weight bearing, and are effective at obtaining bony union. For these reasons, they are effective treatment for nonunions. Their drawbacks include the need to wear a bulky frame for long periods of time and complications of pin site infections, which in this series was 19.5%.

The authors also note that this technique of distraction is appropriate for the stiff hypertrophic nonunion. The technique of distraction is appropriate for a stiff hypertrophic nonunion, but not for an atrophic or pseudarthrotic condition. In fact, in this series, the misdiagnosis of a pseudarthrosis as a hypertrophic nonunion was felt to contribute to the failure in 1 patient.

Careful diagnosis and classification of the type of nonunion is critical when using this technology. Hexapod ring fixtures are an effective method of treatment of hypertrophic, stiff tibial nonunions, but they are technically demanding. The correction must occur at the proper rate, and the fixator must be left in place long enough to gain union. The hexapod external fixator allows high rates of union while avoiding needs for surgical exposures and bone grafting of the nonunion site.

S. A. Sems, MD

Character, Incidence, and Predictors of Knee Pain and Activity After Infrapatellar Intramedullary Nailing of an Isolated Tibia Fracture

Obremskey W, for the SPRINT Investigators (Vanderbilt Orthopaedic Inst, Nashville, TN)

J Orthop Trauma 30:135-141, 2016

Objective.—To study the activity and incidence of knee pain after sustaining an isolated tibia fracture treated with an infrapatellar intramedullary nail at 1 year.

Design.—Retrospective review of prospective cohort.

Setting.—Multicenter Academic and Community hospitals.

Patients.—Four hundred thirty-seven patients with an isolated tibia fracture completed a 12-month assessment on pain and self-reported activity.

Intervention.—Infrapatellar intramedullary nail.

Outcomes.—Demographic information, comorbid conditions, injury characteristics, and surgical technique were recorded. Knee pain was defined on a 1–7 scale with 1 being "no pain" and 7 being a "very great deal of pain." Knee pain >4 was considered clinically significant. Patients reported if they were "able," "able with difficulty," or "unable" to perform the following activities: kneel, run, climb stairs, and walk prolonged. Variables were tested in multilevel multivariable regression analyses.

Results.—In knee pain, 11% of patients reported a "good deal" to a "very great deal" of pain (>4), and 52% of patients reported "no" or "very little" pain at 12 months. In activity at 12 months, 26% and 29% of patients were unable to kneel or run, respectively, and 31% and 35% of patients, respectively, stated they were able with difficulty or unable to use stairs or walk.

Conclusions.—Clinically significant knee pain (>4/7) was present in 11% of patients 1 year after a tibia fracture. Of note, 31%–71% of patients had difficulty performing or were unable to perform routine daily activities of kneeling, running, and stair climbing, or walking prolonged distances (Table 2).

▶ This interesting multicenter study of a clinically relevant question offers great insight useful to the surgeon and patient. The sample size of more than 400 patients is more than adequate to validate the conclusions. That 10% have considerable problems at 1 year is really important to know. That these problem range from kneeling to walking to running to stairs is also relevant. Further, that 30% to 70%, a pretty wide range, have some significant problem of some time is also noteworthy. Finally, it should be recognized that among patients having knee problems at 3 months, a surprising high percentage will continue to have problems at 1 year (Table 2). My take-home message? Because this

TABLE 2.—Distribution of Knee Pain at 3-Month, 6-Month, and 12-Month Follow-Up

Knee Pain Score	3 Mo (n = 393), N (%)	6 Mo (n = 361), N (%)	12 Mo (n = 428), N (%)
1	65 (17)	86 (24)	101 (24)
2	112 (29)	113 (31)	118 (28)
3	104 (26)	81 (22)	103 (24)
4	71 (18)	46 (13)	57 (13)
5	25 (6)	17 (5)	36 (8)
6	9 (2)	10 (3)	7 (2)
7	7 (2)	8 (2)	6 (1)
Average score (SD)	2.9 (1.4)	2.8 (1.4)	2.7 (1.4)

1, no pain; 2, very little pain; 3, some pain; 4, a moderate amount of pain; 5, a good deal of pain; 6, a great deal of pain; 7, a very great deal of pain.

Reprinted from Obremskey W, for the SPRINT Investigators. Character, incidence, and predictors of knee pain and activity after infrapatellar intramedullary nailing of an isolated tibia fracture. *J Orthop Trauma.* 2016;30:135-141, with permission Wolters Kluwer Health, Inc.

is such a good procedure to manage the fracture, is there any opportunity to modify technique to reduce these numbers?

B. F. Morrey, MD

Type III Open Tibia Fractures: Immediate Antibiotic Prophylaxis Minimizes Infection

Lack WD, Karunakar MA, Angerame MR, et al (Loyola Univ Med Ctr, Chicago, IL; Carolinas Med Ctr, Charlotte, NC)
J Orthop Trauma 29:1-6, 2015

Objective.—To examine the association between antibiotic timing and deep infection of type III open tibia fractures.

Design.—Retrospective prognostic study.

Setting.—Level 1 Trauma Center.

Patients.—The study population included 137 patients after exclusions for missing data (13), nonreconstructible limbs (9), and/or absence of 90-day outcome data (3).

Intervention.—An observational study of antibiotic timing.

Main Outcome Measurement.—Deep infection within 90 days.

Results.—Age, smoking, diabetes, injury severity score, type IIIA versus 3B/C injury, and time to surgical debridement were not associated with infection on univariate analysis. Greater than 5 days to wound coverage ($P < 0.001$) and greater than 66 minutes to antibiotics ($P < 0.01$) were univariate predictors of infection. Multivariate analysis found wound coverage beyond 5 days [odds ratio, 7.39; 95% confidence interval (CI), 2.33–23.45; $P < 0.001$] and antibiotics beyond 66 minutes (odds ratio, 3.78; 95% CI, 1.16–12.31; $P = 0.03$) independently predicted infection. Immediate antibiotics and early coverage limited the infection rate (1 of 36, 2.8%) relative to delay in either factor (6 of 59, 10.2%) or delay in both factors (17 of 42, 40.5%).

Conclusions.—Time from injury to antibiotics and to wound coverage independently predict infection of type III open tibia fractures. Both should be achieved as early as possible, with coverage being dependent on the condition of the wound. Given the relatively short therapeutic window for antibiotic prophylaxis (within an hour of injury), prehospital antibiotics may substantially improve outcomes for severe open fractures.

Level of Evidence.—Prognostic Level II. See Instructions for Authors for a complete description of levels of evidence.

► Open fractures are typically considered surgical urgencies or emergencies. Infection after type III open tibia fractures are not uncommon, and many factors play into the development of infection, including time to debridement, level of contamination, method of fixation, type of irrigation, and timing and selection of antibiotics.

This was a retrospective review of a single level 1 trauma center's experience over a 1-year period with 137 open grade 3 tibia fractures. The authors looked at the relationship between antibiotic timing and infection. Univariate logistic regression analysis showed that time to antibiotics and time to wound coverage were the 2 factors associated with subsequent development deep infection within 90 days. In the patients who experienced both delay in administration of antibiotics greater than 66 minutes and delay of wound coverage greater than 5 days, 40% developed an infection, whereas patients who received early antibiotics and early coverage had an infection rate of 2.8%.

In this series, surgical debridement was performed urgently, but more than two-thirds of patients underwent debridement greater than 8 hours from injury. There was no relationship between time to surgery and infection.

Type III open tibia fractures should be treated with immediate antibiotic administration and early wound coverage. Emergent surgical debridement within 8 hours is not mandatory, although unnecessary delays to surgery should be avoided.

Institutions treating type III open tibia fractures should work with their pre-hospital providers and first responders to consider providing early antibiotic treatment to these patients. Institutional Protocols that facilitate the early administration of antibiotics in the field or in the emergency department should be developed if they are not already in place.

S. A. Sems, MD

Autosterilization of Contaminated and Devascularized Bone Fragments Through a Subcutaneous Bone Pouch

Lindvall E, Martirosian A, Morshed S (UCSF, Fresno, CA)

J Orthop Trauma 29:558-562, 2015

Objectives.—The purpose of this article was to present results of cases using a subcutaneous bone pouch technique and to assess the potential "autosterilization" effect that occurs when these contaminated free bone fragments are placed in nontraumatized tissue.

Design.—Retrospective review of prospectively collected data.

Setting.—Community-Based Level 1 Trauma Center.

Patients/Participants.—Eight patients were consented for the described technique, and data were collected over an 8-year period.

Intervention.—Placement of fragments into a surgically created subcutaneous pouch in a nontraumatized tissue zone, followed by delayed, cultured, and attempted reimplantation at the initial injury site.

Main Outcome Measurements.—Culture results after extraction of bone fragments from subcutaneous bone pouch and clinical outcomes after reimplantation into initial open fracture site.

Results.—All 8 cases undergoing this technique resulted in healing of the subcutaneous bone pouch without signs or symptoms of infection at the time of attempted reimplantation or fragment removal. Four of the 8 cases had successful reimplantation and union at the open fracture site.

Conclusions.—Preserving devascularized bone fragments in a subcutaneous pouch in a region of nontraumatized tissue appears to be a safe procedure that allows for an "autosterilization" type of process to occur.

Level of Evidence.—Therapeutic Level IV. See Instructions for Authors for a complete description of levels of evidence.

▶ Orthopedic trauma surgeons occasionally encounter a case in which a decision must be made to save or discard a large, contaminated, devascularized bone fragment. If the decision is made to discard the fragment, a lengthy limb salvage undertaking may occur. If the decision is made to preserve the fragment and place it back into the contaminated wound, there is a significant potential for development of infection. This is a decision that must be made at the time of initial treatment, and it may change the entire course of the patient's treatment.

This study presents a technique using a subcutaneous bone pouch to autosterilize devascularized bone fragments. The authors report on 8 cases in which this technique was used. All 8 cases resulted in healing of the subcutaneous pouch, but only 4 of the 8 cases underwent successful reimplantation of the bony fragment. Of the 4 unsuccessful cases, 3 cases never underwent reimplantation due to recurrent infection at the fracture site, and the fourth case underwent reimplantation with subsequent failure and below-knee amputation.

Cultures of the bone fragment were taken before reimplantation of the bone fragment. All cultures were negative. No patient had a deep wound infection around the bone pouch site.

This technique represents an option for the on-call orthopedic surgeon who encounters a large, devitalized fragment of bone in the setting of an open fracture. A bone pouch is easily made near the iliac crest, and the large fragment may be implanted for later reimplantation. This allows aggressive debridement of the traumatized limb and local wound management. After restoration of soft tissue coverage and treatment of any infection, these large fragments may be reimplanted into the limb.

Placement of a contaminated and the devascularized fragment of bone into a subcutaneous pouch appears to be effective at autosterilizing the bone to allow subsequent reimplantation.

S. A. Sems, MD

Multiplanar Fixation for Patella Fractures Using a Low-Profile Mesh Plate

Lorich DG, Warner SJ, Schottel PC, et al (New York Presbyterian Hosp; Hosp for Special Surgery, NY; Univ of Texas, Houston)

J Orthop Trauma 29:e504-e510, 2015

Patella fractures are challenging orthopaedic injuries. Many commonly used fixation techniques can be ineffective and lead to poor clinical outcomes even with satisfactory reductions and fracture healing. In this investigation, we present the technique of cage plate fixation of patella fractures and the clinical outcomes of 9 initial patients surgically treated at our institution. This technique allows direct visualization of the articular reduction, provides multiplanar fixation, effectively stabilizes inferior pole comminution, and reduces the risk of patella vascular disruption. Using this technique, we have achieved excellent functional and radiographic outcomes.

▶ Myriad techniques are described for the fixation of patellar fractures, with varying reports on their results. Managing the comminution and large forces that are applied across the extensor mechanism has driven surgeons to investigate alternative methods of fixation to the tension band constructs commonly applied to patella fractures. The authors describe an anterolateral cage plate with full lateral parapatellar arthrotomy and full inversion of patella. This technique is lauded by the authors for its reproducibility, generalizability to any fracture type regardless of comminution, strength of construct, ability to achieve direct visualization of the articular reduction, and preservation of inferomedial blood supply. The results reported on their series with 18-month follow-up showed average range of motion from 0 to 143 degrees, and 100% union rate at average of 23 weeks. The authors recommend this technique as a universal technique applicable to all types of patellar fractures.

This technique is attractive in the setting of comminution and poor bone quality, as the construct "traps" the fragments and does not necessarily rely on the strength of screw pull out to maintain the fixation. This technique may also hold promise for the challenging situation of the revision patella fracture fixation. Whether this technique should be applied to all patella fracture patterns is uncertain. In this series, 3 of the 9 patients had simple transverse fracture pattern (34-C1), which have shown good union rates and outcomes with less invasive and hardware intensive techniques.

On initial reports, this appears to be an effective treatment to have in one's skill set, particularly for more comminuted fracture patterns, but it may be more hardware-intensive than necessary for a simple transverse patella fracture.

S. A. Sems, MD

Operatively Treated Meniscal Tears Associated With Tibial Plateau Fractures: A Report on 661 Patients

Stahl D, Serrano-Riera R, Collin K, et al (Scott and White Hosp, Temple, TX; Florida Orthopaedic Inst, Tampa; Univ of South Florida, Tampa)
J Orthop Trauma 2015;29:322-324

Objective.—To describe the incidence and common patterns of lateral meniscal tears detected intraoperatively and surgically treated based on tibial plateau fracture patterns.

Design.—Retrospective analysis of a prospective database.

Setting.—Level One Regional Trauma Center.

Methods.—All tibial plateau fractures in skeletally mature patients treated operatively between 2002 and 2011 were included. All operative notes and radiographs were reviewed to determine type of tibial plateau fracture, mechanism of injury, intraoperative detection of a lateral meniscal tear, and operative repair/partial resection of the meniscus itself. Patients were excluded if there was no mention of a submeniscal arthrotomy, if fracture stabilization was performed percutaneously, or if the fracture was an isolated medial condyle fracture. Statistical analysis was performed using χ^2 analysis and Fisher exact test to determine the overall incidence of lateral meniscal tears and any correlation between meniscal tear and fracture pattern.

Results.—A total of 602 patients were included in the final analysis. Lateral meniscal tears requiring operative repair were detected intraoperatively in 179 patients (30%). This could be broken down into 12% for pure lateral split fractures, 45% for split depression fractures ($P < 0.001$), 18% for pure depression fractures, 22% for bicondylar fractures, and 26% for intraarticular plus shaft fractures. Lateral meniscal tears associated with a split depression fracture pattern were most commonly peripheral rim tears (83%). For all other fracture patterns, the type of meniscal injury was evenly distributed between peripheral and radial tear. Young males demonstrated a statistically higher rate of lateral meniscal tears (33%).

Conclusions.—In our series, the incidence of a lateral meniscal tear detected intraoperatively requiring repair was 30%. These tears occurred more frequently in young males, with peripheral rim tears most commonly associated with split depression fractures. Based on our data, we believe that preoperative imaging for meniscal injury overstates the true incidence of meniscal tears requiring operative intervention.

Level of Evidence.—Prognostic Level IV. See Instructions for Authors for a complete description of levels of evidence.

▶ Many factors predict the outcome of operatively treated tibial plateau fractures, including limb alignment, ligamentous instability, associated meniscal injuries, and articular displacement. Surgical fixation of tibial plateau fractures should address these 4 factors to maximize functional outcomes.

Previous studies using MRI have reported that meniscal injuries associated with tibial plateau fractures occur in 50% and 90% of cases. These studies reported radiographic findings found on MRI, which may not correspond with the need for surgical treatment of the associated meniscal injury.

This study look at a single institution's experience over a 9-year period with meniscal injuries associated with tibia plateau fractures. They found a 30% rate of lateral meniscal tears requiring surgical repair. Further analysis found that split depression fractures had meniscal injuries requiring repair in 45% of cases.

Routine preoperative imaging of the menisci is not necessary in the setting of a tibial plateau fracture. Surgical decision making should be based on plain radiographs, CT scans, and clinical evaluation. The routine preoperative work-up of a tibial plateau fracture does not necessitate obtaining an MRI.

When meniscal injuries that require repair are encountered, surgeons can make a decision at the time of exposure to perform the repair.

This study highlights that the findings on the MRI do not necessarily correlate with need for surgical repair. Many meniscal tears apparent on MRI are not clinically significant and do not require surgical repair. Surgeons treating tibial plateau fractures should expect that 30% of patients will have a meniscal injury requiring surgical repair and that split-depression fractures have an even higher rate of meniscal injury requiring surgical repair. When performing internal fixation of a tibia plateau fracture, surgeons should be prepared to perform meniscal repair and have the necessary equipment and supplies available to perform meniscal repair in every case.

S. A. Sems, MD

Results of Displaced Pediatric Tibial Spine Fractures: A Comparison Between Open, Arthroscopic, and Closed Management

Edmonds EW, Fornari ED, Dashe J, et al (Rady Children's Hosp and Health Ctr, San Diego, CA; Montefiore Med Ctr, Bronx, NY; Boston Univ School of Medicine, MA; et al)

J Pediatr Orthop 35:651-656, 2015

Background.—Displaced tibial spine fractures are frequently treated with surgical reduction and fixation, but no comparison studies have been performed. This study was undertaken to compare fragment reduction and adverse outcomes between open arthrotomy [open reduction and internal fixation (ORIF)], arthroscopy [arthroscopic-assisted internal fixation (AAIF)], and closed management [closed management and casting (CMC)] of pediatric tibial spine fractures.

Methods.—A retrospective review of children treated for displaced tibial spine fractures from 2003 to 2011 was performed after categorizing into the 3 treatment groups. Demographics, mechanism of injury, radiographic measures (plain film and computed tomography), treatment, duration of immobilization and follow-up, final range of motion, and complications were recorded. Families were contacted to obtain long-term Lysholm scores, return to activity, pain, and satisfaction with treatment.

Results.—Seventy-six children (mean age, 12.4 y) met criteria with 29 ORIF, 28 AAIF, and 19 CMC. Radiographic measurements between x-ray and computed tomography scans found a mean error of 1 mm (SD = 1.33 mm; inter-class coefficient = 0.977, $P < 0.001$). Initial fracture displacement was similar between AAIF and ORIF, 10.3 ± 4.4 mm and 10.8 ± 3.9 mm; but, less in CMC group (5.3 ± 2.6 mm). The mean reduction amount was 8.6 ± 4.7, 9.1 ± 4.0, and 2.3 ± 2.6 mm, respectively. A Bonferroni post hoc analysis revealed a difference between surgical and nonoperative reduction ($P < 0.001$), but not between AAIF and ORIF ($P = 0.9$). Arthrofibrosis occurred with equal frequency in surgical cohorts (AAIF 12.5%, ORIF 11.1%), compared with none in the CMC group. Yet, the CMC group had a 16.7% risk for reoperation secondary to instability, loose bodies, or impingement. Twenty-four percent of each cohort was available (at mean 6.0 y) for interview with mean (median) Lysholm score: ORIF 97.4 (99), AAIF 95 (100), and CMC 86 (97.5), $P = 0.35$.

Conclusions.—Open or arthroscopic treatment of displaced tibial spine fractures affords a better reduction than closed management, but with higher risk for arthrofibrosis. Closed management may be successful when displacement is <5 mm, and advanced imaging may not be necessary to delineate the amount of displacement.

Level of Evidence.—Level III—therapeutic study.

▶ This study compared the results of pediatric patients who sustained tibial spine fractures treated with 1 of 3 methods—open reduction and internal fixation (ORIF), arthroscopically assisted internal fixation, and closed reduction and casting—in 76 children with the mean age of 12.4 years.

The study found that arthrofibrosis occurred more commonly in patients treated surgically. However, the nonoperatively treated group was at a higher risk of reoperation for instability, loose bodies, or impingement.

This study also compared the plain x-ray and CT scan measurements of displacement. They found that the displacement measurements were the same whether the fracture was measured on a plain x-ray or CT. This brings into question the need for advanced imaging to evaluate displacement of the tibial spine fracture. Advanced imaging is still useful to evaluate articular extension of the fracture and degree of comminution, which may be difficult to interpret on plain films.

It should be noted that 19 of the 29 patients in the ORIF group were converted from arthroscopic assisted internal fixation. This was the standard protocol for 2 of the surgeons during the study period. The fact that the majority of patients undergoing ORIF also underwent arthroscopy at the time of surgery makes it more difficult to distinguish the underlying reason for subsequent arthrofibrosis—was it the arthroscopic treatment or the open treatment?

The initial displacement of the fracture was greater in the cohorts treated surgically than the nonoperative cohort. The mean displacement in the nonoperatively treated group was 5.3 mm, whereas the operatively treated groups were almost twice that displaced.

The long-term outcomes were available in 18 of the original 76 patients. At a mean of 6 years, there was no difference in pain, Lysholm score, or treatment satisfaction. The authors conclude that minimally displaced fractures with less than 5 mm of elevation can be treated with closed reduction and casting. Surgical intervention should be considered when greater than 5 mm of initial displacement is present. Plain x-rays are as useful as CT in determining displacement of pediatric tibial spine fractures.

S. A. Sems, MD

Which Fixation Device is Preferred for Surgical Treatment of Intertrochanteric Hip Fractures in the United States? A Survey of Orthopaedic Surgeons

Niu E, Yang A, Harris AHS, et al (Stanford Univ, Redwood City, CA)
Clin Orthop Relat Res 473:3647-3655, 2015

Background.—The best treatment for intertrochanteric hip fractures is controversial. The use of cephalomedullary nails has increased, whereas use of sliding hip screws has decreased despite the lack of evidence that cephalomedullary nails are more effective. As current orthopaedic trainees receive less exposure to sliding hip screws, this may continue to perpetuate the preferential use of cephalomedullary nails, with important implications for resident education, evidence-based best practices, and healthcare cost.

Questions/Purposes.—We asked: (1) What are the current practice patterns in surgical treatment of intertrochanteric fractures among orthopaedic surgeons? (2) Do surgical practice patterns differ based on surgeon characteristics, practice setting, and other factors? (3) What is the rationale behind these surgical practice patterns? (4) What postoperative approaches do surgeons use for intertrochanteric fractures?

Methods.—A web-based survey containing 20 questions was distributed to active members of the American Academy of Orthopaedic Surgeons. Three thousand seven-hundred eighty-six of 10,321 invited surgeons participated in the survey (37%), with a 97% completion rate (3687 of 3784 responded to all questions in the survey). The survey elicited information regarding surgeon demographics, preferred management strategies, and decision-making rationale for intertrochanteric fractures.

Results.—Surgeons use cephalomedullary nails most frequently for treatment of intertrochanteric hip fractures. Sixty-eight percent primarily use cephalomedullary nails, whereas only19% primarily use sliding hip screws, and the remaining 13% use cephalomedullary nails and sliding hip screws with equal frequency. The cephalomedullary nail was the dominant approach regardless of experience level or practice setting. Surgeons who practiced in a nonacademic setting (71% versus 58%; $p < 0.001$), did not supervise residents (71% versus 61%; $p < 0.001$), or treated more than five intertrochanteric fractures a month (78% versus 67%; $p < 0.001$) were more likely to use primarily cephalomedullary nails. Of the surgeons who used only cephalomedullary nails, ease of surgical technique (58%) was cited as the primary reason, whereas surgeons who used only sliding hip screws cite familiarity (44%) and improved outcomes (37%) as their primary reasons. Of those who use only short cephalomedullary nails, ease of technique (59%) was most frequently cited. Postoperatively, 67% allow the patient to bear weight as tolerated. Nearly all respondents (99.5%) use postoperative chemical thromboprophylaxis.

Conclusions.—Despite that either sliding hip screw or cephalomedullary nail fixation are associated with equivalent outcomes for most intertrochanteric femur fractures, the cephalomedullary nail has emerged as the preferred construct, with the majority of surgeons believing that a cephalomedullary nail is easier to use, associated with improved outcomes, or is biomechanically superior to a sliding hip screw. The difference between what is evidence-based and what is done in clinical practice may be attributed to several factors, including financial considerations, educational experience, or inability of our current outcomes measures to reflect the experiences of surgeons. The educators, researchers, and policymakers among us must work harder to better define the roles of sliding hip screws and cephalomedullary nails and ensure that the increasing population with hip fractures receives high-quality and economically responsible care.

Level of Evidence.—Level V, therapeutic study.

▶ Geriatric hip fractures are one of the most common injuries encountered in orthopedic trauma. For the standard obliquity intertrochanteric hip fracture, both the sliding hip screw (SHS) and cephalomedullary nail (CMN) have been shown to be equally effective. Despite the data showing equal outcomes between the 2 fixation devices, there has been a dramatic increase in the number of surgeons using the CMN to treat intertrochanteric hip fractures.

This study was a survey of members of the American Academy of Orthopaedic Surgeons (AAOS), and nearly 4000 surgeons responded. It was found that nearly 70% of surgeons used only the CMN, and 13% would use either CMN or SHS. The surgeons most likely to always use a CMN were those in a nonacademic setting, those who did not teach residents, and those who treated more than 5 hip fractures per month. The most common reason they use the CMN was reported to be ease of use. Despite literature showing equivalent outcomes of CMN versus SHS, most surgeons surveyed thought the CMN was a superior construct. Academic centers responsible for training orthopedic surgeons continue to provide exposure to both implants, so the belief that the increase in CMN use is due to lack of experience with SHS in training is not supported by this article.

This study highlights the perplexing situation seen in hip fracture implant selection: despite multiple reports indicating the equality of the implants, the majority of surgeons choose 1 product (which also happens to be more expensive). This may be due to clever and convincing marketing strategies by implant manufacturers, but it also may represent a phenomenon that the literature is unable to capture: surgeons make decisions based on what they experience, not just what they read. In this case, the totality of surgeons in the AAOS experience scenarios that differ from the majority of the published literature, which is superiority and easier use of CMN implants over SHS.

S. A. Sems, MD

Exchange nailing for femoral diaphyseal fracture non-unions: Risk factors for failure

Tsang STJ, Mills LA, Baren J, et al (Royal Infirmary of Edinburgh, UK; Royal Aberdeen Children's Hosp, UK; et al)

Injury 46:2404-2409, 2015

The aim of this study was to identify risk factors for failure of exchange nailing for femoral diaphyseal fracture non-unions. The study cohort comprised 40 patients with femoral diaphyseal non-unions treated by exchange nailing, of which six were open injuries. The median time to exchange nailing from primary fixation was 8.4 months. The main outcome measures were union, number of secondary fixation procedures required to achieve union and time to union. Multiple causes for non-union were found in 16 (40%) cases, with infection present in 12 (30.0%) patients. Further surgical procedures were required in nine (22.5%) cases, one of whom (2.5%) required the use of another fixation modality to achieve union. Union was ultimately achieved with exchange nailing in 34/37 (91.9%) patients. The median time to union after the exchange nailing was 9.4 months. Cigarette smoking and infection were risk factors for failure of exchange nailing. Multivariate analysis found infection to be the strongest predictor of exchange failure ($p < 0.05$). Exchange nailing is an effective treatment for aseptic femoral diaphyseal fracture non-union. However, 50% of patients undergoing exchange nailing in the presence of infection required at least one further procedure. It is important to counsel patients of this so that they can plan for it and do not consider that the first exchange operation has failed.

▶ Intramedullary nail fixation of diaphyseal femoral fractures should result in union in approximately 90% of cases. Unfortunately, this means that 10% of cases will develop a nonunion. The treatment of this nonunion should focus on correctly diagnosing the reason for the nonunion, modifying risk factor that predict failure of nonunion treatment, and developing a surgical plan to gain union.

This study reports the results of 37 patients with femoral diaphyseal now unions treated with exchange nailing. Exchange nailing with or without bone graft had a 22.5% failure rate as a treatment for femoral diaphyseal nonunions in this series. Univariate analysis showed that cigarette smoking and infection predicted failure of exchange nailing.

This article did not clearly describe the diameters of nails that were used in either of the procedures. The technique describes sequential reaming to remove fibrous tissue until healthy bone was seen. However, it is not specifically mentioned how many millimeters larger the new nails were done the old nails.

Exchange nailing of femoral nonunions should ideally not be performed in a patient who continues to use cigarettes. Smoking cessation programs should be implemented before surgical treatment of a femoral nonunion. Serum nicotine and cotinine levels can be monitored to confirm that cigarette smoking cessation was successful.

The rate of exchange nail failure in the setting of known infection was 50% in this series, leading the authors to recommend that in the setting of infection, a staged procedure using local and systemic antibiotic treatment should be considered. An antibiotic cement-coated intramedullary nail can be temporarily placed to provide skeletal stability while delivering local antibiotics. Following systemic treatment with antibiotics, subsequent exchange nailing to a larger diameter nail may be considered.

S. A. Sems, MD

Influence of Femoral Component Design on Retrograde Femoral Nail Starting Point

Service BC, Kang W, Turnbull N, et al (Orlando Health, FL; Univ of Central Florida College of Medicine, Orlando)

J Orthop Trauma 29:e380-e384, 2015

Purpose.—Our experience with retrograde femoral nailing after periprosthetic distal femur fractures was that femoral components with deep trochlear grooves posteriorly displace the nail entry point resulting in recurvatum deformity. This study evaluated the influence of distal femoral prosthetic design on the starting point.

Methods.—One hundred lateral knee images were examined. The distal edge of Blumensaat's line was used to create a ratio of its location compared with the maximum anteroposterior condylar width called the starting point ratio (SPR). Femoral trials from 6 manufacturers were analyzed to determine the location of simulated nail position in the sagittal plane compared with the maximum anteroposterior prosthetic width. These measurements were used to create a ratio, the femoral component ratio (FCR). The FCR was compared with the SPR to determine if a femoral component would be at risk for retrograde nail starting point posterior to the Blumensaat's line.

Results.—The mean SPR was 0.392 ± 0.03, and the mean FCR was 0.416 ± 0.05, which was significantly greater ($P = 0.003$). The mean FCR was 0.444 ± 0.06 for the cruciate retaining (CR) trials and was 0.393 ± 0.04 for the posterior stabilized trials; this difference was significant ($P < 0.001$).

Conclusions.—The FCR for the femoral trials studied was significantly greater than the SPR for native knees and was significantly greater for CR femoral components compared with posterior stabilized components. These findings demonstrate that many total knee prostheses, particularly CR designs, are at risk for a starting point posterior to Blumensaat's line.

▶ Periprosthetic distal femur fractures around a total knee arthroplasty are often treated with either retrograde intramedullary nailing or locked internal fixation. Retrograde femoral nailing offers some advantages compared with locked plating, including smaller incisions and less soft tissue disturbance, and maintains high rates of union and satisfactory functional outcomes. The authors of this study have noticed that often after placing a retrograde femoral nail through a total knee component, the distal femur often has a residual recurvatum deformity likely because the starting point is more posterior than the anterior edge of Blumensaat's line, which is commonly used as the starting point in a native knee.

This study examined 100 perfect lateral native knee images to determine a starting point ratio (SPR), which was defined as the ratio from the anterior femoral cortex to the anterior edge of Blumensaat's line over the maximal anteroposterior condylar width. The SPR was compared with the femoral component ratio (FCR), which was measured as the most anterior aspect of a femoral component that would accommodate the 12-mm driving end of a retrograde femoral nail. The authors studied both cruciate retaining and posterior stabilized implants from 6 manufacturers.

The study found that, compared with the starting point in a native knee, the starting point when attempting a retrograde femoral nail around a total knee arthroplasty and especially in cruciate retaining box designs is often more posterior and may lead to a distal femur recurvatum deformity. This may be important information to consider for preoperative planning and deciding the method of fracture fixation. When using a retrograde intramedullary nail in the treatment of a periprosthetic distal femur fracture, the surgeon should consider using an implant that will accommodate the more posterior starting point of the nail without creating deformity. Nails that have a more aggressive bend in the distal part of the nail may be preferred in this situation to prevent inducing a deformity.

S. A. Sems, MD

Preoperative Testing for Hip Fracture Patients Delays Surgery, Prolongs Hospital Stays, and Rarely Dictates Care

Bernstein J, Roberts FO, Wiesel BB, et al (Univ of Pennsylvania School of Medicine, Philadelphia; Northwestern Univ, Chicago, IL; Georgetown Univ Hosp, Washington, DC)

J Orthop Trauma 30:78-80, 2016

Objectives.—To determine how often preoperative testing is requested for geriatric hip fracture patients, to assess the extent to which preoperative testing is associated with delayed surgery, and to measure the frequency with which preoperative testing changes patient management.

Design.—Retrospective.

Setting.—Academic health system.

Patients.—Two hundred fifty consecutive geriatric hip fracture patients admitted through the emergency department and underwent surgery.

Intervention.—Hip fracture surgery.

Main Outcome Measurements.—The patients were categorized according to whether additional preoperative tests were requested. For each patient, the times of presentation and surgery were recorded, yielding a "time-to-surgery interval." The results of any tests, the actions resulting from testing, and the length of hospital stay were also noted.

Results.—Additional preoperative testing was performed for 67 patients (27%). For those patients, the mean time-to-surgery was 73 hours. For the 183 patients who had no testing, the mean time-to-surgery was 37 hours. Moreover, 42 of the 67 patients with testing (63%) had time-to-surgery greater than 48 hours, compared with only 37 of the 183 (20%) patients without testing. The mean length of stay for tested patients was 12.0 days compared with 9.0 days for nontested patients. In only 2 of the 67 tested patients was further care offered based on the test result.

Conclusions.—Testing was associated with greater time-to-surgery and length of stay. Furthermore, testing rarely influenced management. Patients might be able to have surgery more expeditiously and leave the hospital earlier if testing were deferred.

Level of Evidence.—Prognostic Level II. See Instructions for Authors for a complete description of levels of evidence.

▶ Hip fracture patients are often older and have multiple medical comorbidities. Literature supports early operative intervention with a goal of less than 48 hours to decrease overall mortality. Maximizing medical fitness often requires additional testing which can delay surgery and may lead to longer hospital stays. This study was a retrospective review of 250 geriatric hip fracture patients and looked at patients who received additional preoperative testing. Additional testing was considered those items other than basic labs, chest radiograph, electrocardiogram, and urinalysis. This included items such as echocardiograms, stress testing, electroencephalogram, and endoscopy. About 30% of patients had additional testing, and for these patients, their average time to surgery was almost double compared with those who did not have additional preoperative testing. These patients also had an average of 3 days longer hospital stay. Two of the additional testing patients required further evaluation with cardiac catheterization recommendations before surgery.

Although this study looked at the number of patients undergoing further preoperative studies, they did not evaluate whether there were differences outcomes of the additional testing group and did not comment on whether the delay to time of surgery increased mortality risk in the short term or midterm.

The initial medical management of hip fracture patients should include correction of any readily reversible conditions. Often, the preoperative medical management is diverted toward evaluating and treating chronic or nor readily reversible conditions. To this extent, tests and procedures that do not treat readily reversible or modifiable conditions should be avoided or delayed until after surgical intervention. This series highlighted that a small (2 of 67) number of patients had further treatments based on findings from additional preoperative tests. The tests identified in this study as "additional tests" should be reserved for situations in which the findings will change the course of treatment or when indicated by American Heart Association/American College of Cardiology guidelines.

S. A. Sems, MD

Volume Matters: Returning Home After Hip Fracture

Gozalo P, Leland NE, Christian TJ, et al (Brown Univ, Providence, RI; Univ of Southern California, Los Angeles; Abt Associates Inc., Cambridge, MA; et al)

J Am Geriatr Soc 63:2043-2051, 2015

Objectives.—To examine the effect of the relationship between volume (number of hip fracture admissions during the 12 months before participant's fracture) and other facility characteristics on outcomes.

Design.—Prospective observational study.

Setting.—U.S. skilled nursing facilities (SNFs) admitting individuals discharged from the hospital after treatment for hip fracture between 2000 and 2007 (N = 15,439).

Participants.—Community-dwelling fee-for-service Medicare beneficiaries aged 75 and older admitted to U.S. hospitals for their first hip fracture and discharged to a SNF for postacute care from 2000 to 2007 (N = 512,967).

Measurements.—Successful discharge from SNF to community, defined as returning to the community within 30 days of hospital discharge to the SNF and remaining in the community without being institutionalized for at least 30 days, was examined using Medicare administrative data, propensity score matching, and instrumental variables.

Results.—The overall rate of successful discharge to the community was 31%. Of the 15,439 facilities, the facility interquartile range varied from 0% (25th percentile) to 42% (75th percentile). An important determinant of variation in discharge rate was SNF volume of hip fracture admissions. Unadjusted successful discharge from SNF to community was 43.7% in high-volume facilities (>24 admissions/year), versus 18.8% in low-volume facilities (1–6 admissions/year). This facility volume effect persisted after adjusting for participant and facility characteristics associated with outcomes (e.g., adjusted odds ratio = 2.06, 95% confidence interval = 1.91–2.21 for volume of 25 vs 3 admissions per year).

Conclusion.—In community-dwelling persons with their first hip fracture, successful return to the community varies substantially according to SNF provider volume and staffing characteristics.

▶ Geriatric hip fractures cause significant morbidity and mortality to patients. Many geriatric patients who sustain a hip fracture are unable to return to their prior level of function, independence, and activity. In-hospital care typically involves surgical treatment of the hip fracture, and after the period of acute hospitalization, patients are often discharged to a hospital postacute care center. Skilled nursing facilities are the most common postacute care setting for hip fracture patients.

The authors evaluated Medicare data on more than 500 000 patients aged 75 and older who sustained a hip fracture. Overall, 31% of patients discharged to a skilled nursing facility were able to return to the community within 30 days of discharge from the hospital. Patients discharged to high-volume facilities were nearly twice as likely to be discharged to the community within 30 days as those discharged to low-volume skilled nursing centers.

The authors highlight the fact that there is limited transparency regarding skilled nursing facilities volumes related to hip fracture patients. Surgeons should council hip fracture patients and their families about the relationship between skilled nursing volume and successful return to the community. Surgeons should make it their business to be aware of the hip fracture volumes that facilities in their area treat and provide this information to patients and families when appropriate.

S. A. Sems, MD

Adherence to Preoperative Cardiac Clearance Guidelines in Hip Fracture Patients

Stitgen A, Poludnianyk K, Dulaney-Cripe E, et al (Wright State Univ, Dayton, OH)

J Orthop Trauma 29:500-503, 2015

Objectives.—To identify if preoperative cardiac consultations are made in accordance with the American College of Cardiology (ACC) Foundation and American Heart Association (AHA) guidelines and the delays in care after unnecessary consults.

Design.—Retrospective review.

Setting.—Level 1 trauma center.

Patients/Participants.—A retrospective review of 315 patients with hip fractures admitted over a 2-year period was conducted. After excluding patients younger than 65 years and those admitted by the general surgery trauma service, 266 patients were included.

Intervention.—Criteria meeting the ACC/AHA guidelines for preoperative cardiac consultations.

Main Outcome Measurements.—Time to surgical intervention and total hospital length of stay.

Results.—Of the 266 patients reviewed, 55 patients (21%) received preoperative cardiac consultations, whereas 211 patients did not. Only 16 of the 55 patients (29%) with cardiac consults met the ACC/AHA guidelines, whereas 39 patients received unnecessary cardiac consults. Of the 247 patients (39 with consults and 208 without consults) who did not meet the guidelines, those who received a preoperative cardiac consult had a significantly longer average time to surgery (43.9 vs. 23.1 hours) ($P = 0.005$) and hospital length of stay (7.9 vs. 5.3 days) ($P = 0.010$). There were no significant differences in postoperative complications or disposition.

Conclusions.—Preoperative cardiac consults are frequently overused and lead to delays to surgical intervention and longer hospital length of stay while not revealing any further need for cardiac intervention or changing the rate of adverse events. Stricter adherence to the ACC/AHA guidelines will help decrease surgical delay and hospital length of stay.

Level of Evidence.—Prognostic Level II. See Instructions for Authors for a complete description of levels of evidence.

▶ Hip fractures are a common orthopedic injury with high yearly mortality. Many studies have shown that early surgical intervention within 48 hours improves outcomes. The increasing age of the general population adds additional comorbidities to hip fracture patients, and there must often be a balance between early surgical intervention and optimizing medical comorbidities before surgery. This study was a retrospective review of hip fracture patients to determine whether preoperative cardiac consultation resulted in surgical delay and changes in overall medical outcomes.

The American College of Cardiology (ACC) and American Heart Association (AHA) have developed criteria to determine which patients require preoperative evaluation and possible further testing only if the results may alter treatment or monitoring of the patient. In the review of their institution, the authors found that 70% of their patients who had a cardiology consult preoperatively did not meet AHA/ACC guidelines. In general, those who had a preoperative cardiac consult had a longer hospital stay and longer time to surgery without significantly worse postoperative outcomes.

This study emphasizes the importance of selective preoperative consultations in hip fracture patients. All patients should be evaluated and optimized by medical hospitalists but further subspecialty consultation with a cardiologist should be reserved for those who meet strict ACA/AHA guidelines to avoid surgical delays and increased length of hospital stay.

S. A. Sems, MD

Geriatric trauma G-60 falls with hip fractures: A pilot study of acute pain management using femoral nerve fascia iliac blocks

Mangram AJ, Oguntodu OF, Hollingworth AK, et al (John C. Lincoln North Mountain Hosp, Phoenix, AZ; Valley Surgical Clinics, LTD, Phoenix, AZ)
J Trauma Acute Care Surg 79:1067-1072, 2015

Background.—Hip fractures due to falls cause significant morbidity and mortality among geriatric patients. A significant unmet need is an optimal pain management strategy. Consequently, patients are treated with standard analgesic care (SAC) regimens, which deliver high narcotic doses. However, narcotics are associated with delirium as well as gastrointestinal and respiratory failure risks. The purpose of this pilot study was to determine the safety and effectiveness of ultrasound-guided continuous compartmental fascia iliaca block (CFIB) in patients 60 years or older with hip fractures in comparison with SAC alone.

Methods.—We performed a retrospective study of 108 patients 60 years or older, with acute pain secondary to hip fracture (2012–2013). Patient variables were age, sex, comorbidities, and Injury Severity Score (ISS). Primary outcome was pain scores; secondary outcomes included hospital length of stay, discharge disposition, morbidity, and mortality. Statistical analysis was performed using (IBM SPSS version 22). For group comparison (SAC vs. SAC + CFIB) median test, repeated-measures analysis and Student's *t* test of transformed pain scores were used.

Results.—Sixty-four patients received SAC only, and 44 patients received SAC + CFIB. Each CFIB placement was successful on first attempt without complications. Median time from emergency department arrival to block placement was 12.5 hours (interquartile range, 4–22 hours). Patients who received SAC + CFIB had significantly lower pain score ratings than patients treated with SAC alone. There were no differences in inpatient morbidity and mortality rates. Patients treated with SAC + CFIB were discharged home more often ($p < 0.05$).

Conclusion.—Ultrasound-guided CFIB is safe, practical, and readily integrated into the G-60 service for improved pain management of hip fractures. We are now conducting a prospective randomized control trial to confirm our observations.

Level of Evidence.—Therapeutic study, level IV.

▶ Hip fractures are the most common injury associated with ground-level falls in the geriatric population. Geriatric patients are very susceptible to complications including respiratory depression, nausea, constipation, and delirium due to the administration of opioids. Alternative methods of pain management are often preferred in the hip fracture patient. This study retrospectively reviewed 108 patients with hip fractures, evaluating 2 groups of patients: 1 that was treated with standard analgesic care and a second that was treated with a continuous compartmental fascia iliaca block.

They found that patients treated with a block had lower pain ratings than patients did not receive the block. They also found that patients who received the block or more likely to be discharged home.

The median time from patient arrival in the emergency department to placement of the block was 12.5 hours. The article does not indicate whether these blocks were placed before or after surgical intervention, how the pain levels related to surgical treatment, nor does it explain why there was such a long delay between presentation to the emergency department and block administration.

Fascia iliaca blocks hold significant promise in the management of hip fracture associated pain. This study shows that continuous fascia iliaca block can be safely placed in patients with hip fractures. Surgeons should consider timing and location of block placement as it relates to the timing of the planned surgical procedure and planned surgical incisions.

Consultation and discussion with the anesthesia provider who will be performing anesthesia for the surgical procedure should occur before placement of any regional anesthetics. It is helpful to have a fully formulated anesthesia plan in place before a regional is blocked is given. This may require including the anesthesiologist who will be involved with the procedure in the decision making process when blocks are being placed.

S. A. Sems, MD

Femoral offset following trochanteric femoral fractures: a prospective observational study

Buecking B, Boese CK, Seifert V, et al (Univ of Giessen and Marburg, Germany; et al)

Injury 46:S88-S92, 2015

Background.—Reconstruction of the femoral offset reportedly improves outcome following total hip arthroplasty, but little is known of its influence following hip fractures. We aimed to establish the effect of the femoral offset on the medium-term functional outcome in elderly patients who had sustained trochanteric fractures requiring proximal femoral nailing.

Patients and Methods.—We measured the rotation corrected femoral offset (FO_{RC}) and relative femoral offset (FO_{RL}) on plain anteroposterior radiographs of the hip in 188 patients (58 male, 130 female) with a trochanteric fracture who underwent proximal femoral nailing at our institution. The primary outcome measure was the Harris hip score (HSS) 6 and 12 months postoperatively; the Barthel index was assessed as a secondary outcome.

Results.—The mean FO_{RC} after surgery was 58 mm (± 11 mm), while the mean FO_{RL} was 1.21 (± 0.22). At final follow up, we found significant inverse relationships (Spearman's rank correlation coefficient, ρ) between FO_{RC} and FO_{RL} and the functional outcome assessed by the HSS (FO_{RC}: $\rho = -0.207$, $p = 0.036$; FO_{RL}: $\rho = -0.247$, $p = 0.012$), and FO_{RL} and the Barthel index (FO_{RC}: $\rho = -147$, $p = 0.129$; FO_{RL}: $\rho = -0.192$, $p = 0.046$). A consistent trend was observed after adjustment for confounding variables.

Conclusions.—Our results underline the biomechanical importance of the femoral offset for medium-term outcomes in elderly patients with trochanteric fractures. In contrast with the published findings on total hip arthroplasty, we found an inverse correlation between functional outcome and the extent of the reconstructed femoral offset.

Level of Evidence.—Level I – Prognostic study.

▶ Intertrochanteric hip fractures are one of the most common orthopedic injuries in elderly patients and have a high 1-year mortality risk after fracture. Given the high mortality risk, there has been a strong focus on methods to reduce the short-term mortality. There is also a growing interest in optimizing postoperative outcomes in addition to lowering mortality. Femoral offset is one of the many factors that have been found to be important in the outcomes of total hip arthroplasty (THA). Restoring femoral offset after THA correlates with reduced dislocation, impingement, and limping. Although femoral offset has been well established in THA as an important factor to improve outcomes, it has not been well studied after internal fixation of hip fractures.

This prospective study evaluated trochanteric hip fractures to see how measured femoral offset correlates with subjective hip scores at 6 and 12 months postoperatively. All patients were treated with an intramedullary device placed in a supine position on a fracture table. Measurement of femoral offset was defined as the perpendicular distance between the center of rotation of the femoral head to the long axis of the femoral shaft on an anterior-posterior radiograph at a standardized tube-to-film distance. Mathematical formulas were used to correct for any malrotation and patient size.

Surprisingly, there was a trend toward lower offset and higher functional outcome scores. This is the opposite of what would be expected based on information regarding offset in the total hip literature. Although the study's outcome was not to detect the mechanism for decreased offset, they do offer some suggestions. A valgus reduction of the proximal femur (that produces less offset) increases compression at the fracture site and may increase stability and decrease risk of implant failure. In addition, less offset reduces tension on the iliotibial band and hip abductors which may decrease forces across the fracture site and implants, thus decreasing the risk for fixation failure.

This study suggests that restoring femoral offset in posttraumatic trochanteric hip fractures may not be beneficial in short- and medium-term functional outcomes.

S. A. Sems, MD

Surgical Treatment of Femoral Neck Fractures After 24 Hours in Patients Between the Ages of 18 and 49 Is Associated With Poor Inpatient Outcomes: An Analysis of 1361 Patients in The National Trauma Data Bank

Samuel AM, Russo GS, Lukasiewicz AM, et al (Yale School of Medicine, New Haven, CT)

J Orthop Trauma 30:89-94, 2016

Objective.—To determine (1) the incidence of delayed surgical treatment, (2) risk factors associated with delayed surgical intervention, (3) inpatient adverse events and discharge disposition, and (4) the association of delayed surgery with inpatient adverse events.

Design.—Retrospective cohort study.

Setting.—2011 and 2012 National Trauma Data Bank.

Patients/Participants.—All adult patients younger than 50 years of age with femoral neck fractures.

Intervention.—Not applicable.

Main Outcome Measures.—(1) Time to surgical intervention after inpatient admission, (2) odds ratio (OR) for delayed surgery (later than 24 hours after admission), (3) incidence of inpatient adverse events and discharge disposition, (3) rates of inpatient adverse events and discharge disposition, and (4) OR for occurrence of serious adverse events, minor adverse events, and any adverse events.

Results.—Of a total of 1361 patients, 67.8% of patients underwent surgery within 24 hours of presentation. In multivariate analysis (controlling for patient and injury characteristics), Charlson comorbidity index of 3+ compared with Charlson comorbidity index of 0 (OR: 3.62), pelvic fracture (OR: 2.01), and treatment at an American College of Surgeons level

I trauma center (compared with levels II–IV; OR: 1.56) were associated with delayed surgery. The overall rate of mortality and inpatient adverse events was 0.2% and 12.1%, respectively. Delayed surgery was independently associated with increased occurrence of serious adverse events, minor adverse events, and any adverse events.

Conclusions.—Although a majority of nonelderly patients with femoral neck fractures underwent surgery within the first 24 hours of admission and had good outcomes in the short-term, certain subpopulations have a higher risk of delayed surgery. As delayed surgery is associated with worse outcomes, and short-term and long-term outcomes, efforts should focus on expediting care of these patients.

Level of Evidence.—Prognostic Level II. See Instructions for Authors for a complete description of levels of evidence.

▶ Femoral neck fractures occurring in young patients is considered an urgent or emergent injury thought by most orthopedic surgeons to require early surgical fixation. Reduction and fixation of the femoral neck fracture may preserve or restore blood flow to the femoral head and decrease the risk of avascular necrosis. Prior reports have indicated that fixation of displaced femoral neck fractures earlier than 24 hours was associated with better results, with better hip function and lower rates of avascular necrosis. The authors of this study wanted to see how frequently surgery occurred within 24 hours of presentation to the emergency department. They studied 1361 patients in the National Trauma Data Bank and found that 68% of young femoral neck fractures (18-49) were able to be surgically fixed within 24 hours of presentation. Patients treated within 24 hours had fewer adverse advents, even after controlling for preexisting comorbidities. The patients found to be at risk for delayed surgery were not surprisingly those with higher injury scores, and patients with concomitant pelvic fractures. Patients treated at a level 1 trauma center were more likely to experience delayed surgery, a finding likely related to the associated injuries that were more commonly experienced at level 1 centers. This study does not provide any long-term outcomes or functional outcomes specific to the hip fracture. This study should be considered when deciding on the treatment timing of a young patient with a displaced femoral neck fracture.

S. A. Sems, MD

Surgical Hip Dislocation Is a Reliable Approach for Treatment of Femoral Head Fractures

Massè A, Aprato A, Alluto C, et al (Univ of Turin, Italy; et al)

Clin Orthop Relat Res 473:3744-3751, 2015

Background.—Femoral head fractures are rare injuries; incongruency and instability are indications for surgical intervention. Anterior, posterior, and transtrochanteric surgical approaches have been proposed, but the exposure is limited with classical approaches. Surgical hip dislocation allows for a 360° view of the head and may facilitate a reduction in selected head fractures, but to our knowledge, few studies have reported on the results with this technique. We therefore report on the (1) quality of fracture reduction; (2) modified Harris hip score at a minimum of 2 years (mean, 6 years, range, 26–122 months); and (3) frequency of complications, including avascular necrosis (AVN), arthritis development, and heterotopic ossification, in a case series of patients with femoral head fractures treated with this approach.

Description of Technique.—The procedure involves digastric trochanteric flip osteotomy and safe dislocation of the femoral head, preserving its vessels. Using this technique we are able to reduce all displaced femoral head fractures under direct view. Definitive fixation is performed through this approach with 2.7-mm nonabsorbable screws. The same technique may be used also for Pipkin IV fractures to fix transverse, T-type, posterior wall, or posterior column acetabular fracture.

Methods.—Between 2004 and 2011, we used this approach to manage all displaced femoral head fractures in patients younger than 55 years old. A total of 17 patients were thus treated; of those three were lost to followup before 2 years, and one was excluded from study because of severe preoperative neurological impairment, leaving 13 for analysis here. Patient demographic, injury, and surgical variables as well as complications were recorded and retrospectively evaluated. Radiographic outcome was scored according to Matta's criteria on postoperative radiographs. Outcomes were evaluated with the modified Harris hip score. Minimum followup was 24 months (mean, 77 months; SD, 32.8 months).

Results.—Fracture reduction was anatomic in eight hips and imperfect in five. Mean clinical score was 82 points (SD, 7.7). One patient developed symptomatic femoral head AVN and underwent total hip arthroplasty 4 years after the index procedure; no other patient underwent arthroplasty. Besides this patient, signs of arthritis (Grade I according to Tönnis classification) were found in one patient and heterotopic ossification was recorded in two patients, but neither was symptomatic.

Conclusions.—Our experience with surgical dislocation shows clinical results comparable to previously reported outcomes in femoral head fractures treated with common approaches; we also present a similar rate of AVN and a lower rate of posttraumatic arthritis, but a higher risk of heterotopic ossification. Further case-control studies are necessary to confirm these statements.

Level of Evidence.—Level IV, therapeutic study.

▶ Femoral head fractures are rare injuries, and the literature is lacking evidence for making definitive recommendations for internal fixation of these fractures. Controversy exists in regard to surgical approach and type of surgical fixation. The anterior Smith-Peterson approach and the posterior Kocher-Langenbeck are classical approaches used in the literature, but exposure of the femoral head is often limited in these approaches. Surgical hip dislocation allows for visualization of the entire femoral head and spares the blood supply.

This study looked at one center's experience using a surgical hip dislocation to fix femoral head fractures. Radiographic and functional outcomes were evaluated. Thirteen patients were included in the study over a 7-year period. All surgery was performed by a single surgeon who had experience with surgical hip dislocations. Patients were instructed to be non–weight bearing on the operative extremity for 3 months and avoid hip abduction for 1 month. The outcomes of their study were acceptable. Of the 13 patients, 11 had excellent Harris hip scores, 1 patient developed symptomatic avascular necrosis, and 1 showed radiographic signs of arthritis at mean follow-up. These results were not significantly worse than previous literature examining the standard anterior or posterior surgical approaches.

This study provides additional data about a nontraditional approach to difficult femoral head fractures. The surgical hip dislocation allows complete visualization of the femoral head and permits internal fixation of femoral head fractures to be placed in the mechanically ideal location and direction. Femoral head fractures typically involve a shearing type of injury to the head, and a spherical cap shaped fragment must be reduced to the femoral head. This fragment may appear to be anatomically reduced if it is only visualized over a small area, like the visualization provided by a standard anterior approach. The reductions through the Smith-Peterson approach are challenging and may not be as accurate as the surgical hip dislocation allows. The surgical hip dislocation approach also allows complete visualization of the acetabular labrum and allows debridement of any fragments or comminution that would have remained in the cotyloid fossa had the femoral head not been surgically dislocated. This approach uses techniques and anatomic landmarks that are familiar to the orthopaedic trauma surgeon and should be considered the next time a femoral head fracture is encountered.

S. A. Sems, MD

Open reduction and internal fixation aided by intraoperative 3-dimensional imaging improved the articular reduction in 72 displaced acetabular fractures

Eckardt H, Lind D, Toendevold E (Dept of Trauma, Basel, Switzerland; Skane Univ Hosp, Malmö, Sweden; Rigshospitalet Univ Hosp, Copenhagen, Denmark)

Acta Orthop 86:684-689, 2015

Background and Purpose.—During acetabular fracture surgery, the acetabular roof is difficult to visualize with 2-dimensional fluoroscopic views. We assessed whether intraoperative 3-dimensional (3D) imaging can aid the surgeon to achieve better articular reduction and improve implant fixation.

Patients and Methods.—We operated on 72 acetabular fractures using intraoperative 3D imaging and compared the operative results, duration of surgery, and complications with those for 42 consecutive acetabular fracture operations conducted using conventional fluoroscopic imaging.

Postoperative reduction was evaluated on reconstructed coronal and sagittal images of the acetabulum.

Results.—The fracture severity and patient characteristics were similar in the 2 groups. In the 3D group, 46 of 72 patients (0.6) had a perfect result after open reduction and internal fixation, and in the control group, 17 of 42 (0.4) had a perfect result. The mean difference in postoperative articular incongruity was 0.5 mm (95% CI: 0.4–0.7). In 29 of 72 operations, the intraoperative 3D scans led to intraoperative correction of the reduction and an improved result. The duration of surgery and infection rate were similar in the 2 groups.

Interpretation.—Intraoperative 3D imaging, which is not time-consuming, allowed the surgeon to correct malreductions and screw placement in 29 of 72 operations, leading to better articular reduction and more precise screw placement than in operations where conventional fluoroscopic imaging was used to control the reduction.

▶ Intraoperative 3-dimensional (3D) imaging using a device such as the O-Arm allows the orthopaedic trauma surgeon to evaluate the reduction and hardware positioning during fracture fixation. This study looked at 72 fractures treated using 3D imaging and compared them to 42 fractures treated with conventional imaging.

The authors obtained perfect reductions more commonly when 3D imaging was used, with a mean improvement of 0.54 mm. Although 0.54 mm may not seem like a large difference, the acetabulum has little tolerance for malreduction, and this small difference may have a very significant clinical impact.

One point of concern with this study is how the postoperative evaluations of reduction were performed. In the control group, these images were obtained with a standard CT scan, whereas in the 3D group, the final intraoperative O-Arm scan was used to determine final reduction. This represents the comparison of 2 different imaging modalities. The clarity of the standard CT is greater than the O-Arm, so measuring small differences (like 0.54 mm) may not be accurate.

The average operative time was the same whether 3D imaging was used or not. This is interesting because the authors mention that 35 of the 72 patients had more than 1 scan performed. The average time of each scan was not specified, but it takes between 5 to 10 minutes to set up the 3D imaging machine and perform a scan. Despite the fact that multiple scans were obtained, the operative time was similar whether the 3D scanner was used or not. This indicates that the information obtained from the 3D scan may have been useful to expeditiously correct displacement that was identified. The time spent trying to interpret unclear 2D fluoroscopy images also likely contributed to the equalization of the operative times.

The use of intraoperative 3D imaging resulted in a change in the reduction and fixation of 29 of the 72 patients. This high rate of adjustment based on intraoperative 3D imaging highlights the usefulness of this technology and is the most convincing information in this study that favors the routine use of intraoperative 3D imaging.

The authors mention to specific situations where they found the 3D scan to be helpful. The first is for fixation of posterior column fractures through an anterior approach. When placing "drop-down" screws into the posterior column, the 3D imaging allows the surgeon to confirm that the screw is not in the cotyloid fossa. The second situation is when small posterior wall fragments are encountered. The intraoperative imaging allows the surgeon to assess the specific position of these fragments, which may not be accessible with standard imaging or direct visualization once the hardware is placed. The intraoperative 3D scanner may be the only way to determine the location of small intra-articular fragments once the cortical pieces of the posterior wall have "closed the door" on the construct.

If 3D imaging is available to the orthopedic trauma surgeon, intraoperative use in acetabular fracture fixation should be considered.

S. A. Sems, MD

Knee Injury Associated with Acetabular Fractures: A Multicenter Study of 1273 Patients

Kempegowda H, Maniar HH, Tawari AA, et al (Geisinger Med Ctr, Danville, PA; et al)

J Orthop Trauma 30:48-51, 2016

Objectives.—The purpose of this study was to determine the incidence and pattern of the knee injury associated with acetabular fractures.

Design.—Retrospective cohort study.

Setting.—Three level I and one level II trauma centers.

Patients.—A total of 1273 skeletally mature patients treated at 4 trauma centers between November 2004 and December 2013 for acetabular fractures were retrospectively identified from orthopaedic trauma databases.

Intervention.—Analysis of all acetabular fractures with knee injury regarding type of acetabular fracture, mechanism of injury, energy of injury, pattern of the knee injury, knee examination findings at initial presentation, intraoperative and on follow-up, requirement for surgery/conservative management, and the associated injuries. The clinical data entered during inpatient stay and office visits were analyzed.

Main Outcome Measures.—Incidence and pattern of the knee injury.

Results.—One hundred ninety-three of 1273 patients (15%) were found to have ipsilateral knee symptoms within a period of 1 year from the date of injury. The patterns of knee injury included 56 fractures (29%), 49 ligamentous lesions (25%), and 88 miscellaneous (46%) causes including bone bruises, wounds, and swelling. Associated injuries included 85 patients with ipsilateral hip dislocation (45%), 59 pelvic injuries (31%), 61 extremity injuries (32%), 38 head injuries (20%), 37 chest injuries (20%), 23 abdominal and genitourinary injuries (12%), and 7 injuries of the spine (4%).

Conclusion.—Based on this study, we conclude that knee injuries associated with high-energy acetabular fractures constitute a significant portion of the patient population. Ligament injuries are frequently overlooked and thorough clinical evaluation and utilization of magnetic resonance imaging in selected cases will help in early detection and prevention of long-term complications.

Level of Evidence.—Prognostic Level IV. See Instructions for Authors for a complete description of levels of evidence.

▶ The association between knee injuries and acetabular fractures has been described previously. A well-described mechanism for acetabular fractures is an axial impact on the flexed knee (the dashboard injury). This study looked at 193 patients who had ipsilateral knee injuries associated with acetabular fractures.

The majority of the acetabular fractures included in this study were due to high-energy trauma including fall from great height or motor vehicle accident, so it is not surprising that there is a high likelihood of associated knee injuries. Although most of the bony knee injuries in this setting were found on initial trauma evaluation (96%), only 40% of ligamentous injuries were picked up on initial exam.

Ligamentous injuries were eventually identified in 49 patients. Examination under anaesthesia at time of acetabular fixation was performed in 21 of these 49 patients. Almost all of the knees with missed injuries were not examined under anesthesia.

Knee injuries most commonly occurred in association with fractures involving the posterior wall, posterior column, or combined posterior wall and posterior column. This reinforces the understood mechanism of these fracture patterns due to an axial load to the anterior knee.

A knee exam should be performed on every patient with high-energy trauma and acetabular fracture, and the surgeon should have a low threshold to obtain advanced imaging if there is any clinical suspicion of injury, recognizing that 15% of patients with an acetabular fracture will have an ipsilateral knee injury.

S. A. Sems, MD

Misclassification of Pelvic Ring Injuries in the National Trauma Data Bank

Haws BE, Wuertzer S, Lenchik L, et al (Wake Forest School of Medicine, Winston-Salem, NC)

J Orthop Trauma 29:460-462, 2015

Background.—The American College of Surgeons has advocated for all trauma centers to participate in the National Trauma Data Bank (NTDB); however, no previous study has evaluated the accuracy of coding included in this data bank. The purpose of this study was to determine whether pelvic ring injuries are coded accurately in the NTDB and, if not, how they were misclassified.

Methods.—A retrospective review of all pelvic ring injuries based on Abbreviated Injury Scale (AIS) codes was performed at a single level I academic trauma center from July 2010 to June 2013. Thin-section computed tomography (CT) scans in all patients were reviewed and classified using AIS codes: posterior arch intact, incomplete posterior arch, or complete posterior arch. The surgeon was blinded to the AIS code from the registry. These CT-based classifications were then compared with the pelvic ring injury codes designated in the trauma registry for each patient to evaluate agreement.

Results.—Two hundred thirty-five patients with a mean age of 42 years had pelvic ring injuries in our registry. The agreement between trauma registry codes and CT reclassification was 24% in the intact group, 43% in the incomplete group, and 59% in the complete group. Using only the trauma registry codes, injuries were underclassified in 48% of the incomplete group and 76% of the intact group.

Conclusions.—Many pelvic ring injuries are miscoded and misclassified in the NTDB. The etiology of this misclassification is unclear, but any research data mined from these databases should be regarded cautiously.

▶ Participation in the National Trauma Data Bank is highly recommended for trauma centers by the American College of Surgeons. Individual hospitals are responsible for collecting and submitting a wide variety of data to the National Trauma Data Bank. In return, trauma centers are able to access the data from multiple, comparable institutions for use in quality improvement projects. Institutions can then determine where they are succeeding and where there are falling short in patient care. To truly benefit from participating in this endeavor, accurate data must be submitted to the National Trauma Data Bank. Because individual institutions use a variety of methods to ensure there are submitting accurate data, it is unknown which institutions submit data that has been individually vetted by physicians or medical personnel with the knowledge base and understanding to identify correct diagnosis related to the codes being submitted.

In this article, the authors reviewed the records of all patients with pelvic ring injuries over a 3-year period that were submitted to the data bank. Pelvic ring injury types were derived from Abbreviated Injury Scale scores that were submitted by the author's institution. The method through which the institution compiled and confirmed accuracy of their data was not specified. Abbreviated Injury Scales from the institutional trauma registry were submitted, and from these codes, pelvic ring injury type was determined.

They found that the agreement between computed tomography classification of the injuries (by an orthopaedic trauma surgeon) and the classification submitted to the data bank (by the Abbreviated Injury Scale) was poor. Unfortunately, the shockingly high number of inaccuracies brings into question the usefulness of this entire data bank. Individual institutions may be able to guarantee that they provide accurate data, but if every other institution participating in the data bank do not provide accurate information, their ability to compare their performance and isolate areas that need improvement is severely compromised.

This study represents the experience of a single institution.

This article should motivate physicians who provide care to traumatize patients in several ways. The first is that they should be involved with the methods of data collection and submission for their individual institutions. For this program to work, accurate data are necessary, and the physicians can be the driving force of this.

The second issue involves the integrity of studies produced from databases that collect data based on billing, coding, or any method other than direct input by a qualified health care provider. Articles utilizing data from the National Trauma Data Bank should be reviewed in light of this article, with appropriate levels of skepticism and understanding the potential that any conclusions drawn may be based on wildly inaccurate data.

Finally, surgeons and institutions that base their quality improvement programs on benchmarks derived from the National Trauma Data Bank should be concerned that they are being misled by poor data. Institutions may actually be underperforming in areas in which they scored well relative to similar institutions, while being deficient in benchmarks that appear to show them scoring highly. Institutional quality improvement programs should be weary of this data.

S. A. Sems, MD

Does Removal of the Symphyseal Cartilage in Symphyseal Dislocations Have Any Effect on Final Alignment and Implant Failure?

Lybrand K, Kurylo J, Gross J, et al (Boston Univ Med Ctr, MA; Hennepin County Med Ctr, Minneapolis, MN)

J Orthop Trauma 29:470-474, 2015

Objectives.—To compare final symphyseal alignment, incidence of implant failure, and revision surgery with and without symphyseal cartilage excision in patients with symphyseal dislocations treated operatively.

Design.—Retrospective review.

Setting.—Two academic level 1 trauma centers.

Patients/Participants.—We reviewed the records of 96 patients (89 men, 7 women) who had anterior posterior compression (APC) type 2 and 3 injuries requiring anterior plating. The average age was 46 years, and the average Injury Severity Score was 15.6.

Intervention.—Fifty patients were treated with symphyseal cartilage removal, whereas a second cohort of 46 patients was treated without removal of the symphyseal cartilage at the time of symphyseal open reduction and internal fixation during the same time period in a different center. Operative indications were the same for both centers, with iliosacral screws used only for type 3 injuries. Both centers used 6-hole plates through a rectus sparing approach.

Main Outcome Measurements.—Symphyseal separation was measured radiographically on preoperative and postoperative anteroposterior (AP) and outlet projections. The incidence of implant failure was recorded from the final postoperative radiograph available. Revision surgery was documented.

Results.—The symphyseal space after cartilage excision was less than if retained, which was maintained through union. The incidence of implant failure was statistically lower when symphyseal cartilage was excised. There were 2 revisions of symphyseal fixation in the symphyseal retention group for implant failure versus none when excised.

Conclusions.—Symphyseal cartilage excision led to closer apposition of the symphyseal bodies, which correlated with substantially lower rates of implant failure, and revision surgery.

Level of Evidence.—Therapeutic Level III. See Instructions for Authors for a complete description of levels of evidence.

▶ Anterior-posterior compression injuries result in disruption of the pubic symphysis with some form of posterior pelvic ring injury. Treatment of these injuries consists of restoring the anterior pelvic ring alignment most commonly using a plate bridging the pubic symphysis. Commonly, an open, rectus-sparing approach is used in which the rectus abdominal muscles are elevated from their insertions on the anterior pubic body, retracted laterally, and a plate is placed on the superior service of the superior pubic ramus and pubic bodies. Because this plate bridges the symphysis, it is prone to hardware failure and plate breakage as the symphysis regains its natural mobility with time.

During this procedure, the surgeon is faced with the decision of whether to remove the symphyseal cartilage or not. The symphyseal cartilage is readily accessible during an open approach and can easily be removed with a curette or osteotome. This study looked at 2 patient groups treated at separate level 1 trauma centers. At 1 center, removal of the symphyseal cartilage was standardly performed, while the other center did not remove any symphyseal cartilage. The authors reported radiographic outcomes describing the initial displacement, postoperative reduction, and position at final union. They found that the postoperative space was less in the cartilage excision group than the retention group. The difference in the change in alignment from immediately postoperative to final union was only 0.5 mm different between the 2 groups, with the excision group moving 1.6 mm and the retention group moving 2.1 mm. These authors also found that the incidence of screw loosening or breakage, plate breakage, and implant problems were lower when the cartilage was excised.

In this study, removal of the symphyseal cartilage resulted in fewer implant complications and lower rates of subsequent symphyseal displacement. Removal of the symphyseal cartilage during fixation of symphyseal dislocations should be considered as a useful technique to minimize hardware failure and bony displacement. However, the relationship among implant failure, loosening, and redisplacement of the pubic symphysis with functional outcome remains unclear.

S. A. Sems, MD

Surgical Versus Conservative Treatments for Displaced Midshaft Clavicular Fractures: A Systematic Review of Overlapping Meta-Analyses

Zhao J-G, Wang J, Long L (Tianjin Hosp, China)

Medicine (Baltimore) 94:e1057, 2015

Multiple meta-analyses have been performed to compare surgical and conservative interventions for treating displaced midshaft clavicular fractures. But conclusions are discordant.

The purposes of current study were (1) to conduct a systematic review of meta-analyses comparing surgical and conservative interventions for the treatment of displaced midshaft clavicular fractures, (2) to help decision makers interpret and choose among discordant meta-analyses, and (3) to provide treatment recommendations through the best available evidence.

We searched the Cochrane library, PubMed, and EMBASE databases to identify meta-analyses comparing surgical and conservative treatments for the displaced midshaft clavicular fractures. Two investigators independently scanned titles and abstracts to exclude irrelevant articles and identify meta-analyses that met the eligibility criteria. The methodological quality of the meta-analysis was independently assessed by the two investigators using the Oxford Centre for Evidence-based Medicine Levels of Evidence and the Assessment of Multiple Systematic Reviews (AMSTAR) tool. The Jadad decision algorithm was applied to determine which of the included studies provided the best available evidence.

Six meta-analyses met the eligibility criteria in this systematic review. AMSTAR scores ranged from 5 to 10. The Jadad decision-making tool suggests that the highest quality review should be selected based on the publication characteristics of the primary trials, the methodology of the primary trials, the language restrictions, and whether analysis of data on individual patients was included in the study. As a result, we selected a high-quality Cochrane review.

This systematic review of overlapping meta-analyses comparing surgical and conservative treatments suggests that surgical treatment provides a lower rate of overall treatment failure and a better functional outcome, but is associated with more implant-related complications. Hence, treatment should be individualized, with careful consideration of the advantages and disadvantages of each treatment method and of patient preferences.

▶ Although I am disappointed in it, I include this article in the trauma section. It sets about to resolve the controversy of when to operate on the fractured clavicle. The indications currently are comminuted midshaft fractures with shortening. As might be expected, this study found better functional results with surgery, but with more complications. Nothing new here. So what else could be concluded but to "individualize" each patient in the decision-making process. Nothing new here, it's called determining the risk/benefit ratio. Then I realized that this is a medical journal, and all became clear.

B. F. Morrey, MD

Posttraumatic midshaft clavicular shortening does not result in relevant functional outcome changes: observations in 32 healed, nonoperatively treated fractures

Stegeman SA, de Witte PB, Boonstra S, et al (Leiden Univ Med Ctr, the Netherlands)

Acta Orthop 86:545-552, 2015

Background and Purpose.—Shoulder function may be changed after healing of a nonoperatively treated clavicular fracture, especially in cases of clavicular shortening or mal-union. We investigated scapular orientations and functional outcome in healed clavicular fractures with and without clavicular shortening.

Patients and Methods.—32 participants with a healed nonoperatively treated midshaft clavicular fracture were investigated. Motions of the thorax, arm, and shoulder were recorded by standardized electromagnetic 3D motion tracking. The DASH score and Constant-Murley score were used to evaluate functional outcome. Orientation of the scapula and humerus at rest and during standardized tasks, and strength and function of the affected shoulders were compared with corresponding values for the uninjured contralateral shoulders.

Results.—Mean clavicular shortening was 25 mm (SD 16). Scapula protraction had increased by mean 4.4° in rest position in the affected shoulders. During abduction, slightly more protraction, slightly more lateral rotation, and slightly less backward tilt was found for the affected shoulders. For anteflexion, the scapular orientations of the affected shoulders also showed slightly increased protraction, slightly increased lateral rotation, and slightly reduced backward tilt. Scapulohumeral kinematics, maximum humerus angles, and strength were not associated with the degree of clavicular shortening. All participants had excellent performance on the Constant-Murley score and DASH score.

Interpretation.—Scapulohumeral kinematics in shoulders with a healed clavicular fracture differ from those in uninjured shoulders, but these changes are small, do not result in clinically relevant changes in outcome, and do not relate to the amount of clavicular shortening. These findings do not support routine operative reduction and fixation of shortened midshaft clavicular fractures based on the argument of functional outcome.

▶ Most of the recent literature regarding clavicle fractures deals with techniques of fixation of the comminuted fracture with shortening. This interesting study provides a possible threshold of what might be acceptable shortening form a functional perspective. Using established and validated methodology, the authors demonstrate that a mean of 25-mm shortening is associated with little kinematic or functional deficiencies—in fact, only about 5 degrees of scapular protraction. This offers additional input to define a baseline of what might be an acceptable amount of clavicular shortening, thus avoiding a surgical procedure.

B. F. Morrey, MD

Clinical comparison of two different plating methods in minimally invasive plate osteosynthesis for clavicular midshaft fractures: A randomized controlled trial

Sohn H-S, Shon MS, Lee K-H, et al (Natl Med Ctr, Seoul, Republic of Korea)
Injury 46:2230-2238, 2015

Aim.—The aim of this study was to compare the clinical and radiographic outcomes between two different plating methods (superior vs. anteroinferior) in minimally invasive plate osteosynthesis (MIPO) for acute displaced clavicular shaft fractures.

Materials and Methods.—A prospective, randomized controlled trial was performed in a single centre. Nineteen patients were treated with superior plating and 18 with anteroinferior plating using the MIPO technique. A 3.5-mm locking reconstruction plate was bent preoperatively and applied to either the anteroinferior or superior aspect of the clavicle through two separate incisions. The operating time, time to union, the proportional length difference, complications, and functional outcome of the shoulder joint were evaluated using the Constant score and the University of California Los Angeles (UCLA) score.

Results.—There was no statistically significant difference in the Constant score and UCLA score. The mean time to union was 16.8 weeks for superior plating and 17.1 weeks for anteroinferior plating ($p = 0.866$). The average operation time was 77.2 min in superior plating and 79.4 min in anteroinferior plating ($p = 0.491$). One patient in the superior plating group showed plate failure. Despite no significant difference, one patient had nonunion in the superior plating group ($p > 0.999$).

Conclusions.—From a clinical perspective, although MIPO with anteroinferior plating provides better outcomes especially in complications without statistically significant difference, both plating methods provided satisfactory clinical and radiographic outcomes.

Level of Evidence.—Level I, a single-centre, prospective, randomized controlled trial.

▶ Although surgical treatment of displaced clavicle fractures remains controversial, there has been a trend toward more operative fixation of midshaft clavicle fractures with better evidence indicating that long-term outcomes of shortened fractures treated nonoperatively are not ideal. This well-designed randomized prospective trial adds to the body of literature that shows that either anteroinferior or superior plating techniques are both effective methods of fixation for this fracture type. The authors felt that tissue trauma and complication rates were lower with the anteroinferior plating technique, but this did not bear out in their objective results. Patients had similar Constant scores regardless of the plate location.

This is an operation with high success rates and low complication rates reported, although the number of patients in each group was small (18 and 19, respectively). The limitation of this study is that it is not powered adequately to determine a true difference between the 2 methods because the overall rate of complication with either plating method is low. Additionally, a minimum 1-year follow-up does not allow the authors to decisively comment on the need for reoperation for hardware removal because the majority of elective hardware removal for soft tissue irritation or prominent hardware would likely occur after that time point. At an average of 18.5-month follow-up, 7 of 37 patients had undergone hardware removal, which is consistent with previously published rates of hardware removal. This number may increase with further follow-up.

Surgeons who perform internal fixation of displaced midshaft clavicle fractures should choose the plate location that they prefer based on experience and comfort level. Either location should result in high chances of success with minimal risks of complications.

S. A. Sems, MD

A Cost Analysis of Internal Fixation Versus Nonoperative Treatment in Adult Midshaft Clavicle Fractures Using Multiple Randomized Controlled Trials

Walton B, Meijer K, Melancon K, et al (Louisiana State Univ, New Orleans)
J Orthop Trauma 29:173-180, 2015

Background.—To determine whether the cost of nonoperative treatment, including those who require delayed operative treatment, is less than those receiving initial operative management.

Methods.—We identified 4 recent randomized controlled trials comparing operative and nonoperative treatment of displaced midshaft clavicle fractures in adults with a minimum of 1-year follow-up. A decision tree was then created from these data using reoperation for those treated with surgery or delayed operative treatment of those treated nonoperatively as end points. Actual costs estimated from 2013 Medicare reimbursement rates were applied and adjusted to better reflect private insurance rates. We then performed a 2-way sensitivity analysis to test the stability of our model.

Results.—Based on our decision tree, the expected costs for operative and nonoperative treatment were $14,763.21 and $3112.65, respectively, producing a cost savings of $11,650.56 with nonoperative treatment. After application of a 2-way sensitivity analysis, our model remains valid until delayed operative treatment for nonoperative patients approaches 95% and reoperation after initial operative management falls below 15%.

Conclusions.—From the perspective of a single payer, initial nonoperative treatment of midshaft clavicle fractures followed by delayed surgery as needed is less costly than initial operative fixation.

Level of Evidence.—Economic Level III. See Instructions for Authors for a complete description of levels of evidence.

▶ Surgical treatment of displaced clavicle fractures remains a controversial procedure. Functional outcomes, complications, reoperations, and costs must all be considered when discussing treatment options with a patient. Improved functional outcomes, lower rates of malunion and subsequent shoulder dysfunction are more commonly associated with an atomic reduction and surgical fixation of displaced clavicle fractures. Nonoperative treatment remains an option for less displaced fractures and patients with lower functional expectations for their shoulder.

This study looks at 1 perspective of the clavicle treatment debate: the cost of surgical versus nonsurgical treatment to a single payer. To do this, it reviewed 4 randomized trials and calculated costs based on surgeon, implant, facility, and anesthesia fees, factoring in costs associated with reoperation accounting for the reoperation rate.

Unsurprisingly, it found that surgical treatment is more expensive than nonoperative treatment to a single payer. Operative treatment cost between $10,000 and $11,000 more than nonoperative treatment in a single-payer model. This difference is less than would be expected, given that nonoperative treatment of clavicle fractures generally consist of a few sets of radiographs, a sling, and a few office visits. Meanwhile, surgical costs include facility fees, anesthesia fees, implants, medications, and operating room supplies in addition to the same office visits and radiographs.

This article achieved its stated purpose, which was to evaluate a single-payer perspective. Surgeons reading this article must not try to over-apply the findings to their practice.

It presents a narrow and one-sided perspective of this treatment of clavicle fractures. It does not account for cost to the patient or the impact on patient's quality of life, function, or ability to return to work, earn a salary, and be productive. When all of these factors are accounted for, the financial difference is potentially equalized or actually favors surgical fixation. In a well-written rebuttal to this article, Althausen[1] correctly evaluates the situation, accounting for both cost to the payer and to the patient. When all costs are considered, operative treatment is likely associated with an overall savings to society compared with nonoperative treatment in actively employed patients.

This article was selected for inclusion in the Year Book of orthopedics because of the interesting debate and commentary that accompanied the published article. The article itself presents unsurprising and predictable information, but the commentary does an excellent job of highlighting all of the factors one must consider when treating clavicle fractures. Although surgeons should be aware of the costs to the payer when making decisions regarding surgical treatment of clavicle fractures, the most important factor should be the needs of the patient.

S. A. Sems, MD

Reference

1. Althausen PL. Invited commentary related to: A cost analysis of internal fixation versus nonoperative treatment in adult midshaft clavicle fractures using multiple randomized controlled trials. *J Orthop Trauma*. 2015;29:180-181.

Prognostic Factors for Reoperation After Plate Fixation of the Midshaft Clavicle

Schemitsch LA, Schemitsch EH, Kuzyk P, et al (Univ of Toronto, Ontario, Canada)

J Orthop Trauma 29:533-537, 2015

Objectives.—To determine which prognostic factors were associated with an increased risk for all-cause reoperation in a heterogeneous population of patients treated with primary plate fixation of a midshaft clavicular fracture.

Design.—Retrospective observational study.

Setting.—Single university-affiliated tertiary care Level 1 trauma center.

Patients.—Of 235 consecutive patients with primary plate fixation for a midshaft clavicular fracture. A reviewer extracted data through a retrospective chart review regarding 20 possible prognostic variables and documented reoperations (defined as any surgical procedure after the initial surgery, including implant removal, bone grafts, implant exchanges, or debridement for infection).

Intervention.—Open reduction and internal fixation of the clavicle using straight and precontoured clavicle plates.

Main Outcome Measurements.—Complete 2-year follow-up information was available for 153 of 235 patients (65%). Of these 153 patients included in the analysis, 58 (38%) had reoperations. The preoperative risk factors for 3 specific "reoperation outcomes" were examined: (1) reoperation for implant removal alone; (2) reoperation for nonunion, infection, or fixation failure; and (3) multiple reoperations.

Results.—There was a significant reoperation rate in this patient series (58 of 153 patients, 38%). Although most were for isolated plate removal (42 of 153 patients, 27%), there were a minority of patients who required more complex (16 of 153 patients, 10%) or multiple (8 of 153 patients, 5%) procedures. For these 3 possible outcomes (reoperation for implant removal alone, reoperation for nonunion, infection, or fixation failure, and the need for multiple reoperations), significant risk factors were identified that can assist surgeons in patient selection and predicting reoperation after plate fixation of midshaft clavicle fractures. The significant risk factors for implant removal alone (42 of 153, 27%) were the use of a plate that was not precontoured and patient height <175 cm. The significant risk factors for reoperation for nonunion, infection, or fixation failure (16 of 153, 10%) were illicit drug use, diabetes, and previous surgery of the shoulder. The significant risk factors for multiple reoperations (8 of 153, 5%) were age >55 years and alcohol use >15 drinks per week.

Conclusions.—The use of precontoured plates can decrease the rate of hardware removal after primary fixation of displaced fractures of the midshaft clavicle. Also, specific preoperative prognostic factors may be used to counsel patients, maximize outcomes, minimize serious complications, and limit revision surgery.

Level of Evidence.—Prognostic Level II. See Instructions for Authors for a complete description of levels of evidence.

▶ Internal fixation of clavicle fractures remains controversial, and reoperation is not an uncommon occurrence after surgical treatment. In this retrospective series, 153 patients with a minimum 2-year follow-up were evaluated for reoperation. The authors found that 38% of patients had reoperations. The majority of the operations were for plate removal, but 10% of patients had more complex procedures after their initial surgery.

Bivariate analysis indicated that failure to precontour a plate and patients shorter than 175 cm were risk factors for implant removal. Unsurprisingly, risk factors for nonunion, infection, or fixation failure included drug use, diabetes, and previous shoulder surgery. Age greater than 55 years and alcohol use greater than 15 drinks per week were associated with multiple reoperations.

The reoperation rate in the study is markedly higher than previously published reports. This may be because a minimum follow-up of 2 years was required to be included in this study. Most other reports have required follow-up to 1 year. Additionally, the study looked at a certain single surgical technique, which was superior plating of the clavicle. Anterior-inferior plate positioning is an alternative option for plate location, and this location may leave the plate in a less prominent position. The rate of reoperation may differ between surgical and anterior-inferior plating.

This study identifies that patients that are older, heavier drinkers, diabetic, and illicit drug users, will more often have complex revision surgery following plate fixation of clavicle fractures. When a surgeon identifies a patient who has one of these characteristics, the preoperative discussion and decision-making process should address the higher risk for complex subsequent surgeries. This information should be considered when deciding whether to offer surgical fixation of clavicle fractures to a patient.

S. A. Sems, MD

What Factors are Associated With a Surgical Site Infection After Operative Treatment of an Elbow Fracture?

Claessen FMAP, Braun Y, van Leeuwen WF, et al (Massachusetts General Hosp, Boston; et al)

Clin Orthop Relat Res 474:562-570, 2016

Background.—Surgical site infections are one of the more common major complications of elbow fracture surgery and can contribute to other adverse outcomes, prolonged hospital stays, and increased healthcare costs.

Questions/Purposes.—We asked: (1) What are the factors associated with a surgical site infection after elbow fracture surgery? (2) When taking the subset of closed elbow fractures only, what are the factors associated with a surgical site infection? (3) What are the common organisms isolated from an elbow infection after open treatment?

Methods.—One thousand three hundred twenty adult patients underwent surgery for an elbow fracture between January 2002 and July 2014 and were included in our study. Forty-eight of 1320 patients (4%) had a surgical site infection develop. Thirty-four of 1113 patients with a closed fracture (3%) had a surgical site infection develop.

Results.—For all elbow fractures, use of plate and screw fixation (adjusted odds ratio [OR] = 2.2; 95% CI, 1.0–4.5; $p = 0.041$) and use of external fixation before surgery (adjusted OR = 4.7; 95% CI, 1.1–21; $p = 0.035$) were associated with higher infection rates. When subset analysis was performed for closed fractures, only smoking (adjusted OR = 2.2; 95% CI, 1.1–4.5; $p = 0.023$) was associated with higher infection rates. *Staphylococcus aureus* was the most common bacteria cultured (59%).

Conclusions.—The only modifiable risk factor for a surgical site infection after open reduction and internal fixation was cigarette smoking. Plate fixation and temporary external fixation are likely surrogates for more complex injuries, therefore no recommendations should be inferred from this association. Surgeons should counsel patients who smoke.

Level of Evidence.—Level IV, prognostic study.

▶ This is a review of a large number of elbow fractures asking clinically relevant questions. The key is, knowing that elbow injuries are fraught with complications of stiffness, infection, nerve and would problems, can anything be done to decrease these problems, especially surgical site infection. The conclusion is that smoking is the only risk factor identified as independently correlated with infection. Frankly, I disagree that the problems with hardware are hard to address due to the correlation with the severity of the disease. We have analyzed our experience as well. Use of a plate and screws was associated with a ×10 factor of increased wound-healing problems. This is a modifiable practice by placing the plate off the subcutaneous border or using the AO technique to fix an olecranon osteotomy. For me the message is clear: avoid plates on the olecranon region. It can be done.

B. F. Morrey, MD

Is Prone Position Ideal for Manipulation and Pinning of Displaced Pediatric Extension-type Supracondylar Fractures of Humerus?: A Randomized Control Trial

Venkatadass K, Balachandar G, Rajasekaran S (Ganga Hosp, Coimbatore, Tamilnadu, India)

J Pediatr Orthop 35:672-676, 2015

Background.—Closed reduction and percutaneous pin fixation is the standard of care for displaced supracondylar fractures of humerus in children. Although it is routinely performed in supine position, some authors recommend prone position to be advantageous as it aids in gravity reduction and avoids elbow hyperflexion. This study was conducted to compare the ease of manipulation and pinning, clinical, and radiologic outcomes in supine versus prone position.

Methods.—Fifty-two children with acute, grade III supracondylar humerus fractures without vascular injury were included in the study. They were grouped into prone (n = 26) and supine (n = 26) based on computer-generated block randomization. The duration of procedure, number of radiation exposures, attempts at closed reduction, and attempts at placing the pins were analyzed. Functional and radiologic outcomes were assessed for a minimum follow-up of 1 year.

Results.—There was no significant difference between the 2 groups in the duration of procedure ($P = 0.422$), number of radiation exposure ($P = 0.470$), attempts at closed reduction ($P = 0.904$), and attempts for pinning ($P = 0.745$) and the final clinical and radiologic outcomes. One patient in prone group had cubitus varus of 8 degrees. Functionally, 2 in the supine group and 3 in prone group had poor outcomes.

Conclusions.—There is no significant difference in the ease of reduction and pinning between supine and prone positions. Grossly displaced fractures with skin puckering are difficult to manipulate in prone position. Supine position is ideal for closed reduction and pinning of all patterns of type III supracondylar fractures.

Level of Evidence.—Level I—a prospective randomized study.

▶ Manipulation and pinning of pediatric supracondylar humerus fractures can be performed in either the supine or prone position. The advantage of the supine position includes easier positioning, access to the antecubital fossa for open reduction, and vascular access, whereas the prone position theoretically allows gravity to assist in the reduction, minimizes the need for assistants, and avoids hyperflexion of the elbow and subsequent ulnar nerve irritation. The authors sought to investigate whether prone or supine positioning had an impact on fluoroscopy usage, operating room time, and reduction attempts. No statistically significant differences were found in any outcome. This study was performed as a randomized control trial, and all patients in both study and control groups were operated on by a single surgeon who was familiar and comfortable with both techniques. This study indicates that both positioning method can be effective, and likely the surgeon's comfort and experience with a particular position is more important than the position itself. In light of the data, the senior author did change his protocol such that he performs all pinnings of type 3 supracondylar humerus fractures in a supine position.

If a surgeon trained by performing the operation prone, this study supports that it is safe and effective to continue doing so, but it does not present any data that would suggest switching from one positioning type to the other, especially if a surgeon has a preference and more experience with a particular patient position. The obvious limitation to the prone position is the difficulty with performing an open approach for neurovascular injury or irreducible fracture. This implies that when learning to approach these fractures, there is limited benefit to learning to perform the operation prone if the surgeon is already comfortable with a supine position.

S. A. Sems, MD

Value of a Dedicated Saturday Orthopaedic Trauma Operating Room

Runner R, Moore T Jr, Reisman W (Emory Univ, Atlanta, GA; et al)

J Orthop Trauma 30:e24-e29, 2016

Objectives.—To determine the effect of an additional scheduled operative day on length of stay, distribution of caseload, waiting time to surgery, and direct variable hospital costs.

Design.—Retrospective chart review.

Setting.—Urban level 1 trauma center.

Patients.—Consecutive operative tibia and femur fractures admitted from November 1, 2009, to October 31, 2011.

Intervention.—Addition of a dedicated Saturday orthopaedic trauma operating room.

Main Outcome Measurements.—Length of stay, distribution of caseload, and waiting time to surgery.

Results.—The overall length of stay for all trauma patients admitted with femur or tibia fractures was significantly reduced by 2.7 days from a mean of 14.0–11.3 days (*P* value 0.018). Additionally, there was a trend toward shorter waiting time to surgery (average reduction of 25.1 hours) for patients admitted on a Friday (48.6 vs. 23.5 hours, *P* value 0.06). Furthermore, there was an increase in the number of cases performed on Saturdays by 59% (6.2% of the total caseload), whereas the originally disproportionally high number of cases on Mondays was appropriately reduced by 33% (6.7% of the total caseload). The estimated direct variable cost savings per year for the hospital was $1.13 million.

Conclusions.—Overall, these findings support the continuation of a dedicated Saturday orthopaedic trauma operating room and can provide the foundation for other departments with similar circumstances to negotiate for more dedicated operative time on weekends to improve efficiency.

Level of Evidence.—Therapeutic Level III. See Instructions for Authors for a complete description of levels of evidence.

▶ Orthopaedic surgeons who provide on-call services on weekends need access to a dedicated orthopaedic trauma operating room to efficiently care for patients. Too often, surgeons must compete with other surgical specialties for weekend operating room access. This is suboptimal because it often delays care of the injured patient, something that results in poor outcomes and increased costs of caring for patients.

This article shows how both hospitals and patients benefit from having a dedicated orthopedic trauma operating room available on the weekend. The authors studied their institution, which is a busy level 1 urban trauma center, and found that in the years after adding a dedicated trauma room, patient length of stay decreased by about 3 days, and patients were able to go to surgery a day sooner. This should result in decreased overall costs to the hospital, as well as improved performance in the metrics reported to the National Trauma Data Bank.

Certain orthopedic trauma patients (ie, hip and femoral shaft fractures) have fewer complications and overall better mortality when able to undergo surgery sooner rather than later. If the hospital does not have dedicated orthopedic operating rooms on the weekends, all emergent and trauma cases, regardless of specialty, must share available resources, which can delay time to surgery for all those involved. This article found a direct benefit to patients as a decreased length of stay and time to surgery. This in turn decreased the overall cost of the hospital stay by more than $1 million. The cost to dedicate an orthopedic trauma operating room was just over $100,000 per year at this institution. The authors concluded that adding an orthopedic trauma operating room on the weekend was beneficial to both hospital and patients. In addition to being a sound financial decision, hospital administrators should provide surgeons access to a dedicated weekend operating room for orthopaedic trauma to improve the care of injured patients.

S. A. Sems, MD

Determination of Radiographic Healing: An Assessment of Consistency Using RUST and Modified RUST in Metadiaphyseal Fractures

Litrenta J, Tornetta P III, Mehta S, et al (Boston Med Ctr, MA; Hosp of the Univ of Pennsylvania, Philadelphia; et al)

J Orthop Trauma 29:516-520, 2015

Objective.—To determine the reliability of the Radiographic Union Scale for Tibia (RUST) score and a new modified RUST score in quantifying healing and to define a value for radiographic union in a large series of metadiaphyseal fractures treated with plates or intramedullary nails.

Design.—Healing was evaluated using 2 methods: (1) evaluation of interrater agreement in a series of radiographs and (2) analysis of prospectively gathered data from 2 previous large multicenter trials to define thresholds for radiographic union.

Intervention.—Part 1: 12 orthopedic trauma surgeons evaluated a series of radiographs of 27 distal femur fractures treated with either plate or retrograde nail fixation at various stages of healing in random order using a modified RUST score. For each radiographic set, the reviewer indicated if the fracture was radiographically healed. Part 2: The radiographic results of 2 multicenter randomized trials comparing plate versus nail fixation of 81 distal femur and 46 proximal tibia fractures were reviewed. Orthopaedic surgeons at 24 trauma centers scored radiographs at 3, 6, and 12 months postoperatively using the modified RUST score above. Additionally, investigators indicated if the fracture was healed or not healed.

Main Outcome Measures.—The intraclass correlation coefficient (ICC) with 95% confidence intervals was determined for each cortex, the standard and modified RUST score, and the assignment of union for part 1 data. The RUST and modified RUST that defined "union" were determined for both parts of the study.

Results.—ICC: The modified RUST score demonstrated slightly higher ICCs than the standard RUST (0.68 vs. 0.63). Nails had substantial agreement, whereas plates had moderate agreement using both modified and standard RUST (0.74 and 0.67 vs. 0.59 and 0.53).

Union.— The average standard and modified RUST at union among all fractures was 8.5 and 11.4. Nails had higher standard and modified RUST scores than plates at union. The ICC for union was 0.53 (nails: 0.58; plates: 0.51), which indicates moderate agreement. However, the majority of reviewers assigned union for a standard RUST of 9 and a modified RUST of 11, and >90% considered a score of 10 on the RUST and 13 on the modified RUST united.

Conclusions.—The ICC for the modified RUST is slightly higher than the standard RUST in metadiaphyseal fractures and had substantial agreement. The ICC for the assessment of union was moderate agreement; however, definite union would be 10 and 13 with over 90% of reviewers assigning union. These are the first data-driven estimates of radiographic union for these scores.

▶ Determination of radiographic healing has been a challenging area of orthopedics since the beginning of the x-ray era. Postoperative decisions such as weight-bearing progression, discontinuation of external support devices and casts, and recommendations regarding activity modification and return to work are often based on the radiographic appearance of fracture healing. The Radiographic Union Scale for Tibia (RUST) score for assessment of diaphyseal tibial fractures treated with IM nailing has tried to bring a level of objectivity to this assessment. The purpose of this study was to attempt to improve upon the RUST score by modifying it based on the characterization of fracture callous, and to generalize the results to other bones and regions.

The authors proposed a modified RUST score that takes into account whether the callous is simply present or if it is bridging the fracture gap. This allows higher interclass correlation, implying that the modified score is more easily interpreted similarly by different surgeons. The authors did show that an objective scoring system achieves interclass correlation in the metadiaphyseal region in both the femur and tibia, effectively generalizing the results to other bones and opening the door for further future studies of this nature to evaluate other areas of bony healing.

The other weakness of the RUST that the authors attempted to address in an objective fashion was the lack of a strict cutoff score that had high probability of union. The authors propose that more than 90% of surgeons believe a fracture is united with a RUST score of 10 and a modified RUST score of 13 and advocate that this should be used as the cutoff for union.

S. A. Sems, MD

12 Orthopedic Oncology

Introduction

I welcome readers to the Oncology section of the YEAR BOOK of Orthopedics, 2016. As in previous years, I have sought to bring together a collection of articles which will be of use to the practicing tumor surgeon and to also include articles of general interest which can be passed on to interested colleagues or trainees.

The chapter begins with general articles which will be of use to trainees and also can serve as contemporary updates for tumor surgeons. I have specifically included articles on the evolving field of computer navigation and quality of life in cancer survivors in this area. Subsequent articles include manuscripts on primary bone tumors and tumor reconstruction techniques. The chapter closes with articles on soft tissue sarcomas, metastatic disease, and benign conditions to round out the coverage of oncology. I hope this collection will be useful to surgeons as they stay abreast of the field of orthopedic oncology.

Peter S. Rose, MD

General

The evolving role of computer-assisted navigation in musculoskeletal oncology

Young PS, Bell SW, Mahendra A (Glasgow Royal Infirmary, United Kingdom)
Bone Joint J 97-B:258-264, 2015

We report our experience of using a computer navigation system to aid resection of malignant musculoskeletal tumours of the pelvis and limbs and, where appropriate, their subsequent reconstruction. We also highlight circumstances in which navigation should be used with caution.

We resected a musculoskeletal tumour from 18 patients (15 male, three female, mean age of 30 years (13 to 75) using commercially available computer navigation software (Orthomap 3D) and assessed its impact on the accuracy of our surgery. Of nine pelvic tumours, three had a biological reconstruction with extracorporeal irradiation, four underwent endoprosthetic replacement (EPR) and two required no bony reconstruction. There were eight tumours of the bones of the limbs. Four diaphyseal tumours underwent biological reconstruction. Two patients with a sarcoma of the proximal femur and two with a sarcoma of the proximal humerus underwent extra-articular resection and, where appropriate, EPR. One soft-tissue sarcoma of the adductor compartment which involved the femur was resected and reconstructed using an EPR. Computer navigation was used to aid reconstruction in eight patients.

Histological examination of the resected specimens revealed tumour-free margins in all patients. Post-operative radiographs and CT showed that the resection and reconstruction had been carried out as planned in all patients where navigation was used. In two patients, computer navigation had to be abandoned and the operation was completed under CT and radiological control.

The use of computer navigation in musculoskeletal oncology allows accurate identification of the local anatomy and can define the extent of the tumour and proposed resection margins. Furthermore, it helps in reconstruction of limb length, rotation and overall alignment after resection of an appendicular tumour.

▶ This group from Glasgow reports on intraoperative navigation for tumor resection and reconstructions. This article is significant in that little has been written directly on the role of navigation in assisting in the reconstruction as well as the resection of tumors. The authors have a reasonable experience they put forth (18 attempted resections under navigation and 8 reconstructions). In 2 cases, the authors had to abandon the navigation. One was a morbidly obese patient in whom they could not adequately register the tracking probe. The other required a conversion intraoperatively to more traditional techniques because of apparent navigation error. In the ultimate analysis, this was due to surgeon error in the planning.

The system that the authors used is a Stryker system that allows preoperative merging of magnetic resonance and CT scanning. This is useful in that this capability is not universally available. In the United States, different navigation packages are available. The most commonly employed is tied to an intraoperative CT scanner that is designed for spine surgery. Tumor surgeons have often adapted it because it is frequently already in place at their institutions. It does lack the capabilities of the navigation software that these authors report on allows.

Where to place this article in clinical context? The authors have been forthright about their experience, and I applaud them for this. Navigation continues to be an evolving and interesting topic. Its use in the extremities is probably less critical than its use in the axial skeleton. This series is useful for its discussion of the specific capabilities of the navigation software that this group employs as well as a frank discussion of the limitations and challenges that they encountered employing this in their clinical practice. Whether this will become standard of care in North American practice remains to be seen; since its inception, strong proponents of navigation have predicted that it will supplant more traditional methods of tumor resection. This has yet to occur. At present I think this is a useful tool for surgeons to be familiar with and to consider as they approach patients with difficult cases. Probably the most critical issue in considering navigation for tumor resection is to define the goals of navigation. If the goals of navigation are to allow a surgeon to come closer and closer to a tumor, I personally feel this is a bad idea. However, if navigation is used to allow one to more reliably obtain what we consider to be traditional and appropriate oncologic margins, that is probably a good use for it in 2016.

P. S. Rose, MD

Current Concepts in the Biopsy of Musculoskeletal Tumors: AAOS Exhibit Selection

Traina F, Errani C, Toscano A, et al (Istituti Ortopedici Rizzoli, Bologna, Italy)
J Bone Joint Surg Am 97:e7(1-6), 2015

Background.—A musculoskeletal tumor biopsy can involve fine needle aspiration, core needle biopsy, or incisional biopsy. Controversy regarding the diagnostic yield of these biopsy techniques continues. The purpose of this article is to summarize the current concepts in the biopsy of musculoskeletal tumors.

Methods.—We performed a literature review of clinical articles reporting on the biopsy of bone and soft-tissue primary tumors. Clinical articles were excluded on the basis on abstract content if they represented case reports, review or opinion articles, or technique descriptions. Eighteen of the thirty-nine articles that remained were excluded because the results did not indicate the diagnostic accuracy of the various biopsy techniques. Thus, twenty-one articles with diagnostic data on the biopsy of bone and soft-tissue tumors were included in this review.

Results.—Core needle biopsy appeared to be more accurate than fine needle aspiration, and incisional biopsy appeared to be more accurate than both of these techniques, but the differences did not reach significance. Incisional biopsy was more expensive than the percutaneous biopsy methods. In deep musculoskeletal tumors, incorporation of ultrasonography or computed tomography for guidance is easy and safe and can be useful for increasing the accuracy of the biopsy. Advantages of a percutaneous technique compared with an incisional one are the low risk of contamination and the minimally invasive nature. Certain anatomic locations and histologic types were associated with diagnostic difficulty. Vertebral tumors had the lowest diagnostic accuracy regardless of the biopsy technique. Myxoid, infection, and round cell histologies were associated with the lowest diagnostic accuracy.

Conclusions.—The current literature has not clarified the optimal biopsy technique for the diagnosis of bone and soft-tissue tumors. However, core needle biopsy is usually preferable to incisional biopsy because of the low risk of contamination and the low cost. In addition, the use of imaging guidance increases the diagnostic accuracy of musculoskeletal biopsies and reduces the risk of complications. If the result of a percutaneous biopsy is nondiagnostic, a small incisional biopsy should be performed.

Level of Evidence.—Diagnostic Level IV. See Instructions for Authors for a complete description of levels of evidence.

▶ This is an excellent article from the AAOS exhibit section published in the JBJS on the role and results of biopsy of musculoskeletal tumors. An article of this nature provides a compilation of the literature for an oncologic surgeon to readily access. Probably more importantly, it is an excellent and readable article which can be given to trainees and colleague as they deal with biopsy of tumors. The authors provide a nice table of relevant studies and the results and break-out biopsies into both bone and soft tissue biopsies.

As such, this is a useful article to be included in the Year Book, primarily to share with colleagues and trainees. However, it is a reasonable reference for surgeons involved in the day-to-day delivery of oncologic care in the evaluation of new patients who require biopsies.

P. S. Rose, MD

Fluoroscopic Radiation Exposure: Are We Protecting Ourselves Adequately?

Hoffler CE, Ilyas AM (Thomas Jefferson Univ, Philadelphia, PA)
J Bone Joint Surg Am 97:721-725, 2015

Background.—While traditional intraoperative fluoroscopy protection relies on thyroid shields and aprons, recent data suggest that the surgeon's eyes and hands receive more exposure than previously appreciated. Using a distal radial fracture surgery model, we examined (1) radiation exposure to the eyes, thyroid, chest, groin, and hands of a surgeon mannequin; (2) the degree to which shielding equipment can decrease exposure; and (3) how exposure varies with fluoroscopy unit size.

Methods.—An anthropomorphic model was fit with radiation-attenuating glasses, a thyroid shield, an apron, and gloves. "Exposed" thermoluminescent dosimeters overlaid the protective equipment at the eyes, thyroid, chest, groin, and index finger while "shielded" dosimeters were placed beneath the protective equipment. Fluoroscopy position and settings were standardized. The mini-c-arm milliampere-seconds were fixed based on the selection of the kilovolt peak (kVp). Three mini and three standard c-arms scanned a model of the patient's wrist continuously for fifteen minutes each. Ten dosimeter exposures were recorded for each c-arm.

Results.—Hand exposure averaged 31 μSv/min (range, 22 to 48 μSv/min), which was 13.0 times higher than the other recorded exposures. Eye exposure averaged 4 μSv/min, 2.2 times higher than the mean thyroid, chest, and groin exposure. Gloves reduced hand exposure by 69.4%. Glasses decreased eye exposure by 65.6%. There was no significant difference in exposure between mini and standard fluoroscopy.

Conclusions.—Surgeons' hands receive the most radiation exposure during distal radial plate fixation under fluoroscopy. There was a small but insignificant difference in mean exposure between standard fluoroscopy and mini-fluoroscopy, but some standard units resulted in lower exposure than some mini-units. On the basis of these findings, we recommend routine protective equipment to mitigate exposure to surgeons' hands and eyes, in addition to the thyroid, chest, and groin, during fluoroscopy procedures.

▶ This is an interesting article that I have included in the YEAR BOOK this year because radiation exposure is known to be associated with the development of malignancy, and orthopedic oncologists are often asked about these issues by their colleagues. This particular article in the *American Journal of Bone and Joint Surgery* studies radiation exposure to surgeons using a distal radius fracture model. Although this is not a technique that many orthopedic oncologists will commonly perform, the principles of radiation safety hold true and are relevant to clinical practice and consultation with colleagues.

Interestingly, the natural assumption that a mini C-arm would have a lower radiation exposure than a standard C-arm was not universally true. The authors compared 3 mini C-arms and 3 standard C-arms from different manufactures.

Not surprisingly, in the model that was employed, the surgeon's hands received the highest doses of radiation. Shielded gloves are available, and other basic precautions can be taken for surgeons who wish to minimize their exposure to radiation of the hands. The next highest organ group exposed was the surgeons' eyes. Additionally, exposure to the eyes was the dose most dramatically reduced by basic shielding compared with the reduction in exposure in other areas seen by basic shielding.

Where to place this study in clinical context? Oncologists can use this both to inform their own practice and to counsel their colleagues. The implicit assumption that a mini C-arm has lower radiation exposure, and thus lower risk to surgeons and other personnel in the operating room, is shown to be incorrect in this setting. Additionally, this report highlights the danger to surgeon's eyes from radiation exposure and the easy methods of shielding that are available.

P. S. Rose, MD

Cured of Primary Bone Cancer, But at What Cost: A Qualitative Study of Functional Impairment and Lost Opportunities

Fauske L, Bruland OS, Grov EK, et al (Norwegian Radium Hosp, Oslo, Norway; Oslo and Akershus Univ College of Applied Sciences, Norway; et al)

Sarcoma 2015:10, 2015

Purpose.—Our study aims to explore how former cancer patients experience physical and psychosocial late effects 3–7 years after they underwent treatment for primary bone sarcoma in the hip/pelvic region. A qualitative, phenomenological, and hermeneutic design was applied.

Methods.—Sarcoma survivors ($n = 10$) previously treated at Oslo University Hospital, Norwegian Radium Hospital were selected to participate. In-depth and semistructured interviews were conducted. The interviews were analysed using inductive thematic analysis.

Results.—The participants reported that the late effects had three core spheres of impact: "their current daily life," "their future opportunities," and "their identity." They expressed negative changes in activity, increased dependence on others, and exclusion from participation in different areas. Their daily life, work, sports activities, and social life were all affected. Several of their experiences are similar to those described by people with functional impairment or disability.

Conclusion.—Patients cured of bone cancer in the hip/pelvic region pay a significant price in terms of functional impairment, practical challenges, exclusion from important aspects of life, and loss of previous identity. It is important to appreciate this in order to help bone cancer survivors who struggle to reorient their life and build a secure new identity.

▶ Surgeons are grateful when patients with pelvic and other proximal sarcomas survive their malignancies. As well, we have all been gratified to see patients achieve meaningful employment and a vigorous life after they are cured of their disease. However, this certainly does come at a price, and this interesting article from Norway helps to quantify that. The authors interviewed 10 long-term sarcoma survivors to explore how their identity and daily lives had changed 3 to 7 years after treatment for their sarcomas. The goal was to report the physical and psychosocial affects that patients experienced late.

Note that some of this is specific to aspects of Norwegian society, but most of this generalizes to patients who are seen in North American practice. The results are fairly sobering. Although patients overall appear to be doing well, the descriptions and data that are recorded highlight the significant changes (both good and bad) that these patients have experienced in their lives.

I have included this article in the YEAR BOOK to highlight this area for surgeons to consider. Although it is easy to focus on clean scans and appropriate x-rays, this aspect of survivorship in cancer patients is important. Additionally, the National Cancer Institute (NCI) is now requiring survivorship programs to be implemented in NCI cancer centers. Articles like this highlight the important need for ongoing support of patients after they have been cured of their malignancies and also the challenges that they face that we may be able to address preemptively for them.

P. S. Rose, MD

Primary Bone Tumors

Does amputation offer any survival benefit over limb salvage in osteosarcoma patients with poor chemonecrosis and close margins?

Reddy KIA, Wafa H, Gaston CL, et al (Royal Orthopaedic Hosp, Birmingham, UK)

Bone Joint J 97-B:115-120, 2015

A poor response to chemotherapy (≤ 90% necrosis) for osteosarcomas leads to poorer survival and an increased risk of local recurrence, particularly if there is a close margin of excision. We evaluated whether amputation confers any survival benefit over limb salvage surgery (LSS) with narrow margins in patients who respond poorly to chemotherapy.

We only analysed patients with an osteosarcoma of the limb, a poor response to chemotherapy and close margins on LSS (marginal/intralesional) or primary amputation: 360 patients (36 LSS (intralesional margins), 197 LSS (marginal margins) and 127 amputations) were included. Local recurrence developed in 13 (36%) following LSS with intralesional margins, and 39 (20%) following LSS with marginal margins. There was no local recurrence in patients who underwent amputation. The five-year survival for all patients was 41% (95% confidence interval (CI) 35 to 46), but for those treated by LSS with marginal margins was 46.2% (95% CI 38 to 53), 36.3% (95% CI 27 to 45) for those treated by amputation, and 28% (95 CI 14 to 44) for those treated by LSS with intralesional margins. Patients who had LSS and then developed local recurrence as a first event had the same survival as those who had primary amputation without local recurrence. Prophylactic adjuvant radiotherapy was used in 40 patients but had no discernible effect in preventing local recurrence.

Although amputation offered better local control, it conferred no clear survival benefit over LSS with marginal margins in these patients with a poor overall prognosis.

▶ This report from the Birmingham group compares the survival of 127 patients with poor chemotherapy necrosis and amputations to 233 patients who had a poor histologic response to chemotherapy and a less than wide limb salvage oncologic margin. This is a relevant topic because the survival of patients with osteosarcoma is known to be correlated with the response to chemotherapy. Additionally, the risk of local recurrence is known to be correlated with the response to chemotherapy and the quality of the surgical margin. Finally, local recurrence is associated with death from disease. It is not clear, however, if the influence of margin as a prognostic factor is relevant to overall survival or only to the development of local recurrence in this scenario. Essentially, it is unclear whether patients with aggressive tumors and a poor response to chemotherapy should be amputated because of the elevated risk of local recurrence.

These authors were retrospectively reviewing a series of patients accrued over many years with varying chemotherapy regimens. However, they were all treated at an excellent center in the UK National Health Service. Surprisingly, amputation did not provide a clear survival benefit, although it did provide much better local control (see Fig 1 in the original article). No local recurrence was seen in patients with amputation, but local regional recurrence was seen in a large percentage of patients who had less than wide margins.

Where to put this article in clinical context? Although it suffers from the flaws of a retrospective study, it is unlikely that a prospective randomized trial will ever be designed to answer this question in a meaningful manner. As such, studies of this nature are likely the best we are going to have in the near- to intermediate-term future on which to base patient treatment. In this setting, it appears that any survival benefit gained from amputation is small at best in patients with a poor response to chemotherapy. Although there certainly may be benefits for local control, it is probably not currently reasonable to promote amputation in these patients as a way to significantly improve overall survival.

P. S. Rose, MD

Age, Tumor Characteristics, and Treatment Regimen as Event Predictors in Ewing: A Children's Oncology Group Report

Marina N, Granowetter L, Grier HE, et al (Stanford Univ, Palo Alto, CA; Langone Med Ctr, NY; Dana Farber & Boston Children's Hosp, MA; et al)
Sarcoma 2015:927123, 2015

Purpose.—To associate baseline patient characteristics and relapse across consecutive COG studies.

Methods.—We analyzed risk factors for LESFT patients in three randomized COG trials. We evaluated age at enrollment, primary site, gender, tumor size, and treatment (as randomized).We estimated event-free survival (EFS, Kaplan-Meier) and compared risk across groups (log-rank test). Characteristics were assessed by proportional hazards regression with the characteristic of interest as the only component. Confidence intervals (CI) for RR were derived. Factors related to outcome at level 0.05 were included in a multivariate regression model.

Results.—Between 12/1988 and 8/2005, 1444 patients were enrolled and data current to 2001, 2004, or 2008 were used. Patients were with a median age of 12 years (0—45), 55% male and 88% Caucasian. The 5-year EFS was 68.3% ± 1.3%. In univariate analysis age, treatment, and tumor location were identified for inclusion in the multivariate model, and all remained significant ($p < 0.01$). Since tumor size was not collected in the last study, the other two were reanalyzed. This model identified age, treatment, tumor location, and tumor size as significant predictors.

Conclusion.—Age > 18 years, pelvic tumor, size > 8 cms, and chemotherapy without ifosfamide/etoposide significantly predict worse outcome. AEWS0031 is NCT00006734, INT0091 and INT0054 designed before 1993 (unregistered) (Fig 2).

► I have included this article from the Children's Oncology Group (COG) on Ewing's sarcoma in the Year Book for several reasons. First, it provides an

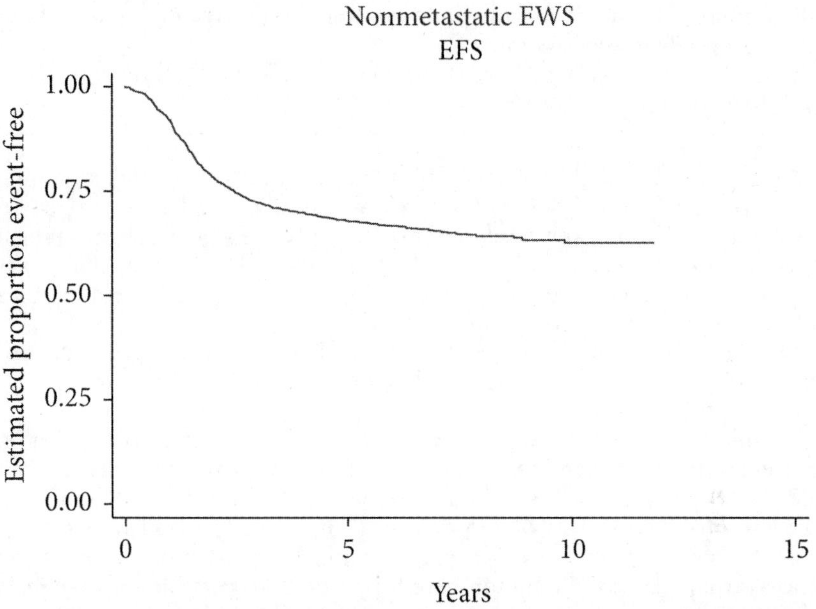

FIGURE 2.—EFS for 1444 patients enrolled in consecutive COG trials. The 5-year EFS for the group was 68.32% ± 1.3%. EFS = event-free survival; COG = Children's Oncology Group. (Reprinted from Marina N, Granowetter L, Grier HE, et al. Age, tumor characteristics, and treatment regimen as event predictors in Ewing: a children's oncology group report. *Sarcoma.* 2015;2015:927123, with permission from Hindawi Publishing Corporation.)

excellent summary of results for patients treated on COG protocols from 1988 through 2005 (1444 patients). Additionally, it identifies risk factors for poor outcome. This includes an excellent discussion of the current treatment of Ewing's sarcoma and an up-to-date reference bibliography for surgeons to refer to.

Five-year event-free survival was 68% (Fig 2). Not surprisingly, age greater than 18 years, pelvic tumor location, long axis dimension of greater than 8 cm, and chemotherapy not including ifosfamide/etoposide were predictors of significantly worse outcome in this patient population. Thankfully, the addition of ifosfamide, etoposide, and the use of interval compression chemotherapy appears to provide a clear benefit in these patients. Other risk factors (age, location, and size) are not modifiable.

This article provides an excellent summary of current treatment in Ewing's sarcoma as well as the results of recent COG trials. As such, it is an important and readable article for surgeons who care for children with this malignancy.

P. S. Rose, MD

High-grade focal areas in low-grade central osteosarcoma: high-grade or still low-grade osteosarcoma?

Righi A, Paioli A, Dei Tos AP, et al (Rizzoli Inst, Bologna, Italy; et al)

Clin Sarcoma Res 5:23, 2015

Background.—High-grade foci (grade 3 according to Broder's grading system) are sometimes detected in low-grade (grade 1 and 2) central osteosarcoma. The aim of this study was to retrospectively evaluate the clinical outcome in patients upgraded to high grade (grade 3) after a first diagnosis of low-grade osteosarcoma, following the detection of high-grade areas (grade 3) in the resected specimen.

Methods.—Of the 132 patients with a diagnosis of low-grade central osteosarcoma at surgical biopsy at our Institute, 33 patients were considered eligible for the study.

Results.—Median age was 37 (range 13–58 years). Location was in an extremity in 29 patients (88%). Post-operative chemotherapy was given in 22 (67%) patients. Follow-up data were available for all patients, with a median observation time of 115 months (range 4–322 months). After histological revision, areas of high-grade (grade 3) osteosarcoma accounting for less than 50% of the tumor were found in 20 (61%) patients, whereas the majority of the tumor was composed of a high-grade (grade 3) component in 13 (39%) patients. In the 20 cases of low-grade osteosarcoma with high-grade foci (grade 3) in less than 50% of the tumor, 9 patients did not receive adjuvant chemotherapy; only one of them died, of unrelated causes. In the adjuvant chemotherapy group (11 out of 20 patients), one patient developed multiple lung metastases and died of disease 39 months after the first diagnosis. In the other 13 cases of low-grade osteosarcoma with high-grade foci (grade 3) in more than 50% of the tumor, 12 patients received adjuvant chemotherapy: 2 had recurrence, 4 developed multiple lung metastases and 3 died of disease. The only patient who did not receive chemotherapy is alive without disease 232 months after complete surgical remission.

Conclusion.—Our data indicate that patients with a diagnosis of low-grade osteosarcoma where the high-grade (grade 3) component is lower than 50% of the resected specimen, may not require chemotherapy, achieving high survival rates by means of complete surgical resection only.

▶ Patients with low-grade osteosarcoma are generally treated by surgical resection alone, while those with high-grade osteosarcoma benefit from chemotherapy. This is well established in clinical experience and in the oncologic literature. However, these authors from the Rizzoli Institute collected a series of cases in which patients had a preoperative biopsy of a low-grade osteosarcoma and therefore went to immediate surgical resection. At the time of analysis of the resected specimen, they identified 33 patients (of 132 who were treated for low-grade central osteosarcoma) who had high-grade foci within their tumors. They subsequently divided these into those who had very small focal areas and those in whom the majority of the tumor was high grade.

Interestingly, in the patients who had only focal areas of high-grade tumor, some were treated with chemotherapy and some were not. Both did well. In those in whom the majority of the tumor was high grade (and the biopsy was a clear result of sampling error), chemotherapy and standard treatment was performed.

This is an interesting study in that traditional teaching has been at the highest grade area of a tumor defines the ultimate grade of the tumor, even if that area is small. These authors challenge that dogma and demonstrate in a limited series of patients that focal high-grade zones within a predominant background of low-grade osteosarcoma may have a better prognosis than previously thought and may not require chemotherapy.

This is the only report of this nature of a series of this size that I am aware. It must therefore be interpreted in context, but it raises a provocative question for surgeons and other physicians who treat these patients.

P. S. Rose, MD

The Identification of Prognostic Factors and Survival Statistics of Conventional Central Chondrosarcoma

Nota SPFT, Braun Y, Schwab JH, et al (Harvard Med School, Boston, MA; et al)

Sarcoma 2015:623746, 2015

Introduction.—Chondrosarcomas are malignant bone tumors that are characterized by the production of chondroid tissue. Since radiation therapy and chemotherapy have limited effect on chondrosarcoma, treatment of most patients depends on surgical resection. We conducted this study to identify independent predictive factors and survival characteristics for conventional central chondrosarcoma and dedifferentiated central chondrosarcoma.

Methods.—A systematic literature review was performed in September 2014 using the Pubmed, Embase, and Cochrane databases. Subsequent to a beforehand-composed selection procedure we included 13 studies, comprising a total of 1114 patients.

Results.—The prognosis of central chondrosarcoma is generally good for the histologically low-grade tumors. Prognosis for the high-grade chondrosarcoma and the dedifferentiated chondrosarcoma is poor with lower survival rates. Poor prognostic factors in conventional chondrosarcoma for overall survival are high-grade tumors and axial/pelvic tumor location. In dedifferentiated chondrosarcoma the percentage of dedifferentiated component has significant influence on disease-free survival.

Conclusion.—Despite the fact that there are multiple prognostic factors identified, as shown in this study, there is a need for prospective and comparative studies. The resulting knowledge about prognostic factors and survival can give direction in the development of better therapies. This could eventually lead to an evidence-based foundation for treating chondrosarcoma patients.

▶ These authors present a systematic review of the literature focusing on outcomes of central chondrosarcoma. Readers should immediately know that these authors use the term "central chondrosarcoma" not to mean axial malignancies. Rather, they define a central chondrosarcoma as one that has arisen within the intramedullary cavity of the bone and distinguish it from a "peripheral chondrosarcoma," which rises from an exostosis. This nomenclature is reasonable, but it is also easily confused with a common tendency to refer to peripheral chondrosarcomas as those arising in the extremity and central chondrosarcomas being those that arise within the axial skeleton.

The results are largely as expected. Higher-grade tumors and axial location portended poor outcome. My primary reason for including this article in the Year Book is because of the bibliography it includes. The authors have identified 13 total studies with more than 1000 patients from which they base their analysis. Reviewing the bibliography from this article is probably of similar use as the article itself for a practicing surgeon to be sure that he or she is aware of appropriate references for this disease process. The conclusions the authors drew are already accepted in the literature, and thus the article is reasonable but not earth shattering in and of itself.

P. S. Rose, MD

What is the Proportion of Patients With Multiple Hereditary Exostoses Who Undergo Malignant Degeneration?

Czajka CM, DiCaprio MR (Albany Med Ctr, Slingerlands, NY)

Clin Orthop Relat Res 473:2355-2361, 2015

Background.—Multiple hereditary exostoses is an autosomal-dominant skeletal disorder that has a wide-ranging reported risk of malignant degeneration to chondrosarcoma.

Questions/Purposes.—The aims of our study were to use a large, web-based survey approach to characterize (1) the demographic distribution of patients with multiple hereditary exostoses, (2) the number of surgeries performed related to one's diagnosis of multiple hereditary exostoses, and (3) the proportion of survey respondents who described experiencing malignant degeneration in a large international, heterogeneous cohort of patients with multiple hereditary exostoses.

Methods.—An anonymous web-based survey was distributed to several online support groups and social media networks designed to support and educate patients with multiple hereditary exostoses and their families. The survey collected demographic and epidemiologic data on 779 respondents. Data were recorded to assess respondents' disease burden and the rate of malignant degeneration.

Results.—Females represented a slightly greater proportion of those with multiple hereditary exostoses who responded (56% female; 419 of 742 patients). Median age for all respondents was 28 years (range, <1–85 years). Median age for males was 25 years (range, <1–85 years), while median age for females was 29 years (range, <1–82 years). The mean age at diagnosis of male and female respondents was in the mid-first decade (5.4 years ± 7.2 years). The mean number of surgeries a patient had undergone was 7.3 (± 7.1 surgeries). The proportion of respondents who experienced malignant transformation was 2.7% (21 of 757 respondents), at a mean age of 28.6 years (± 9.3 years). The most common sites of malignant change from benign exostoses included the pelvis (eight of 21 respondents) and scapula (four of 21 respondents).

Conclusions.—In the largest and most geographically diverse study of patients with multiple hereditary exostoses of which we are aware, we found the proportion of patients with multiple hereditary exostoses who have undergone malignant degeneration to be consistent with those reported in prior studies. Our study perhaps more accurately assessed the proportion of patients who undergo malignant transformation of multiple hereditary exostoses. As with prior studies on this topic, the proportion of malignant change may be expected to represent a high-end estimate as recruitment and selection bias likely predisposes for patients with more severe disease, whereas patients with lesser disease may be unaware of their diagnosis. In discussing the sequelae of multiple hereditary exostoses, clinicians perhaps might use this study to offer an unspecific statement of risk of malignant degeneration of multiple hereditary exostoses among the population at large.

Level of Evidence.—Level IV, prognostic study.

▶ This article by authors in the Albany Medical Center in New York is interesting for several reasons. First, it nominally gives us more information on the risk of malignant degeneration in patients with multiple hereditary exostoses (MHE). The authors identified a rate of malignant transformation of 2.7% of 757 respondents. The mean age at time of malignant transformation was 28.6 years. These data are interesting in that previous studies have had wide variation in the estimation of malignant degeneration. As well, it appears to have a younger age than most studies.

However, the most interesting thing about this article is the methods through which the authors came to their conclusion. They identified patients with MHE from Internet sites devoted to this condition, and their study is based on an Internet survey of patients. This has the strength in allowing them to have a large patient population from which to draw their study. It has a number of obvious drawbacks as well, however. Most important, there is no way to clinically verify any of the information provided for patients, and there is a clear selection bias in who responded.

MHE is a rare and generally identifiable condition such that there probably is not tremendous clinical ambiguity as to whether patients have the condition and as to whether they have had malignant transformation from it. It will be interesting to see whether similar studies using this methodology appear and are accepted in the literature. Additionally, it will be interesting to see whether studies of this nature can be validated for their accuracy and faithfully report data on patient populations with rare conditions.

P. S. Rose, MD

Can local recurrence of a sacral chordoma be treated by further surgery?

Xie C, Whalley N, Adasonla K, et al (The Royal Orthopaedic Hosp Foundation Trust, Birmingham, United Kingdom)

Bone Joint J 97-B:711-715, 2015

The purpose of this study was to evaluate the long-term outcome of patients with a sacral chordoma and the surgical management of locally recurrent disease.

Between October 1990 and August 2013 we operated on 54 consecutive patients with a sacral chordoma. There were 34 men and 20 women with a mean age of 60 years (25 to 86). The mean maximum diameter of the tumour was 9.3 cm (3 to 20).

The mean follow-up was 7.8 years (2 months to 23.4 years). The disease-specific survival was 82% at five years, 57% at ten years and 45% at 15 years. The local recurrence-free survival was 49% at five years, 37% at ten years and 20% at 15 years. Local recurrence occurred in 30 patients (56%) at a mean of 3.8 years (3 months to 13 years) post-operatively.

Survival after the treatment of recurrence was 89% at two years, 56% at five years and 19% at ten years. Of nine patients who had complete resection of a recurrence, one died after 72 months and eight remain disease-free. Incomplete resection of recurrent disease resulted in a survival of 54% at two years and 36% at five years.

For 12 patients with a local recurrence who were treated palliatively, survival was 81% at two years and 31% at five years.

A wide margin of resection gave the best chance of long-term survival and complete resection of local recurrence the best chance of control of disease.

▶ Chordoma is known by all to be a difficult tumor to treat with a predilection for local and regional recurrence. Once patients develop recurrence, it is even more difficult to know how to treat them. There is a natural pessimism that can set in among both doctors and patients in this clinical scenario.

This group from Birmingham, England, reports their experience with sacral chordomas. Significantly, they reaffirmed that the primary prognostic factor for survival and local recurrence is the extent of the margin achieved at the initial surgery. Additionally, they did demonstrate improved overall survival for patients treated with wide resection of recurrences.

There is obviously a selection bias that comes into a modest sample in which treatments are not assigned randomly. However, this article does add to our understanding for the need for aggressive surgical intervention for this disease process. Additionally, it suggests that it is not futile to attempt to treat recurrent chordomas in a similarly aggressive fashion. Although advanced radiation therapy regimens hold the potential to decrease our reliance on aggressive surgery for this disease process, at this time, surgery remains the primary treatment for this tumor worldwide.

P. S. Rose, MD

Tumor Reconstruction

Extendible Prostheses for Children After Resection of Primary Malignant Bone Tumor: Twenty-seven Years of Experience

Schinhan M, Tiefenboeck T, Funovics P, et al (Med Univ of Vienna, Austria)
J Bone Joint Surg Am 97:1585-1591, 2015

Background.—Endoprosthetic replacement in children following resection of a malignant bone tumor still is controversial because of the high number of reoperations. The aim of this study was to evaluate the long-term outcome with respect to limb-lengthening potential, satisfaction rate, and complications after implantation of extendible devices.

Methods.—Seventy-one patients with a sarcoma in an extremity who had been followed for more than twenty-four months (mean, 131.6 months; range, 27.2 to 281.8 months) after tumor resection and prosthetic reconstruction with an extendible device were analyzed. The mean age at the time of the operation was ten years (range, four to sixteen years). The complication-free survival rate was evaluated with competing-risk analysis. Clinical outcomes and complications were rated with use of the Musculoskeletal Tumor Society (MSTS) score and a failure mode classification for segmental tumor endoprostheses, respectively.

Results.—Twelve of seventy-one patients died of their disease. The overall MSTS score averaged 87.8% (range, 23.3% to 100%). The most common mode of failure was soft-tissue failure (46%), followed by structural failure (28%), infection (17%), and aseptic loosening (8%); only 2% of the children had local recurrence. An average of 4.4 lengthening operations per patient were required for an average limb elongation of 70.8 mm (range, 0 to 224 mm). An average of 2.5 operations (range, zero to eleven) per patient were performed for complications.

Conclusions.—Although limb lengthening with an extendible endoprosthesis seems to be effective, many children have related complications. These data will be a source of preoperative information for children and parents, and will provide a benchmark for further clinical improvements.

Level of Evidence.—Therapeutic Level IV. See Instructions for Authors for a complete description of levels of evidence (Fig 2).

▶ This article represents the largest report of extendible prostheses used in children with long-term follow-up (until the children have reached skeletal maturity). It comes out of Professor Windhager and Kotz's group in Vienna, the group

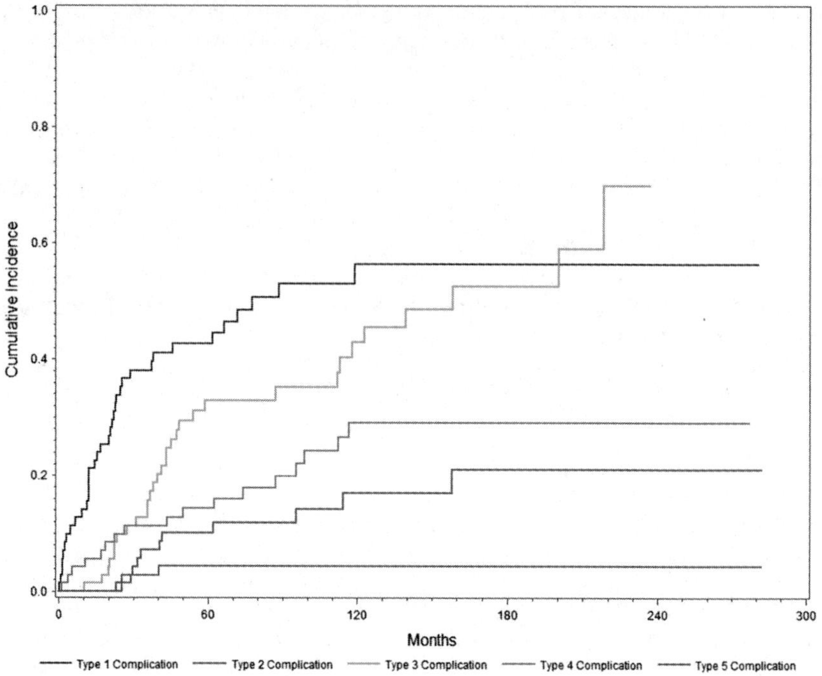

FIGURE 2.—Competing-risk analyses of all complications. The cumulative incidence of a complication was estimated to be 0.73 (95% confidence interval [CI] = 0.63 to 0.85) after five years and 0.87 (95% CI = 0.77 to 0.98) after ten years. The cumulative incidence after five and ten years was estimated to be 0.43 (95% CI = 0.33 to 0.56) and 0.56 (95% CI = 0.45 to 0.71), respectively, for a type-1 complication (soft-tissue failure); 0.10 (95% CI = 0.05 to 0.21) and 0.17 (95% CI = 0.09 to 0.31), respectively, for a type-2 complication (aseptic loosening); 0.33 (95% CI = 0.23 to 0.46) and 0.43 (95% CI = 0.32 to 0.56), respectively, for a type-3 complication (structural failure); 0.14 (95% CI = 0.08 to 0.25) and 0.29 (95% CI = 0.19 to 0.44), respectively, for a type-4 complication (infection); and 0.04 (95% CI = 0.01 to 0.13) for a type-5 complication (tumor progression) after five and ten years. (Reprinted from Schinhan M, Tiefenboeck T, Funovics P, et al. Extendible prostheses for children after resection of primary malignant bone tumor: twenty-seven years of experience. *J Bone Joint Surg Am.* 2015;97:1585-1591, with permission from The Journal of Bone and Joint Surgery, Incorporated.)

that pioneered this technique as the technology for it became available several decades ago. The authors report on 71 patients (12 of whom died) at long-term follow-up.

The results are mixed. Ultimately, most patients achieved good function with a reported Musculoskeletal Tumor Society score of 88%. However, complications were frequent (see Fig 2). Interestingly, soft tissue complications were the most frequently seen complications in patients. Structural failure, infection, and loosening were also frequently seen. Children required an average of 4.4 operations for lengthening and an average of 2.5 operations (and as many as 11) for the treatment of complications.

Where to put the study in clinical context? It is clear that advances in technology can allow extendible prostheses to be used with reasonable success in young children with extremity bone tumors. Newer generations of prostheses hold the potential to decrease the complication rate with noninvasive expansion mechanisms and improved design and metallurgy. However, these technologies are most likely to decrease infectious and mechanical complications; they will have a less direct effect on soft tissue failures (the most frequent complication seen in this series).

As such, surgeons and families need to decide carefully whether to embark on such a long and extensive course of action when treating a child with a primary bone tumor. Rotationplasty (a viable option in any child who undergoes an extendible prosthesis) or amputation remain excellent functional options for children. Although these too can have complications, it appears the complication profile is likely much lower with these options. Functional outcome is generally excellent with these as well.

This is a great study for surgeons who treat children with bone tumors to be aware of. It establishes the current standard for expected outcomes and complications with these devices.

P. S. Rose, MD

Argyria following the use of silver-coated megaprostheses: no association between the development of local argyria and elevated silver levels

Glehr M, Leithner A, Friesenbichler J, et al (Med Univ of Graz, Austria)
Bone Joint J 95-B:988-992, 2013

The aims of this study were to evaluate the incidence of local argyria in patients with silver-coated megaprostheses and to identify a possible association between argyria and elevated levels of silver both locally and in the blood. Between 2004 and 2011, 32 megaprostheses with silver coatings were implanted in 20 female and 12 male patients following revision arthroplasty for infection or resection of a malignant tumour, and the levels of silver locally in drains and seromas and in the blood were determined. The mean age of the patients was 46 years (10 to 81); one patient died in the immediate post-operative period and was excluded.

Seven patients (23%) developed local argyria after a median of 25.7 months (interquartile range 2 to 44.5). Patients with and without local argyria had comparable levels of silver in the blood and aspiration fluids. The length of the implant did not influence the development of local argyria. Patients with clinical evidence of local argyria had no neurological symptoms and no evidence of renal or hepatic failure. Thus, we conclude that the short-term surveillance of blood silver levels in these patients is not required.

► The U.S. Food and Drug Administration may be poised to approve for U.S. distribution of European implants that incorporate a silver coating in an attempt to decrease the risk of surgical-site infection. One concern that has been raised with regard to this is the risk of argyria, a blue or bluish gray discoloration of the skin related to silver exposure. Additionally, there is a natural concern that elevated silver levels may lead to organ damage (particularly renal or hepatic injury). Although this article was published in the European literature in

2013, I have included it in this issue of the YEAR BOOK because of its relevance to potential new implants in the U.S. market.

These authors from Graz, Austria, report 7 or 32 patients (23%) developing local argyria at a median 25.7 months after implantation of their prostheses. Argyria arose as soon as 2 months after implantation. Patients with argyria did not demonstrate elevated silver ion concentrations in blood and joint aspiration fluids compared with those without argyria. Additionally, no end organ toxicity was observed at admittedly short follow-up.

Where to place this study in clinical context? The authors demonstrate no clear association between the development of local argyria and elevated silver levels in a modest population of patients at short-term follow-up. If these prostheses do become available for use in North America, surgeons are cautioned that a 23% rate of local argyria is certainly significant. Additionally, although we can be thankful that no end organ damage or other systemic effects were observed in this study, it contains a small number of patients and a short clinical follow-up. As such, surgeons should be aware of this possibility as they select implants and counsel their patients regarding these implant options.

P. S. Rose, MD

Resurfaced Allograft-Prosthetic Composite for Proximal Tibial Reconstruction in Children: Intermediate-Term Results of an Original Technique

Campanacci L, Alì N, Casanova JMPS, et al (Rizzoli Orthopaedic Inst, Bologna, Italy; Centro Hospitalar e Universitário de Coimbra, Portugal; et al)

J Bone Joint Surg Am 97:241-250, 2015

Background.—Reconstruction of the proximal part of the tibia in children with megaprostheses or standard composite devices removes the distal femoral physis, and osteoarticular allografts have a high incidence of mechanical failure. We evaluated the results of an alternative original technique for proximal tibial reconstruction after tumor resection.

Methods.—Nineteen children, ranging in age from six to sixteen years, who underwent surgical resection and reconstruction with a resurfaced allograft-prosthetic composite were retrospectively reviewed at a mean follow-up time of seventy-eight months. Eighteen children had high-grade sarcoma (fourteen had osteosarcoma and four had Ewing sarcoma), and one child had an aggressive giant cell tumor of the proximal part of the tibia. Surgical resection and its complications, disease-free survival of the patients, implant survival, and functional results according to the Musculoskeletal Tumor Society scoring system were analyzed at the time of the latest follow-up.

Results.—In all patients, wide surgical margins were obtained and no local recurrence was observed. At the time of the latest follow-up, nine of the eighteen patients with a high-grade malignant tumor were continually disease-free, another six had had metastases but had no evidence of disease, and three had died of the disease. The patient with a giant cell tumor was continually disease-free after 168 months. The mean implant survival was sixty-eight months (range, six to 188 months). The major complications were one deep infection; two nonunions, which healed after surgical revision; and six allograft fractures. Limb-length discrepancy was the most frequent complication but, following contralateral epiphysiodesis, resulted in a mean discrepancy of 1.9 cm at the time of the latest follow-up. At the time of the latest follow-up, eight patients had a Musculoskeletal Tumor Society score deemed as excellent or good.

Conclusions.—In children and young teenagers with bone tumors of the proximal part of the tibia requiring an intraarticular resection, knee reconstruction with a resurfaced allograft-prosthetic composite may represent a valid alternative to conventional megaprostheses or to osteoarticular allograft.

▶ Limb salvage of proximal tibial tumors in young children is challenging for any number of reasons. Prosthetic replacement requires violation of the distal femoral physis and worsens an already developing leg-length discrepancy. Osteoarticular allografts that will demonstrate congruency to the femoral articulation are difficult to obtain. These authors invented a technique in which a tibial allograft is resurfaced with the bearing of a rotating platform knee that is then mated directly against the articular cartilage of the distal femur in proximal tibial limb salvage. This is an attempt to allow reasonable congruency with the distal femur and to decrease the risk of allograft fracture and collapse when treating these tumors in children.

This series represents the intermediate-term follow-up in a series of 19 children. The results are reasonable given the population under treatment. Surgeons and patients/families have to recognize that limb salvage treatment in children of this nature involves a series of procedures. Thus, the initial reconstruction is probably best recognized as a "bridging" to skeletal maturity. In this sense, this technique represents an improvement over previous methods.

Specifically, allograft fracture was seen in one-third of patients. However, in a previous series, allograft fractures were seen in 80% of patients. Thus, this new technique appears to improve on that outcome. Other allograft-related complications (infection, nonunion) are present as would be expected in such a series.

Where to place this article in clinical context? The authors are applauded for inventing a unique technique to address a clinical problem in the treatment of children with proximal tibial tumors. Although complications remain frequent, this provides an advance in the care of these children. This technique (and potentially future refinements of it) appears to be our current best option if distal femur physeal preservation is sought in limb salvage treatment of these patients.

P. S. Rose, MD

The mechanical effects of extracorporeal irradiation on bone

Gupta S, Cafferky D, Cowie F, et al (Univ of Strathclyde, Glasgow, UK)
Bone Joint J 97-B:1152-1156, 2015

Extracorporeal irradiation of an excised tumour-bearing segment of bone followed by its reimplantation is a technique used in bone sarcoma surgery for limb salvage when the bone is of reasonable quality. There is no agreement among previous studies about the dose of irradiation to be given: up to 300 Gy have been used.

We investigated the influence of extracorporeal irradiation on the elastic and viscoelastic properties of bone. Bone was harvested from mature cattle and subdivided into 13 groups: 12 were exposed to increasing levels of irradiation: one was not and was used as a control. The specimens, once irradiated, underwent mechanical testing in saline at 37°C.

The mechanical properties of each group, including Young's modulus, storage modulus and loss modulus, were determined experimentally and compared with the control group.

There were insignificant changes in all of these mechanical properties with an increasing level of irradiation.

We conclude that the overall mechanical effect of high levels of extracorporeal irradiation (300 Gy) on bone is negligible. Consequently the dose can be maximised to reduce the risk of local tumour recurrence.

▶ Extracorporeal irradiation of tumor-laden bone is commonly performed in many areas of the world for rapid reconstruction and to avoid the need for allografts. These authors studied the effects of increasing doses of radiation on the biomechanical properties of bone using a model evaluating cow tibia. In summary, they did not find any significant change in the mechanical strength of the bone as tested.

On face value, this result seems reasonable, but it is a superficial evaluation of this problem. Posttreatment fracture is a recognized and frequent complication after limb salvage using extracorporeal irradiation. This study is useful for the discussion that it brings but also has several significant limitations; I see 2 primary limitations. One is that the specimens they analyzed had been previously frozen after harvest. Thus, we do not know if there has been a decrease in their strength from the freezing, which might mask or overpower the decrease in the strength from radiation. Additionally, the authors had only a single control and did not take the opportunity to use left/right controls (radiating one side and using the other from the same animal as an inherent control).

More to the point, when this technique is applied clinically, it is in bone laden with tumor, which is almost always inherently weaker as well. The inherent weakness of the bone may or may not be affected by the extracorporeal irradiation. However, the high rate of fracture seen when these techniques are put into clinical practice highlights that careful laboratory studies such as this probably do not tell the full story of the risk that patients assume when these techniques are used. As such, I think there is value in bringing this article into the Year Book for several reasons. The discussion and the information is reasonable subject to its limitations. However, it also bears caution on the part of surgeons employing this to keep in mind that this does not tell the full story of weakness of bones after extracorporeal irradiation and replantation. Otherwise, we would not expect to see the high risk of fractures that is observed in this clinical setting.

P. S. Rose, MD

Osteocartilaginous Transfer of the Proximal Part of the Fibula for Osseous Overgrowth in Children with Congenital or Acquired Tibial Amputation: Surgical Technique and Results

Fedorak GT, Watts HG, Cuomo AV, et al (Shriners Hosps for Children Honolulu, HI; Shriners Hosps for Children, Los Angeles, CA; Univ of North Carolina, Chapel Hill; et al)

J Bone Joint Surg Am 97:574-581, 2015

Background.—Osseous overgrowth is a common problem in children after tibial transcortical amputation. We present the results of forty-seven children (fifty tibiae) treated for tibial osseous overgrowth with an autologous osteocartilaginous cap from the proximal part of the ipsilateral fibula.

Methods.—We reviewed the records of all patients who underwent amputation at a single pediatric hospital from 1990 to 2011. All patients who had been followed for a minimum of two years after undergoing osteocartilaginous capping with the proximal part of the ipsilateral fibula to treat established tibial overgrowth were included. Patients with acquired and congenital amputations were compared.

Results.—Fifty tibiae in forty-seven patients met our inclusion criteria. There were thirty-one acquired and nineteen congenital amputations. The mean age at surgery was 7.6 years (range, 2.1 to 15.6 years), and the mean duration of follow-up was 7.2 years (range, 2.2 to 15.4 years). Five tibiae (10%) in four patients had recurrence of the overgrowth at a mean of 5.4 years (range, 2.8 to 7.6 years) after the osteocartilaginous transfer. There was no significant difference in the results between children with an acquired amputation and those with a congenital amputation.

Conclusions.—At a mean of 7.2 years after autologous osteocartilaginous capping with the proximal part of the fibula, 90% of the limbs had not had recurrent overgrowth. This is a safe and effective treatment of long-bone overgrowth following either congenital or acquired amputation in children.

Level of Evidence.—Therapeutic Level IV. See Instructions for Authors for a complete description of levels of evidence.

▶ Terminal overgrowth following transcortical amputation is well recognized in pediatric patients; the younger the patient, the more severe this development is likely to be. These authors from the Los Angeles Shriners Hospital retrospectively report the use of an osteocartilaginous transfer of the proximal fibula in children who have established amputations and terminal overgrowth to prevent further overgrowth.

Overall, they found this procedure was largely successful. Only 10% of the patients had further overgrowth. Interestingly, the lateral collateral ligament was released and not repaired in this study, and they had no episodes of varus instability noted.

These children were undergoing amputations for nononcologic indications. Thankfully, most children can be treated with limb salvage or limb shortening (rotationplasty) procedures for malignancies; however, there remains the potential for amputation as we approach children with locally advanced tumors. As such, I think this is a valuable article to include in the oncology section to highlight this issue. Additionally, the discussion that is included is quite good and reviews the literature on primary capping procedures to minimize the risk of overgrowth at the time of definitive amputation surgery. Surgical oncologists who care for children with bone tumors should be familiar with this technique, and it is well illustrated in this article.

P. S. Rose, MD

The vascularised fibular graft for limb salvage after bone tumour surgery: a multicentre study

Hilven PH, Bayliss L, Cosker T, et al (LUMC, Leiden, The Netherlands)

Bone Joint J 97-B:853-861, 2015

Vascularised fibular grafts (VFGs) are a valuable surgical technique in limb salvage after resection of a tumour. The primary objective of this multicentre study was to assess the risk factors for failure and complications for using a VFG after resection of a tumour.

The study involved 74 consecutive patients (45 men and 29 women with mean age of 23 years (1 to 64) from four tertiary centres for orthopaedic oncology who underwent reconstruction using a VFG after resection of a tumour between 1996 and 2011. There were 52 primary and 22 secondary reconstructions. The mean follow-up was 77 months (10 to 195).

In all, 69 patients (93%) had successful limb salvage; all of these united and 65 (88%) showed hypertrophy of the graft. The mean time to union differed between those involving the upper (28 weeks; 12 to 96) and lower limbs (44 weeks; 12 to 250). Fracture occurred in 11 (15%), and nonunion in 14 (19%) patients.

In 35 patients (47%) at least one complication arose, with a greater proportion in lower limb reconstructions, non-bridging osteosynthesis, and in children. These complications resulted in revision surgery in 26 patients (35%).

VFG is a successful and durable technique for reconstruction of a defect in bone after resection of a tumour, but is accompanied by a significant risk of complications, that often require revision surgery. Union was not markedly influenced by the need for chemo- or radiotherapy, but should not be expected during chemotherapy. Therefore, restricted weight-bearing within this period is advocated.

▶ The advent of vascularized bone grafts in the treatment of patients after oncologic resection is well established. However, these remain relatively rare procedures, and few centers have a large number of cases for analysis. These authors from Europe performed a multicenter trial pooling together data on 74 consecutive patients who had undergone vascularized free fibular grafting at 4 orthopedic oncology referral centers. Fifty-two of these were primary reconstructions, and 22 were salvage reconstructions.

These results provide reasonable data to use when counseling patients and expected outcomes. The authors demonstrated successful limb salvage in 93% of patients and ultimate union of the graft in all these patients. As well, 88% of grafts demonstrated hypertrophy at mean follow-up of 77 months. This is particularly important because this technique is often used for the treatment for children and young adults.

However, 47% of patients experienced at least 1 significant complication. Not surprisingly, complications were greater in lower extremity applications, pediatric patients, and patients who did not have bridging osteosynthesis constructs. A third of patients required revision surgery for these complications.

Ultimately, this is a successful and durable technique, but it should not be undertaken lightly. This report of a wealth of experience from 4 centers sets the background for the expected outcomes and complication rates in this patient population. As such, this is an excellent reference article for surgeons to have as they consider patients for this technique.

P. S. Rose, MD

What Are the Functional Results and Complications From Allograft Reconstruction After Partial Hemipelvectomy of the Pubis?

Karim SM, Colman MW, Lozano-Calderón SA, et al (Massachusetts General Hosp, Boston)

Clin Orthop Relat Res 473:1442-1448, 2015

Background.—In patients undergoing hemipelvectomies including resection either of a portion of the pubis or the entire pubis from the symphysis to the lateral margin of the obturator foramen while sparing the hip (so-called Dunham Type III hemipelvectomies), reconstructions typically are not performed given the preserved continuity of the weight-bearing axis and the potential complications associated with reconstruction. Allograft reconstruction of the pelvic ring may, however, offer benefits for soft tissue reconstruction of the pelvic floor and hip stability, but little is known about these reconstructions.

Questions/Purposes.—(1) What is the postoperative functional status after allograft reconstruction of Type III pelvic defects? (2) What are the rates of hernia, infection, and hip instability?

Methods.—In this case series, we reviewed all patients with Type III pelvic resections (with or without anterior acetabular wall resections) who underwent allograft reconstruction between 2005 and 2013 at one center (N = 14). During the period in question, reconstruction was the general approach used in patients undergoing these resections; during that time, three other patients were treated without reconstruction as a result of either surgeon preference or the patient choosing to not have reconstruction after a discussion of the risks and benefits. Of the 14 patients treated with reconstruction, complete followup was available at a minimum of 1 year in 11 (other than those who died before the end of the first year; median, 19 months; range 16–70 months among those surviving), one was lost to followup before a year, and two others had partial telephone or email followup. Patient demographics, disease status, functional status, and complications were recorded. For a portion of the cohort (four patients) later in the series, we used a novel technique for anterior acetabular wall reconstruction using the concave cartilaginous surface of a proximal fibula allograft; the others received either a long bone (humerus or femur) or hemipelvis graft. Seven patients died of disease; two had local recurrence, and five died of metastatic disease.

Results.—All patients remained ambulatory Pain at 12 months after surgery was reported as none in five, mild in two, moderate in two, and severe in one. Operative complications included infection in two, symptomatic hernia in one, hip instability in one, dislocated total hip arthroplasty on the first postoperative day in one, and graft failure in one.

Conclusions.—Allograft reconstruction after Type III pelvic resections can provide functional reconstruction of the pelvic ring, pelvic floor, and, in certain patients with partial anterior acetabular resections, the resected anterior acetabulum. This has implications in preventing the occurrence of hernia and hip instability in this patient population that is classically not reconstructed, although longer-term outcomes in a larger number of patients would help to better delineate this because infection, hernia, hip instability, and graft nonunion still remain concerns with this approach. The most important unanswered question remains whether, on balance, any benefits that may accrue to these patients as the result of reconstruction are offset by a relatively high likelihood of undergoing secondary or revision surgery.

Level of Evidence.—Level IV, therapeutic study.

► Most surgeons do not provide bony reconstruction after a type III internal hemipelvectomy. Traditional teaching has been either to accept a visceral hernia in the area or to provide a soft tissue reconstruction to minimize this. Bony reconstruction has seldom been done in this area. These authors from Massachusetts General Hospital present an intriguing series of 14 patients who underwent type III pelvic resections from 2005 to 2013 and were reconstructed with allografts. The authors purport that this provides an improved functional outcome.

This is an interesting article and one that I have had patients identify and bring to me before type III internal hemipelvectomies. As such, it is something that has found its way into the medical literature and also into the domain of some patients, and it is thus worthwhile for surgeons to be familiar with it.

The technique is interesting; the results are not rigorous, but that is understandable with a retrospective series of a rare problem. The most striking result is the complication profile that is reported. Six patients had major complications requiring reoperation. The authors included patients who had a portion of the medial acetabulum resected, and thus, hip instability contributed to some of their complications. These patients are probably generally better referred to as a type II/III internal hemipelvectomy.

Where to place this study in clinical context? At this time, I do not think the standard of care is to provide a reconstruction of an anterior pelvic resection of this nature. However, the point the authors make is well taken, and this article comes from an established and respected group. As well, given the current dissemination of medical literature to the lay public via the Internet, patients may well ask surgeons about this technique and whether it is suitable for them. As such, it is important for oncologic pelvic surgeons to be familiar with it even if their familiarity makes them chose not to select it for their patient population.

P. S. Rose, MD

Total Femur Replacement After Tumor Resection: Limb Salvage Usually Achieved But Complications and Failures are Common

Sevelda F, Schuh R, Hofstaetter JG, et al (Med Univ of Vienna, Austria; Orthopaedic Hosp Speising, Vienna, Austria)

Clin Orthop Relat Res 473:2079-2087, 2015

Background.—Primary bone or soft tissue tumors of the femur sometimes present with severe and extensive bone destruction, leaving few limb-salvage options other than total femur replacement. However, there are few data available regarding total femur replacement and, in particular, regarding implant failures.

Questions/Purposes.—We asked: (1) What are the revision-free and overall implant survival rates of conventional total femur replacements in patients treated for sarcoma of the femur or soft tissues? (2) What are the revision-free and overall implant survival rates of expandable total femur replacements in skeletally immature patients? (3) Using the comprehensive International Society of Limb Salvage failure-mode classification, what types of complications occur with conventional and expandable total femur replacements?

Patients and Methods.—Our retrospective, single-center cohort study was based on data prospectively collected for 50 patients who received a total femur replacement after tumor resection for indications other than carcinoma or metastatic disease. Of the 50 patients, six (12%) were lost to followup before 6 months. Ten of the remaining 44 patients received expandable implants. The mean followup was 57 months (range, 1–280 months) and 172 months (range, 43–289 months) for patients who underwent conventional and expandable total femur replacements, respectively. For implant survival, competing risk analyses were used.

Results.—At 5 years, revision-free implant survival of conventional total femur replacements was 48% (95% CI, 0.37–0.73), and overall implant survival was 97% (95% CI, 0.004–0.20). Five-year revision-free implant survival of expandable total femur replacements was 30% (95% CI, 0.47–1.00) and overall implant survival was 100%. With conventional total femur replacements soft tissue failures occurred in 13 of 34 patients, structural failures in three, infection in six, and local tumor progression in one. No patient had aseptic loosening with conventional total femur replacements, but hip disarticulation occurred in two patients owing to extensive wound-healing problems and infection. With expandable total femur replacements soft tissue failure, aseptic loosening, and infection occurred in one patient each of 10, and structural failures in three of 10 (two periprosthetic fractures, one loosening of an enhanced tendon anchor). No hip disarticulations were performed. Additionally expandable total femur replacement-related failures included hip instability in eight of 10 patients, contractures attributable to massive scar tissue in six, and defect of the implant's expansion mechanism in four patients.

Conclusions.—Although the indications for total femoral resection are rare, we think that total femur replacement is a reasonable treatment option for reconstruction of massive femoral bone defects after tumor resection in adults and skeletally immature patients, and results in limb salvage in most patients.

Level of Evidence.—Level IV, therapeutic study.

▶ This article from Vienna details the institutional experience in 50 total femurs placed in children and adults for primary bone tumor resection (the authors exclude cases placed for metastatic disease). Allowing for 6 patients lost to follow-up, they report on 10 pediatric patients treated with expandable implants and 34 adult patients with static implants.

The article is well written, and the results are sobering. The requirement for secondary amputation was rare in this series. However, the rate of revision was quite high (greater than 50% at 5 years in conventional implants and 70% at 5 years in expandable implants). The authors tabulated their failures using the Henderson/International Society of Limb Salvage classification.

The information presented is detailed and comes from an acknowledged excellent group. Similarly, the discussion is well written. Obviously the authors are reporting on a heterogeneous group of patients accrued over several decades. Thus, the details of their results may not be immediately translated into all aspects of clinical practice (for example, their early prostheses are no longer manufactured). However, this is an excellent tabulation of the experience, honestly reported, from an expert and experienced center. As surgeons consider the role of total femur replacement in patients, this article is worth reading to understand what reasonable outcomes patients should expect from this reconstruction option.

P. S. Rose, MD

Soft Tissue Sarcomas

Unplanned Excision of Soft-Tissue Sarcomas: Current Concepts for Management and Prognosis

Pretell-Mazzini J, Barton MD Jr, Conway SA, et al (Univ of Miami Miller School of Medicine, FL)

J Bone Joint Surg Am 97:597-603, 2015

- Biopsy, staging, preoperative imaging and planning, as well as surgical treatment of soft-tissue sarcomas, are best carried out in specialized sarcoma centers, with the support of a multidisciplinary tumor board.
- Tumor bed excision is recommended after most unplanned excisions, with a goal of obtaining complete tumor removal with an appropriately wide margin of resection.
- The surgical resection area tends to be more extensive during tumor bed excision than during primary resection because of the need to resect potential areas of contamination, resulting in the need for more reconstructive procedures (flaps and skin grafts) and wider radiation fields.
- Unplanned excisions are associated with an increased rate of local recurrence related to residual disease and positive margins after tumor bed excision, a deep location, and certain histologic subtypes, such as malignant peripheral nerve sheath tumor, myxofibrosarcoma, and dermatofibrosarcoma protuberans.
- While adjuvant radiation therapy has not been found to mitigate the risk of local recurrence in unplanned excisions, it is generally utilized in the treatment of unplanned excisions as it is in the treatment of primary soft-tissue sarcomas.
- Given the surgical and oncologic sequelae of unplanned excisions, prevention through the diffusion of concepts by means of provider education on how to approach soft-tissue masses, which can be potential soft-tissue sarcomas, is the best strategy.

▶ This is a current concepts review published in the *Journal of Bone and Joint Surgery* that provides a nice literature-supported overview of the treatment of patients who have undergone unplanned excision of soft tissue sarcomas. This article is valuable for practicing tumor surgeons in several ways.

First, this article contains an up-to-date review of the literature and synthesis of the available clinical information to help guide evidence-based practice. Although firm practice guidelines often do not exist for all aspects of sarcoma care, a current concepts review of this nature provides relevant advice in the care of patients.

Second, patients with implant excision are often frustrated and question the need for and nature of further treatments that are advised. Although this is a relatively technical article, a highly educated patient may find this valuable as a justification for recommended treatment.

Finally, an article of this nature is readily distributed to nononcologic colleagues as well as residents and fellows to advise of the implications and treatment decisions surrounding patients who undergo unplanned excision of soft tissue sarcomas. As such, I think it is a valuable addition to the YEAR BOOK for surgeons to review.

P. S. Rose, MD

Primary and secondary angiosarcomas: a comparative single-center analysis

Hillenbrand T, Menge F, Hohenberger P, et al (Univ of Heidelberg, Mannheim, Germany)

Clin Sarcoma Res 5:14, 2015

Background.—Angiosarcomas (AS) are rare vascular malignancies. They are subdivided into primary (PAS) and secondary angiosarcomas (SAS). The objective was to compare the characteristics of AS subtypes.

Methods.—Eighteen PAS and ten SAS patients treated at our institution between 2004 and 2012 were included in this study.

Results.—Median age of PAS and SAS patients was 52.9 and 64.2 years, respectively ($p = 0.1448$). The percentage of women was 27.8% for PAS, but 80.0% for SAS ($p = 0.0163$). While PAS occurred throughout the body, the majority of SAS arose from the breast ($p = 0.0012$). All SAS were radiation-induced with a median latency of 7.7 years. The majority of patients with PAS and SAS underwent surgery as primary or recurrence treatment ($p > 0.95$). Local recurrence was developed by 27.8% of PAS and 50.0% of SAS ($p = 0.4119$). 61.1% of PAS metastasized, but only 40.0% of SAS ($p = 0.4328$). Median overall survival for PAS and SAS was 19 and 57 months, respectively ($p = 0.2306$).

Conclusion.—Radical surgery remains the mainstay of both primary and recurrence treatment. SAS show a high local recurrence rate, while PAS tend towards developing early metastases. Overall, prognosis is poor for both groups.

▶ I included this in the YEAR BOOK because it provides a nice discussion of a rare malignancy. Angiosarcomas are encountered in orthopedic oncology generally in 3 scenarios. The first is as a classic deep-seated soft tissue sarcoma; the second is in the setting of lymphedema of the limb; and the third is as a postradiation sarcoma, often following breast-conserving therapy for breast cancer. This article provides a comparison between 18 primary angiosarcomas located in a variety of locations (including visceral), and secondary angiosarcoma patients (primarily following breast cancer treatment).

These results confirm that aggressive surgical resection remains the cornerstone of treatment for patients with either primary or secondary angiosarcoma. Both tumors showed an aggressive course. Secondary angiosarcomas had a high rate of local recurrence (50%) but a lower rate of metastasis compared with primary angiosarcomas. Median survival for patients with primary angiosarcomas was only 19 months, whereas those with secondary angiosarcomas was 57 months.

Where to place this article in clinical context? The authors have put together a reasonable series of a rare condition and provided a nice comparison between patients presenting with primary and secondary disease. These results confirm the role of aggressive surgery and also provide a nice discussion to inform clinicians as they treat these patients. Unfortunately, because this tumor is a rare disease process, our overall literature experience with it remains limited.

P. S. Rose, MD

Intraoperative Radiotherapy in the Management of Locally Recurrent Extremity Soft Tissue Sarcoma

Tinkle CL, Weinberg V, Braunstein SE, et al (Univ of California, San Francisco)

Sarcoma 2015:913565, 2015

Purpose.—To investigate the efficacy and morbidity of limb-sparing surgery with intraoperative radiotherapy (IORT) for patients with locally recurrent extremity soft tissue sarcoma (ESTS).

Methods and Materials.—Twenty-six consecutively treated patients were identified in a single institution retrospective analysis of patients with locally recurrent ESTS treated with IORT following salvage limb-sparing resection from May 2000 to July 2011. Fifteen (58%) patients received external beam radiotherapy (EBRT) prior to recurrence (median dose 63 Gy), while 11 (42%) patients received EBRT following IORT (median dose 52 Gy).The Kaplan-Meier product limit method was used to estimate disease control and survival and subsets were compared using a log rank statistic, Cox's regression model was used to determine independent predictors of disease outcome, and toxicity was reported according to CTCAE v4.0 guidelines.

Results.—With a median duration of follow-up from surgery and IORT of 34.9 months (range: 4 to 139 mos.), 10 patients developed a local recurrence with 4 subsequently undergoing amputation. The 5-year estimate for local control (LC) was 58% (95% CI: 36–75%), for amputation-free was 81% (95% CI: 57–93%), for metastasis-free control (MFC) was 56% (95% CI: 31–75%), for disease-free survival (DFS) was 35% (95% CI: 17–54%), and for overall survival (OS) was 50% (95% CI: 24–71%). Prior EBRT did not appear to influence disease control (LC, $p = 0.74$; MFC, $p = 0.66$) or survival (DFS, $p = 0.16$; OS, $p = 0.58$). Grade 3 or higher acute and late toxicities were reported for 6 (23%) and 8 (31%) patients, respectively. The frequency of both acute and late grade 3 or higher toxicities occurred equally between patients who received EBRT prior to or after IORT.

Conclusions.—IORT in combination with oncologic resection of recurrent ESTS yields good rates of local control and limb-salvage with acceptable morbidity. Within the limitations of small subsets, these data suggest that prior EBRT does not significantly influence disease control or toxicity.

▶ Locally recurrent soft tissue sarcoma is a difficult clinical problem. These authors from San Francisco report a retrospective analysis of 26 consecutively treated patients at a single institution who had intraoperative radiotherapy in combination with external beam radiotherapy in the treatment of locally recurrent soft tissue sarcoma.

The results showed moderate success at best, but readers must acknowledge recurrent sarcoma can be a difficult problem to treat. The 5-year local control rate was only 58%, and 19% of patients required amputation. Metastasis free control was 56% and disease-free survival at 5 years was only 35%. Overall survival was 50%. The authors reported that 23% of patients had significant acute toxicity, and 31% of patients had significant late toxicities associated with this treatment.

Where to put this study in clinical context? Locally recurrent soft tissue sarcoma can be difficult to treat and often ultimately requires amputation. These results highlight both the benefit and limitations of advanced radiation techniques (including intraoperative radiotherapy) in achieving further control. Surgeons faced with patients with difficult locally recurrent soft tissue sarcomas may wish to strongly consider the addition of intraoperative radiotherapy (or referral to a center where this is available). However, patients should be cautioned that the outcome remains uncertain, and the complication profile of such treatment is high. An amputation rate of only 19% is impressive given the adverse presenting characteristics of these patients.

Note that the availability of intraoperative radiotherapy is increasing around the country as mobile units become available (rather than cumbersome fixed units, which are available at a limited number of institutions). Still, the adoption of this technology is relatively limited to major tumor centers at this time.

P. S. Rose, MD

Should High-grade Extraosseous Osteosarcoma Be Treated With Multimodality Therapy Like Other Soft Tissue Sarcomas?

Fan Z, Patel S, Lewis VO, et al (Peking Univ Cancer Hosp & Inst, Beijing, China; Univ of Texas MD Anderson Cancer Ctr, Houston)
Clin Orthop Relat Res 473:3604-3611, 2015

Background.—Extraosseous osteosarcoma is rare, and the most appropriate therapy is unclear because there are few studies regarding its treatment. The effectiveness of radiation and chemotherapy remains uncertain owing to conflicting results in previous reports.

Questions/Purposes.—To review our experience with contemporary multimodality treatment, we asked: (1) What is the disease-specific survival and local relapse-free survival? (2) Does American Joint Commission on Cancer (AJCC) stage, tumor size, or location relate to disease outcome? (3) Does radiation therapy improve local control or survival? (4) Do doxorubicin and ifosfamide improve local control or survival?

Methods.—Between 1990 and 2012, we treated 40 patients for localized, high-grade extraosseous osteosarcoma. In this retrospective study, we could determine the status of 36 patients (90%) either to death or for a minimum of 24 months of followup; four (10%) were lost to followup before 24 months. There were 11 patients with AJCC Stage IIA and 25 with Stage III disease. All patients underwent wide surgical excision. Of the patients with Stage IIA disease, four received radiation and none received chemotherapy. Of the patients with Stage III disease, six received radiation, seven were treated with chemotherapy, and six received radiation and chemotherapy. During the study period, high-dose doxorubicin and ifosfamide was the preferred chemotherapy regimen for patients younger than 60 years with normal cardiac and renal function. Local relapse-free survival and disease-specific survival were determined by Kaplan-Meier analysis using a prospectively maintained institutional database supplemented by information from the institutional tumor registry. The Cox proportional hazard model was used to determine the effect of various factors on local recurrence and patient survival.

Results.—At 5 years, local relapse-free survival was 47% (95% CI, 27%–64%), and disease-specific survival was 53% (95% CI, 35%–68%). In multivariate analysis, AJCC stage, which depends on tumor size, was the strongest predictor of local relapse-free survival (hazard ratio [HR] = 0.17, $p = 0.02$), while tumor depth was the best predictor of disease-specific survival (HR = 5.6, $p = 0.02$). Radiation improved local relapse-free survival (HR = 0.30, $p = 0.03$) but not disease-specific survival in multivariate analysis. A regimen of doxorubicin and ifosfamide was associated with better local relapse-free survival for patients with Stage III disease (HR = 0.16, $p = 0.04$) but not disease-specific survival (HR = 0.32, $p = 0.08$).

Conclusions.—With the limited number of patients in our study, it appears that extraosseous osteosarcoma behaves differently than osteosarcoma of bone. Multimodality treatment that includes doxorubicin and ifosfamide-based chemotherapy, radiation, and surgery may be a valid therapeutic strategy for Stage III disease, but larger, prospective studies will be needed to verify our preliminary observations.

Level of Evidence.—Level III, therapeutic study (Fig 3).

▶ Extraosseous osteosarcoma is a rare tumor; clinical uncertainty exists as to whether this should be treated along osteosarcoma protocols (with chemotherapy and wide surgical resection) or along soft tissue sarcoma protocols (with adjuvant radiotherapy and consideration of adjuvant chemotherapy for

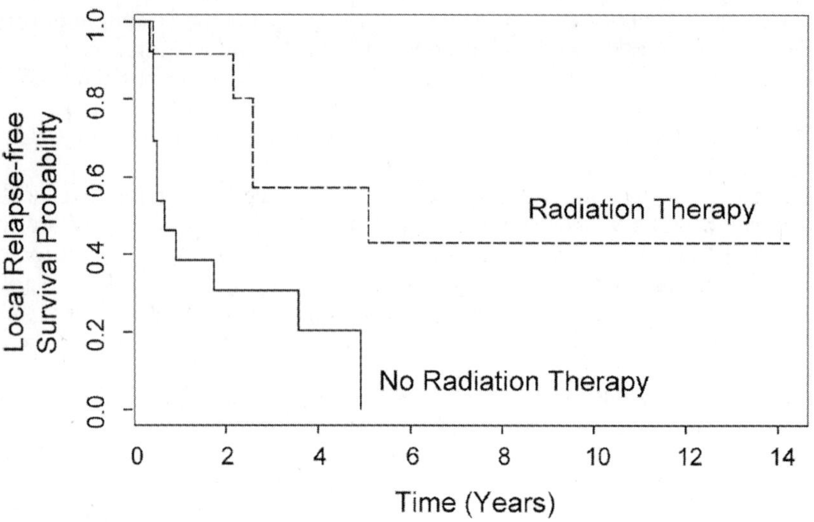

FIGURE 3.—Radiation therapy was the strongest predictor for local relapse in Stage III disease in multivariate analysis. Kaplan-Meier analysis (univariate) showed that patients receiving radiation had 4- and 5-year local relapse-free survival rates of 57% (95% CI, 33%−100%) for both years while patients not receiving radiation had 4- and 5-year local relapse-free survival rates of 21% (95% CI, 7%−64%) and 0% (95% CI not derivable), respectively (log-rank test, $p = 0.01$). (Reprinted from Fan Z, Patel S, Lewis VO, et al. Should high-grade extraosseous osteosarcoma be treated with multimodality therapy like other soft tissue sarcomas? *Clin Orthop Relat Res.* 2015;473:3604-3611, with permission from The Association of Bone and Joint Surgeons.)

high-risk patients). Unfortunately, this is a rare enough tumor that there are no significant series in the literature which addressed this.

This article reports a series of 40 patients treated at the M.D. Anderson Cancer Center over a period of 22 years (this highlights the rarity of this condition if a major cancer center treats fewer than 2 patients per year with it). The authors retrospectively reviewed a series of patients who had been treated with several treatment protocols. That is obviously a limitation of this study, but again, the rarity of the condition and evolving treatments make a study that is hard to conduct practically.

The overall results must be interpreted with caution, but they do suggest that extraosseous osteosarcoma behaves more like a high-grade soft tissue sarcoma with osteoblastic differentiation and histology than a classic osteosarcoma of bone. Radiotherapy (seldom used in the management of osteosarcoma of bone) was the strongest predictive factor to avoid local recurrence in this population (see Fig 3). As such, the authors recommend multimodal therapy including radiation and adjuvant chemotherapy in the treatment of this disease.

Where to place this in clinical context? This is a rare tumor, but given the available data, it seems reasonable to treat this more along the lines of an aggressive soft tissue protocol than a bony protocol given the current evidence. A larger series of patients may be accumulated through multi-institutional efforts. This is probably the only practical way to obtain greater data on this topic; until then, this article serves as a reference for the treatment of patients with this disease process. Additional commentary on this article can be found in Clinical Orthopaedics and Related Research.[1]

P. S. Rose, MD

Reference

1. Miller BJ. CORR Insights: Should high grade extraosseous osteosarcoma be treated with multi-modal therapy like other soft tissue sarcomas? *Clin Orthop Relat Res*. 2015;473:3612-3613.

Homogenous Good Outcome in a Heterogeneous Group of Tumors: An Institutional Series of Outcomes of Superficial Soft Tissue Sarcomas

Francescutti V, Sanghera SS, Cheney RT, et al (Roswell Park Cancer Inst, Buffalo, NY; et al)

Sarcoma 2015:1-7, 2015

Introduction.—Superficial soft tissue sarcomas (S-STS) are generally amenable to wide excision. We hypothesized that local recurrence (LR) should be low, even without radiation therapy (RT), and sought to examine the contribution of depth to LR and OS.

Methods.—Patients with S-STS were retrospectively reviewed. Demographics, tumor features, treatment received, and outcomes were analyzed.

Results.—103 patients were identified. Median age was 55 years; 53% of patients were female. Tumor site was 39% in trunk, 38% in the lower extremity, 14% in the upper extremity, and 9% in other locations. The most common histology was 36% leiomyosarcoma. Median tumor size was 2.8 cm (range 0.2—14 cm). Sixty-six percent of tumors were of intermediate/high grade. RT was administered preoperatively in 6% of patients and postoperatively in 15% of patients. An R0 resection was accomplished in 92%. At a median follow-up of 34.2 months (range 2.3—176), 9 patients had a LR (8.7%). Tumor size and grade were not associated with LR. OS was not associated with any tumor or patient variables on univariate analysis.

Conclusions.—LR was low for S-STS, even with large or high grade tumors and selective use of RT. Surgical resection alone may be adequate therapy for most patients. Superficial location seems to supersede other factors imparting a good prognosis for this group of tumors.

▶ Superficial soft tissue sarcomas are encountered with reasonable frequency in clinical practice. However, only 6 previous reports have clearly reported them as a separate entity with discrete outcome data. Thus, these authors from the Roswell Park Cancer Institute report on 103 patients with superficial soft tissue sarcomas seen over their recent history.

Good outcomes were observed. Despite the fact that only 25% of patients had any radiotherapy administered, the local recurrence rate was less than

9%. Additionally, overall survival was approximately 93%. The authors were aggressive in obtaining a wide margin (defined as greater than 2 cm including their deep margin).

It has long been recognized that superficial soft tissue sarcomas seem to have improved outcome compared with traditional deep tissue sarcomas. This has often been attributed to earlier detection (small size at diagnosis) as well as a preponderance of low-grade lesions. In this series, the majority of patients had intermediate- and high-grade tumors.

Where to place this in clinical context? This study combined with the previous reported information on superficial soft tissue sarcomas highlights both the importance of an aggressive surgical posture and also the favorable long-term outcome. The ability to manage patients without radiotherapy certainly simplifies their treatment and minimizes their morbidity. Although this article does not break tremendous new ground, it does provide an up-to-date discussion and literature review of the field for surgeons who treat soft tissue sarcomas to reference.

P. S. Rose, MD

Metastatic Disease

Intramedullary Nailing of Femoral Diaphyseal Metastases: Is it Necessary to Protect the Femoral Neck?

Moon B, Lin P, Satcher R, et al (Anderson Cancer Ctr, Houston, TX)
Clin Orthop Relat Res 473:1499-1502, 2015

Background.—Intramedullary nailing is the accepted form of treatment for impending or pathologic fractures of the femoral diaphysis. Traditional teaching promotes the use of a cephalomedullary nail so that stabilization is provided for the femoral neck in the event that a future femoral neck metastasis develops. However, that approach may add cost, surgical time, blood loss, and added radiation exposure to staff members, and there is limited evidence in the literature that supports this practice.

Questions/Purposes.—The purpose of our study was to evaluate the incidence of femoral neck metastases in patients who underwent femoral nailing of diaphyseal metastases.

Patients and Methods.—Retrospective analysis of our Musculoskeletal Oncology database identified 145 femoral nailings performed for metastatic disease, myeloma, or lymphoma of the femoral diaphysis between 2001 and 2011. Average patient age was 59 years. One hundred forty-one patients underwent 145 femoral nailings (four were bilateral). One hundred forty-four of the nails used were cephalomedullary implants and one was a flexible nail. Thirty-six (25%) femurs had sustained a pathologic fracture and 109 (75%) femurs were treated as impending fractures. Eighty-four patients received either preoperative or postoperative radiation therapy. Average radiographic followup was 13 months and average postoperative survival was 16 months. Of the 141 patients in this series, 121 (86%) are known to have died at a median of 9 months (range, 0.1–133 months) after surgery. The latest followup radiographs were obtained at a median of 5 months after the femoral nailing (range, 0–119 months). Of the 90 patients with documented dates of death and radiographic followup greater than zero months, 76 (84%) had radiographs available within a year of death. Thirty-one patients had zero months radiographic followup. The median survival for this group of patients was only 0.9 months (range, 0.1–12 months).

Results.—No patients (0%) in this series had femoral neck metastases develop postoperatively.

Conclusion.—Despite traditional teaching that supports the use of cephalomedullary implants when treating metastatic disease of the femur, we were unable to identify a single patient who had femoral neck metastasis after surgery on the femur. Our findings do not support the use of cephalomedullary implants in this patient population for the sole purpose of prophylactic femoral neck stabilization; however, this series was relatively small, and the experiences of other centers will be needed to come to a more-complete sense of the frequency of what in all likelihood is a rare event.

Level of Evidence.—Level IV, therapeutic study.

▶ Standard teaching in the management of metastatic disease to the femur has been to place a long cephalomedullary nail. Some recent work by Damron and colleagues has questioned the need to place a long stem implant after hemiarthroplasty. In their work, the development of new metastases in a patient who previously had been shown to only have proximal femoral metastases was a rare event. This article from the M.D. Anderson Cancer Center expands further on this theme. The authors specifically review 141 patients treated with cephalomedullary nails for present or impending pathologic fractures of the femoral diaphysis. During follow-up, they did not identify any new lesions present in the femoral neck. As such, they propose performing standard nailing in these patients to limit surgical time and radiation exposure to the patient and staff.

I have specifically included this study in the Year Book because of its arguably provocative message. At present, I do not believe this should move standard practice away from performing a cephalomedullary nail. The increased surgical time to place a proximal femoral lag screw is very little in experienced hands. Proposing diminished radiation exposure to the patient as a benefit is of no clinical significance in someone who by definition will be treated with therapeutic radiation to minimize the risk of local tumor progression. There is some reasonable thought that one can decrease radiation exposure to surgeons and room staff, but this too is fairly modest provided standard protective measures can be followed. Additionally, it is hard to say with certainty that no patients in this series would have (or could have) developed femoral neck metastases because follow-up is somewhat incomplete and the imaging is done by plain film radiographs. Certainly metastases near an implant can be difficult to view on plain film radiographs, and it would also not be economical to provide advanced imaging of all patients.

This is an interesting article and one that openly challenges the dogma of metastatic disease. Note the authors excluded from this analysis patients who had peritrochanteric metastatic disease for which few would argue that cephalomedullary rod would be equal to a standard rod. At present, I think a cephalomedullary rod remains the default implant option for patients having intramedullary (as opposed to arthroplasty) treatment of metastatic disease in the femur. That said, we may in the future find these authors have been prescient in raising this issue. Additional commentary on this article can be found in Clinical Orthopaedics and Related Research.[1]

P. S. Rose, MD

Reference

1. Scarborough M. CORR insights: intramedullary nailing of femoral diaphyseal metastases: is it necessary to protect the femoral neck? *Clin Orthop Relat Res.* 2015;473:1503-1504.

Are Allogeneic Blood Transfusions Associated With Decreased Survival After Surgery for Long-bone Metastatic Fractures?

Janssen SJ, Braun Y, Ready JE, et al (Massachusetts General Hosp — Harvard Med School, Boston; Brigham and Women's Hosp, Boston, MA)
Clin Orthop Relat Res 473:2343-2351, 2015

Background.—Previous studies have shown that perioperative blood transfusion increases cancer recurrence and decreases patient survival after resection of primary malignancies. The question arises whether this association also exists in patients with already disseminated disease undergoing surgery for metastatic long-bone fractures.

Purposes.—We sought to determine whether perioperative allogeneic blood transfusion is associated with decreased survival after operative treatment of long-bone metastatic fractures after accounting for clinical, laboratory, and treatment factors. Secondarily, we aimed to identify potential factors that are associated with decreased survival.

Methods.—We included 789 patients in our retrospective study who underwent surgery at two institutions for a pathologic or impending metastatic long-bone fracture. We used multivariable Cox proportional hazards regression model analysis to assess the relationship of perioperative allogeneic blood transfusion with survival, and accounted for patient age, sex, comorbidities, BMI, tumor type, fracture type and location, presence of other bone and visceral metastases, previous radiotherapy and systemic therapy, preoperative embolization, preoperative hemoglobin level, treatment type, anesthesia time, blood loss, duration of hospital admission, year of surgery, and hospital.

Results.—Considering transfusion as an "exposure," and comparing patients who received transfusions with those who did not, we found that blood transfusion was not associated with decreased survival after accounting for all explanatory variables (hazard ratio [HR] 1.06; 95% CI, 0.87–1.30; $p = 0.57$). Evaluating transfusion in terms of dose-response, we found that patients who received more transfusions had lower survival compared with those who had fewer transfusions after accounting for all explanatory variables (HR per unit of blood transfused, 1.07; 95% CI, 1.02–1.12; $p = 0.005$). We found that age (HR, 1.02; 95% CI, 1.01–1.02; $p < 0.001$), comorbidity status (HR, 1.06; 95% CI, 1.01–1.10; $p = 0.014$), duration of hospital stay (HR, 1.02; 95% CI 1.00–1.03; $p = 0.021$), tumor type (HR, 1.71; 95% CI, 1.44–2.03; $p < 0.001$), and visceral metastases (HR, 1.59; 95% CI, 1.34–1.88; $p < 0.001$) were independently associated with survival.

Conclusion.—We found that exposure to perioperative allogeneic blood transfusion does not decrease survival, with the numbers available. However, our sample size might have been insufficient to reveal a small but potentially relevant effect. Our results do suggest a dose-response relationship; patients who received more transfusions had lower survival compared with those with fewer transfusions. Risk of death increased by 7% per unit of blood transfused.

Level of Evidence.—Level III, prognostic study.

▶ Metastatic bone disease is a common clinical presentation that orthopaedic oncologists and many general orthopaedic surgeons deal with. A number of studies in the literature have suggested that patients have diminished survival from primary tumors if they have perioperative blood transfusions; researchers have hypothesized that this may be due to an immunomodulatory effect on patients dealing with primary malignancies. Thus, it is a clinically relevant question to ask whether blood transfusion is associated with a decreased survival in patients being treated for long-bone metastases.

This group reviewed 789 patients treated in the Harvard System. In summary, considering blood transfusion as an exposure (yes or no), patients who received transfusions had equivalent survival to those who did not receive a transfusion. Evaluating transfusion in a dose-response manner, greater numbers of units transfused was associated with a lower survival.

Where to place this study in clinical context? Patients being treated for metastatic disease are fundamentally being treated palliatively, with the goal to maximize both the duration and the quality of their life. These patients often have a preoperative anemia and undergo surgeries that place them at risk for significant perioperative anemias. Given these data, surgeons are certainly justified in having a reasonable transfusion policy. Additionally, withholding a transfusion is not seen as a benefit to patient survival in this setting.

Whether there is a true transfusion risk in patients being treated for primary sarcomas is unclear at this time, acknowledging that this is a level III study. It does report a large cohort of well-documented patients and provides a reasonable answer to a relevant clinical question that surgeons deal with on a daily basis. Additional commentary on this article can be found in Clinical Orthopaedics and Related Research.[1]

P. S. Rose, MD

Reference

1. Randall RL. CORR insights: are allogeneic blood transfusions associated with decreased survival after surgery for long-bone metastatic fractures? *Clin Orthop Relat Res*. 2015;473:2352-2354.

Thromboembolism After Intramedullary Nailing for Metastatic Bone Lesions

Shallop B, Starks A, Greenbaum S, et al (Jefferson Med College, Philadelphia, PA; Albert Einstein Med College, Bronx, NY; et al)
J Bone Joint Surg Am 97:1503-1511, 2015

Background.—The risk of venous thromboembolism (VTE) in patients undergoing intramedullary nailing for skeletal metastatic disease is currently undefined. The purpose of our study was to determine the risk of thromboembolic events, to define the risk factors for VTE, and to define the rate of wound complications in this population.

Methods.—A retrospective review of surgical databases at three National Cancer Institute (NCI)-designated cancer centers identified 287 patients with a total of 336 impending or pathologic long-bone fractures that were stabilized with intramedullary nailing between February 2001 and April 2013. Statistical analysis was performed utilizing multivariable logistic regression and Fisher exact tests.

Results.—The overall rate of VTE was twenty-four (7.1%) of the 336; thirteen (3.9%) were pulmonary embolism (PE), and eleven (3.3%), deep venous thrombosis (DVT). In two patients, adequate anticoagulation data were not available. We found no significant relationship between the type of anticoagulant used and VTE. There was a significant positive correlation found between lung-cancer histology and the development of VTE ($p < 0.001$) or PE ($p < 0.001$). The absence of radiation therapy approached significance ($p = 0.06$) with respect to decreased overall VTE risk. Wound complications were documented for 11 (3.3%) of the operations.

Conclusions.—There is a high rate of VTE among those with skeletal metastatic disease who undergo intramedullary nailing, even while receiving postoperative thromboembolic prophylaxis. Current anticoagulation protocols may be inadequate. Wound-complication risk with anticoagulant use in this population is low and should not be a deterrent to adequate anticoagulant use for this population.

Level of Evidence.—Prognostic Level IV. See Instructions for Authors for a complete description of levels of evidence.

▶ Intramedullary rodding is standard for many patients with impending or present metastatic long bone fracture, and these patients are known to have many risk factors for developing thromboembolic disease postoperatively. However, no standard prophylactic treatment regimen is currently accepted for this patient population, and the exact incidence of thromboembolic disease is not defined. These authors pooled patients reviewed retrospectively from 3 cancer centers to determine the risk of thromboembolic disease in 287 patients undergoing 336 surgical procedures.

It should be noted that each center had a similar surgical technique but different anticoagulation protocols that generally lasted for 2 weeks postoperatively. Thromboembolic disease was defined as a symptomatically detected venous thrombosis or pulmonary embolism within 90 days of the operative procedure. The authors noted 7.1% of patients had thromboembolic complications, and this appeared to be independent of the anticoagulation regimen that was used. Additionally, the time course of these events was such that half of them fell beyond 2 weeks postoperatively.

Where to place this study in clinical context? This certainly underestimates the risk of thromboembolic disease in this patient population because these cases were identified retrospectively and only in patients who were symptomatic and who were known to the authors. Each center ultimately will determine their own protocol and individualize it to specific patients. However, based on these results, it seems reasonable to conclude that prophylactic anticoagulation is important in this patient population and that it should extend beyond 2 weeks. A reasonable and empiric protocol might be to treat all patients for a minimum of 4 weeks postoperatively based on these results. Certainly, if patients are thrombocytopenic or initiate chemotherapy before that time frame, consideration must be given to altering such a protocol because of the interactions it may have on other aspects of their care.

P. S. Rose, MD

Benign Tumors

Does pathological fracture affect the rate of local recurrence in patients with a giant cell tumour of bone? A meta-analysis

Salunke AA, Chen Y, Chen X, et al (Natl Univ Health System, Singapore)
Bone Joint J 97-B:1566-1571, 2015

We investigated whether the presence of a pathological fracture increased the risk of local recurrence in patients with a giant cell tumour (GCT) of bone. We also assessed if curettage is still an appropriate form of treatment in the presence of a pathological fracture. We conducted a comprehensive review and meta-analysis of papers which reported outcomes in patients with a GCT with and without a pathological fracture at presentation. We computed the odds ratio (OR) of local recurrence in those with and without a pathological fracture.

We selected 19 eligible papers for final analysis. This included 3215 patients, of whom 580 (18.0%) had a pathological fracture. The pooled

OR for local recurrence between patients with and without a pathological fracture was 1.05 (95% confidence interval (CI) 0.66 to 1.67, $p = 0.854$). Amongst the subgroup of patients who were treated with curettage, the pooled OR for local recurrence was 1.23 (95% CI 0.75 to 2.01, $p = 0.417$).

A *post hoc* sample size calculation showed adequate power for both comparisons.

There is no difference in local recurrence rates between patients who have a GCT of bone with and without a pathological fracture at the time of presentation. The presence of a pathological fracture should not preclude the decision to perform curettage as carefully selected patients who undergo curettage can have similar outcomes in terms of local recurrence to those without such a fracture.

▶ A significant number of patients with giant cell tumors of bone will present with pathologic fractures. Previous literature has suggested that patients with pathologic fracture are at increased risk of recurrence due to contamination of the joint and/or soft tissue envelope. Thus, a school of thought has developed in some circles that these patients are better treated with resection and reconstruction. These authors provide a meta-analysis of 19 papers totalling more than 3000 patients with giant cell tumor to specifically analyze the rate of local recurrence in patients with and without pathologic fracture and who were and were not treated with curettage as their initial treatment.

The results demonstrated that the odds ratio for local recurrence was similar with or without a pathologic fracture. Additionally, in patients treated with curettage, the odds ratio for local recurrence was similar if pathologic fracture was or was not present.

How to implement this in clinical practice? I would suggest that a conclusion that curettage of any pathologic fracture of giant cell tumor has an equal result to patients without pathologic fractures is not warranted. Readers must remember that this is a pooled analysis of previously published articles. Within those studies (which were not randomized), patients were carefully selected for their treatment operation. Thus, a reasonable conclusion from this article is that curettage does not need to be avoided in patients with a pathologic fracture if the surgeon feels a successful operation can be done. This difference is significant, and it is important to recognize that not all patients with pathologic fractures will be good candidates for curettage, and not all pathologic fractures are the same.

With this in mind, this is a useful article for surgeons to be aware of because it contradicts the traditional teaching in some regions that any significant pathologic fracture required resection. For this reason, I have deliberately included it in the YEAR BOOK but present its results with the preceding caveats.

P. S. Rose, MD

Incidence Trends in the Diagnosis of Giant Cell Tumor of Bone in Sweden Since 1958

Rockberg J, Bach BA, Amelio J, et al (IMS Health (Pygargus), Stockholm, Sweden; Amgen Inc., Thousand Oaks, CA; Amgen Ltd, Uxbridge, England; et al)

J Bone Joint Surg Am 97:1756-1766, 2015

Background.—The Swedish Cancer Registry (founded in 1958) constitutes a unique resource for epidemiological studies of giant cell tumor of bone with potential for use for population-based studies of incidence over time. The aim of this study was to provide what we believe is the first modern population-based assessment of the incidence trends of giant cell tumor, a unique osteoclastogenic lytic stromal tumor with both benign and malignant histological forms, and to compare the findings with data from the same registry on osteosarcoma, a tumor that may display similar histological characteristics.

Methods.—Cases were identified with use of codes for pathological bone tumor (International Classification of Diseases [ICD]-7 196). Specific morphological coding distinguishes benign (PAD 741) from malignant giant cell tumor (PAD 746) and osteosarcoma (PAD 766).

Results.—During the period of 1958 to 2011, 4625 bone tumors were reported, including 505 giant cell tumors (383 benign and 122 malignant) and 1152 osteosarcomas. From 1958 to 1982 the ratio of malignant to benign giant cell tumors was 1.3, whereas from 1983 to 2011 the ratio inverted to 0.09, suggesting a change in the reporting or diagnosis of malignant or benign cases. Cases of giant cell tumor diagnosed from 1983 to 2011 displayed an age and sex distribution (median age at diagnosis, 34.0 years; 54% female) that were consistent with those in large published case series but differed from those in 1958 to 1982 (median age at diagnosis, 31.5 years; 48% female). The most current data (1983 to 2011) showed the giant cell tumor incidence in Sweden to be 1.3 per million per year, while the osteosarcoma incidence was 2.3 per million per year.

Conclusions.—Early Swedish Cancer Registry data (1958 to 1982) revealed a higher proportion of malignant giant cell tumors than seen in large sequential case series and a distinct age and sex profile compared with more recent data (1983 to 2011). This likely represents changes in the diagnostic workup and introduction of multidisciplinary review of giant-cell-containing tumors around 1982. Recent data may reflect the impact of expert centralized biopsy and multidisciplinary case review and more comprehensive reporting of benign giant cell tumors.

▶ This is an interesting study looking at the longitudinal trend in the diagnosis of giant cell tumors in a national health system from 1958 through 2011. The authors draw on and expanding the original population-based giant cell tumor study performed by Larsson in 1975. They are able to draw from the Swedish Cancer Registry, a national tumor registry that has faithfully recorded all tumors since its inception in this national health system; this setting allows greater fidelity in the ascertainment of data than would typically be seen in a North American study.

Most striking, the authors saw a strong shift in their data in 1982. This time frame corresponds to a change in the diagnostic work-up and an increase in the multidisciplinary review of these tumors within Sweden's National Health System.

Where to place this study in clinical context? The recent data (1983-present) that the authors report is probably very representative of what is seen in contemporary North American practice. Although the ethnic background in Sweden does not mirror that of the United States or Canada, the ethnic variations in giant cell tumor are relatively modest. Thus, the data shown likely apply well to current practice if it is restricted to the past few decades.

Additionally, and more importantly, the results presented in this article highlight the critical nature of expert (rather than purely local) review in the diagnosis and treatment of rare conditions. The authors saw a sharp drop in the number of tumors that were declared malignant once multidisciplinary and centralized review was instituted. This virtually certainly implies misdiagnosis in the past because there are no plausible reasons to think that the overall disease process under study would have changed.

As such, this article serves as a reasonable reference for the contemporary characteristics of giant cell tumor. Additionally, it highlights the importance of a true team approach and expert review when reviewing and treating rare conditions.

P. S. Rose, MD

Risk Factors for Pulmonary Metastases from Giant Cell Tumor of Bone

Chan CM, Adler Z, Reith JD, et al (Univ of Florida, Gainesville; Newport Orthopaedic Inst, Newport Beach, CA)

J Bone Joint Surg Am 97:420-428, 2015

Background.—Giant cell tumor (GCT) of bone is a rare, benign, aggressive bone tumor with an unusual capacity to metastasize to the lung. It was the goal of this study to identify patient and treatment-specific variables associated with the development of pulmonary metastases of GCT of bone.

Methods.—From 1980 to 2009, 291 patients with benign GCT of bone were treated at our institution, and 167 were followed for at least two years. Eleven (6.6%) of these 167 patients developed biopsy-confirmed pulmonary metastasis. All patients were evaluated relative to nine patient, disease, and treatment-specific variables.

Results.—We identified four properties of benign GCT of bone associated with an increased risk of metastasis on univariate analysis: age at diagnosis, axial location of the primary GCT, primary Enneking stage-3 disease, and local recurrence. Multivariate analysis showed local recurrence to be an independent risk factor for pulmonary metastasis (adjusted odds ratio, 7.42).

Conclusions.—There is an increased risk of pulmonary metastasis of GCT of bone in patients who are younger, present with Enneking stage-3 disease, develop local recurrence, and/or present with axial disease. The mode of treatment was not found to be associated with the development of pulmonary metastasis.

Level of Evidence.—Prognostic Level IV. See Instructions for Authors for a complete description of levels of evidence.

▶ Physicians have long recognized that giant cell tumors can yield pulmonary metastases. This does not necessarily imply a malignant character to these pulmonary metastases, and the outcome of patients with this disease process has been quite varied in the literature. These authors from the University of Florida–Gainesville draw on large institutional experience treating giant cell tumor of bone to report the prevalence of biopsy-confirmed pulmonary metastases and risk factors in identifying these patients.

The authors found 6.6% of patients who were followed for at least 2 years developed pulmonary metastases. Younger age at diagnosis (25 years on average), axial tumor location, Enneking stage 3 disease, and local recurrence all increased the risk of pulmonary metastases. On multivariate analysis, only local recurrence remained an independent risk factor.

Where to place this study in clinical context? In my mind, this study highlights the importance of evaluating patients for pulmonary metastases. The more difficult issue that the authors do not discuss is the long time interval to develop pulmonary metastasis. Only 1 of their patients had pulmonary metastasis at presentation. The rest all developed them in follow-up, and 2 developed them more than 10 years after initial diagnosis. This places treating surgeons in a difficult situation. There are not established surveillance protocols to detect the development of pulmonary metastases from giant cell tumors over time. Additionally, few surgeons follow patients with giant cell tumors beyond 5 years provided they have healed without recurrence. These issues are not defined in this article, and each surgeon and center will need to develop appropriate protocols in following their patients.

Thankfully, in this series, all patients with pulmonary metastases were alive at last follow-up despite being treated by a variety of mechanisms. To this end, the ideal treatment for pulmonary metastasis in this setting has not been defined.

P. S. Rose, MD

Chondroblastoma of Bone in the Extremities: A Multicenter Retrospective Study

Xu H, Nugent D, Monforte HL, et al (Peking Univ, Xicheng District, Beijing, People's Republic of China; Univ of Florida College of Medicine, Gainesville; All Children's Hosp, St. Petersburg, FL; et al)

J Bone Joint Surg Am 97:925-931, 2015

Background.—Chondroblastoma is a rare benign cartilage tumor that commonly occurs in children and adolescents. This study was designed to review the epidemiologic characteristics and outcomes of surgical management in a large series of patients with extremity chondroblastoma.

Methods.—We performed a multicenter retrospective analysis of 199 patients with extremity chondroblastoma. Clinical data, radiographic images, histological findings, treatment, and outcome were analyzed.

Results.—There were 145 male patients and fifty-four female patients with a mean age of 18.0 years. The most commonly involved bone was the proximal part of the tibia (fifty-five patients [27.6%]), followed by the proximal part of the femur (fifty-two patients [26.1%]) and the distal part of the femur (thirty-eight patients [19.1%]). Prior to presentation, 73.4% (146 of 199 patients) experienced pain. The mean duration of pain and other symptoms was 8.7 months. The physis was open in 25.7%, it was closing in 22.2%, and it was closed in 52.1% of the patients at the time of presentation. One hundred and twenty-six patients had at least twenty-four months of follow-up; their mean follow-up duration was 62.1 months (range, twenty-four to 190 months). Initial treatment was curettage for 119 patients (94.4%) and en bloc resection for seven patients (5.6%). The local recurrence rate was 5.0% after curettage and 0% after resection. The only significant factor related to recurrence was the location of the lesion in the proximal part of the humerus ($p = 0.001$).

Conclusions.—Chondroblastoma occurs most frequently in the proximal part of the tibia and the proximal part of the femur with significant male predilection. In this series, recurrence was most frequent in the proximal part of the humerus. Our results suggest that curettage and bone-grafting provide favorable local control and satisfactory functional outcome for patients with this disease.

Level of Evidence.—Therapeutic Level IV. See Instructions for Authors for a complete description of levels of evidence.

▶ This article represents the largest series of chondroblastoma ever reported. Combining series from the Moffitt Cancer Center and Peking University Hospital, these authors report 199 cases of extremity chondroblastoma. Several points come out of the article that are clinically relevant for practicing surgeons.

No cases of malignant transformation or "benign" pulmonary metastases were observed. These are recognized but rare complications, and this study of nearly 200 patients with none of these events observed helps to quantify just how uncommon these phenomena are. The authors do not comment in detail on surveillance for pulmonary metastases at presentation and over follow-up, so it is possible that 1 or 2 cases slipped through.

The recurrence rate was only 5%. This is the lowest recurrence rate of chondroblastoma that I am aware of, and this is the largest series ever published. This probably provides a floor estimate as to the recurrence rate in typical clinical practice. The complication rate was modest. The authors stress their recognized difficulty of treating chondroblastoma around the hip.

As surgeons approach these patients, this study now becomes the reference for the management and outcome of this entity given its large size and reasonable documentation. The recurrence rate seems low; time will tell whether this is an artefact or if it can be reproduced in other series.

P. S. Rose, MD

The effect of surgical synovectomy and radiotherapy on the rate of recurrence of pigmented villonodular synovitis of the knee: an individual patient meta-analysis

Mollon B, Lee A, Busse JW, et al (Univ of Toronto, Ontario, Canada)

Bone Joint J 97-B:550-557, 2015

Pigmented villonodular synovitis (PVNS) is a rare proliferative process of the synovium which most commonly affects the knee and occurs in either a localised (LPVNS) or a diffuse form (DPVNS). The effect of different methods of surgical synovectomy and adjuvant radiotherapy on the rate of recurrence is unclear. We conducted a systematic review and identified 35 observational studies in English which reported the use of surgical synovectomy to treat PVNS of the knee.

A meta-analysis included 630 patients, 137 (21.8%) of whom had a recurrence after synovectomy. For patients with DPVNS, low-quality evidence found that the rate of recurrence was reduced by both open synovectomy (odds ration (OR) = 0.47; 95% CI 0.25 to 0.90; $p = 0.024$) and combined open and arthroscopic synovectomy (OR = 0.19, 95% CI = 0.06 to 0.58; $p = 0.003$) compared with arthroscopic surgery. Very low-quality evidence found that the rate of recurrence of DPVNS was reduced by peri-operative radiotherapy (OR = 0.31, 95% CI 0.14 to 0.70; $p = 0.01$). Very low-quality evidence suggested that the rate of recurrence of LPVNS was not related to the surgical approach.

This meta-analysis suggests that open synovectomy or synovectomy combined with perioperative radiotherapy for DPVNS is associated with a reduced rate of recurrence. Large long-term prospective multicentre observational studies, with a focus on both rate of recurrence and function, are required to confirm these findings.

▶ All surgeons who deal with pigmented villonodular synovitis (PVNS) recognize the challenges that recurrent disease entails. These authors provide a meta-analysis reviewing 630 previously published cases, 137 of which had a recurrence after synovectomy. They specifically evaluated the effect of synovectomy and radiotherapy on outcomes.

As expected in a pooled analysis of previously published series of varying quality, the strength of the conclusions is modest. However, evidence does clearly support the role of open or combined open and arthroscopy synovectomy in the treatment of diffuse PVNS. Additionally, the available evidence indicates that the rate of recurrence is reduced with the use of perioperative radiotherapy.

Where to place this article in clinical context? Diffuse, and particularly recurrent diffuse, PVNS remains a problem we have not solved. This article highlights the best available evidence for its treatment. Additionally, in an era of tight external review of medical decisions, this article provides firm support for the use of radiotherapy in patients. As such, it is important for practitioners who see these patients to be familiar so that they are aware of the available options and the evidence supporting them. This can be translated directly into clinical practice and also used to support treatment decisions.

P. S. Rose, MD

Article Index

Chapter 1: Basic Science

Chapter 2: General Orthopedics

Chapter 3: Forearm, Wrist, and Hand

Chapter 4: Elbow

Chapter 5: Shoulder and Elbow

Chapter 6: Spine

Chapter 7: Total Hip Arthroplasty

Chapter 9: Foot and Ankle

Chapter 10: Sports Medicine

Chapter 11: Trauma and Amputation

Author Index

R

S

T

U

V

W

X

Y

Z